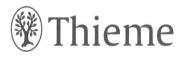

Guide to Periodontal Treatment Solutions for General Dentistry

Tobias K. Boehm, DDS, PhD
Associate Professor
College of Dental Medicine
Western University of Health Sciences
Pomona, California, USA

Sam Chui, DDS, FAGD
Assistant Professor
College of Dental Medicine
Western University of Health Sciences
Pomona, California, USA

315 illustrations

Thieme
New York • Stuttgart • Delhi • Rio de Janeiro

Library of Congress Cataloging-in-Publication Data is available with the publisher.

© 2020. Thieme. All rights reserved.

Thieme Medical Publishers New York
333 Seventh Avenue
New York, New York 10001 USA
+1 800 782 3488
customerservice@thieme.com

Georg Thieme Verlag KG
Rüdigerstrasse 14, 70469 Stuttgart, Germany
+49 [0]711 8931 421, customerservice@thieme.de

Thieme Publishers Delhi
A-12, Second Floor, Sector-2, Noida-201301
Uttar Pradesh, India
+91 120 45 566 00, customerservice@thieme.in

Thieme Publishers Rio de Janeiro,
Thieme Publicações Ltda.
Edifício Rodolpho de Paoli, 25º andar
Av. Nilo Peçanha, 50 – Sala 2508,
Rio de Janeiro 20020-906 Brasil
+55 21 3172-2297

Cover design: Thieme Publishing Group
Typesetting by DiTech Process Solutions, India

Printed in USA by King Printing Company, Inc.   5 4 3 2 1

ISBN 978-1-62623-800-8

Also available as an e-book:
eISBN 978-1-62623-801-5

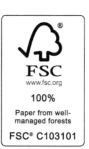

Contents

Contents

Contents

Videos

Preface

Dentistry has transformed with advances in technology, new business models, and demographic and cultural shifts. However, the traditional focus on caries and periodontal disease management remains as important as ever. This requires current dental students to be nimble, proactive learners who can independently work on clinical cases, collaborate across disciplines, and propose intelligent solutions to treatment challenges. At the same time, dental students are more likely to practice outside of a specialty-based dental school clinic, so they may have limited access to specialists and other experts who can guide them through clinical challenges.

Often, these challenges are caused by common periodontal diseases, which complicate restorative dental treatment and cause premature tooth loss. However, periodontal disease diagnosis and treatment are rarely simple and not easily grasped by dental students. Since periodontal specialist faculty may not be readily available for guidance and traditional textbooks in periodontology are too unwieldy for easy reference, we intended to provide a concise guide to periodontal treatment.

The focus of this book is to provide a "how-to" approach to periodontal treatment for a 2nd or 3rd year dental student who has just started practicing dentistry and a dental student gaining experience in periodontal surgery as part of a surgical elective. This book may also serve as a quick introductory guide for a resident who has just started his/her postdoctoral specialist program prior to more in-depth learning.

In Chapter 1, we have provided a summary of the foundational scientific knowledge that underpins periodontal treatment. The rest of the book has been arranged in a logical sequence mirroring the manner in which patients with periodontal disease are treated. Chapters 2 to 4 depict how to assess a patient and provide thought processes for diagnosis, treatment planning, prognosis, and extraction decisions. Chapter 5 deals with nonsurgical treatment aimed at reducing periodontal inflammation, and in Chapters 6 to 9 surgical approaches to address residual deep pockets, furcations, mucogingival defects, and tooth mobility have been discussed.

Each chapter is preceded by a detailed clinical case and a case commentary that previews key aspects of the chapter. These can be used either as a pre-class assignment for a flipped classroom approach or case-based learning in small groups moderated by a facilitator. This is followed by basic foundational knowledge or detailed "how-to" instructions to augment clinical teaching. For review purposes, we have summarized key clinical pearls at the end of each chapter along with detailed case-based NDBE-style questions and explanations of answer choices. We have also suggested research activities and recent literature that can be used to hone evidence-based dentistry skills. Key terminology is highlighted in **bold** where first introduced in the chapters.

In summary, we hope that this guide to periodontal treatment will be a simple, accessible reference source for dental students and residents facing their first clinical challenges. While we attempt to share the knowledge that we wished we had as dental students, we would also like to encourage students to continue to seek out knowledge from different instructors, mentors, and practitioners since "not all knowledge is found in one school."[1]

Safety Warnings:

- Medications and local anesthetics used in periodontal treatment can trigger severe allergic reactions or side effects in some patients.

- Do not perform periodontal surgery on patients with severe, uncontrolled medical conditions until the patient's medical condition has been adequately controlled. Consult with the patient's medical specialists if necessary to develop a pre and postoperative management plan that addresses the patient's medical needs.

- Do not perform periodontal surgery on a patient with a high risk of infective bacterial endocarditis or other severe infection risk without providing antibiotic prophylaxis.

- Consider the risk of osteonecrosis of the jaw in patients who received bisphosphonates or other treatments that affect bone, and carefully weigh benefits and risks of periodontal surgery.

Tobias K. Boehm, DDS, PhD
Sam Chui, DDS, FAGD

---

[1] "A'ohe pau ka 'ike i ka hālau ho'okahi", Hawaiian proverb, recorded and translated by K. Maly (2001)

Acknowledgments

I would like to thank the co-author of this book, Dr. Sam Chui, for providing his views as a senior dentist, developing the key takeaway messages, and helping maintain the focus on the needs of dental students.

I would also like to thank all the contributors as their work greatly adds to the usefulness of this book. The chapter on extraction decisions greatly benefited from the work of Dr. Hardev Singh who is one of the foremost exodontia specialists at Western University of Health Sciences and has great insights on typical problems that students and faculty encounter with extractions. Dr. Jeffrey Elo who is a fountainhead of oral maxillofacial surgery has provided the figures in this chapter. I would like to thank Dr. Jeffrey Lloyd for his insights on occlusion and additional restorative knowledge provided in Chapter 9. A special thank you to Dr. Daniel Melker who has provided the section on biologic shaping and helped me finally grasp this concept. I would like to express my heartfelt gratitude to Dr. Clara Kim and Ms. Josephine Franc for providing figures and feedback throughout the work.

I am indebted to the Western University of Health Sciences Pumerantz Library. I could not have researched, referenced, and read the hundreds of articles used in the preparation of this book without their institutional subscriptions of scientific journals, antique book collection, and interlibrary loan services.

I also owe thanks to the reviewers of this book brought together by Thieme and the following individuals who volunteered to function as "test dental students" while reading the drafts of this book:

- Dr. Scott Lee of Minnesota, who is now a periodontal resident at Mayo Clinic.
- Dr. Umair Ahmed of California, who is an international dentist pursuing postdoctoral training.

I would like to thank Ms. Delia DeTurris of Thieme who initially approached me to write this textbook and then pushed this project towards completion. Likewise, the entire Thieme staff involved in the production of this book deserve due acknowledgment. This book would not have been possible without their constant cooperation.

My heartfelt thanks to Ms. Natalie L. Boehm, who also volunteered as a "test dental student" while reviewing this book, finding and providing various outside perspectives from a patient, legal, or overall health perspective, and for her encouragement throughout the process of writing this book.

Lastly, I owe gratitude to all who made writing this book possible. Even though there are just two editors and a few contributors, there are too many individuals who in some way have contributed to this book: my children, parents, teachers, professors, friends, co-workers, and many others.

Tobias K. Boehm, DDS, PhD

1 Background: Periodontal Disease Mechanisms and Wound Healing

Abstract

Periodontal diseases are one of the most common diseases in adults. Signs of mild periodontal inflammation are usually present in adults, and 10 to 60% of middle-aged adults have severe enough periodontal disease that requires treatment.

For diagnosis, it is helpful to understand the appearance of healthy periodontal tissues. This chapter begins with a description of periodontal health and reviews the contribution of microbes and immune system to the cellular changes that lead to the signs and symptoms of periodontal diseases. This is followed by reviews of periodontal wound healing and tooth development, and their influences on periodontal disease and treatment.

Keywords: structure, microbes, cells, development

1.1 Learning Objectives

- Recognize normal anatomy of healthy periodontal tissue.
- Describe the contribution of microbes to the periodontal disease process.
- Describe cellular and molecular events that lead to clinical signs and symptoms of periodontal disease.
- Describe how periodontal tissue recovers from injury caused by bacteria or tissue trauma.
- Describe how tooth development influences periodontal disease and treatment.

1.2 Case

A 25-year old healthy female dental student is seen for a periodontal exam as part of a clinical peer-to-peer exercise. See ▶ Fig. 1.1 for clinical presentation and ▶ Fig. 1.2 for radiographic presentation. She is currently satisfied with her dental condition, but had minor restorative treatment in the past and receives routine preventive dental care. She brushes and flosses regularly at least twice a day. These are the findings:

- *Soft tissue exam*: No pathology other than the presence of small lingual tori.
- *Tooth condition*: Small occlusal and interproximal amalgam restorations, and a slightly chipped maxillary incisor.
- *Periodontal measurements*: Probing depths less than 5 mm, no bleeding on probing, no clinical attachment loss, furcation involvement, tooth mobility, and gingival recession. The gingiva is coral pink with patches of light pink on the maxilla, firmly attached to underlying hard tissue and stippled. The gingival margin follows the contours of the teeth in a scalloped fashion, and no plaque or calculus is present.

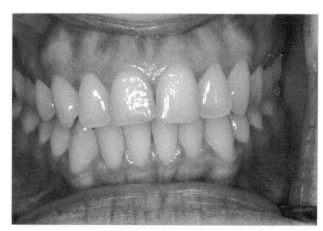

Fig. 1.1 Clinical presentation for case.

Fig. 1.2 Radiographic series for case.

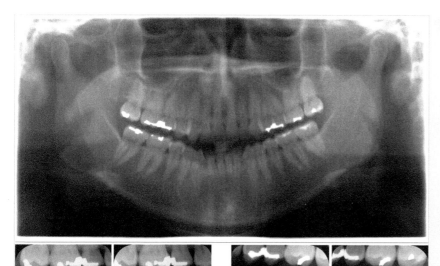

Findings in the periodontal chart are as follows:

Maxilla facial		1	2	3	4	5	6	7	8	9	10	11	12	13	14	15	16
	PD		323	323	323	323	323	312	222	212	212	312	212	212	313	334	
	BOP																
	CAL		000	000	000	000	000	000	000	000	000	000	000	000	000	000	
	GR																
	MGJ		767	767	768	635	678	989	983	379	989	976	556	667	656	656	
	Furc																
	PLQ		0	0	0	0	0	0	0	0	0	0	0	0	0	0	
Maxilla lingual	PD		324	323	324	323	223	112	111	111	112	112	212	212	213	224	
	BOP																
	CAL		000	000	000	000	000	000	000	000	000	000	000	000	000	000	
	GR																
	Furc																
	Mobil																
	PLQ		0	0	0	0	0	0	0	0	0	0	0	0	0	0	

Mandible lingual		32	31	30	29	28	27	26	25	24	23	22	21	20	19	18	17
	PD		324	323	212	212	211	111	111	111	111	212	212	212	312	313	
	BOP																
	CAL		000	000	000	000	000	000	000	000	000	000	000	000	000	000	
	GR																
	MGJ		999	999	876	756	656	656	656	656	656	656	667	888	999	999	
	Furc																
	PLQ																
Mandible facial	PD		324	223	212	212	211	112	212	212	213	212	212	313	323	323	
	BOP																
	CAL		000	000	000	000	000	000	000	000	000	000	000	000	000	000	
	GR																
	MGJ		635	535	535	535	647	656	644	457	757	656	646	656	655	433	
	Furc																
	Mobil																
	PLQ		0	0	0	0	0	0	0	0	0	0	0	0	0	0	

Abbreviations: BOP, bleeding on probing (1), suppuration (2); CAL; clinical attachment level; Furc, furcation involvement (Glickman class); GR, gingival recession; MGJ, position of the mucogingival junction from margin; Mobil, tooth mobility (Miller grade); PD, probing depths; PLQ, plaque level (0 = none, 5 = heavy).

What can be learned from this case?

This dental student displays a good example of **periodontal health**. The description of the gingiva matches characteristics of periodontal health. Periodontal health is most commonly seen in young, healthy adults who receive frequent preventive care and practice effective oral hygiene.

The case illustrates what periodontal health looks like, and clinical data matches many elements of periodontal health as shown in ▶ Table 1.1.

Most patients' periodontal disease experience will fall somewhere on a spectrum of periodontal disease between perfect periodontal health and severe disease, matching all characteristics listed in ▶ Table 1.1. The challenge for a clinician is to decide whether a patient has sufficient signs and symptoms of the disease to warrant treatment.

1.3 Periodontal Health

1.3.1 Characteristics of Healthy versus Diseased Periodontal Tissues

As seen in the previous case, periodontal health means absence of signs and symptoms of periodontal disease. No signs of inflammation are present in any area of the gingiva (see ▶ Fig. 1.1), and all gingival landmarks are easily visible and in normal proportion to each other. Landmarks and areas of gingiva and mucosa are named as shown in ▶ Fig. 1.3.

1.3.2 Healthy, but Reduced Periodontium

The case described in this chapter demonstrates a healthy periodontium in an individual who likely never experienced severe periodontal disease, as the tissues are intact with no evidence of gingival recession, attachment loss, and bone loss. It is possible to achieve periodontal health after periodontal therapy, but here the tissues may show signs of past disease activity. This

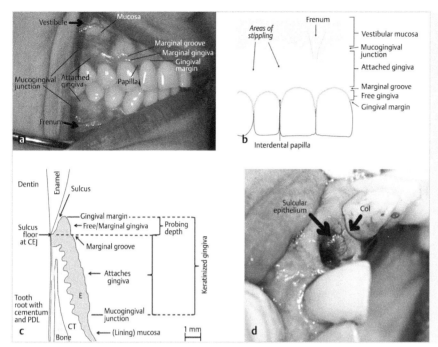

Fig. 1.3 (a) Oblique facial view of gingiva in patient seen in the preceding case with the different gingival landmarks and areas labeled. (b) Diagram of gingival landmarks. Healthy gingiva usually contains patches of stippling in the attached gingiva zone. (c) Diagram of a cross-section of healthy gingiva and periodontium attaching up to the cemento-enamel junction (CEJ). E = epithelium, CT = connective tissue. (d) Atraumatic extraction of a periodontally involved tooth reveals a depression in the interdental papilla called a "col," which forms around wide interproximal contact points. Periodontal disease also produced the rough, pebbly epithelial surface that lined the extracted tooth. This is the sulcular epithelium that normally adapts tightly to the tooth surface inside the periodontal sulcus.

Table 1.1 Findings in periodontal health vs. periodontal disease

		Healthy	Diseased
Symptoms		None	May complain about: Pain or soreness Receding gums Longer appearing teeth Loose teeth Red, swollen gum tissue Bleeds when brushing/eating
Gingival appearance/ signs of periodontal disease	Color	Coral—pink May have racial pigment	**Erythematous** ("red," "beefy red") May have slightly purple/bluish hue
	Firmness	Firm	Spongy, boggy, soft
	Shape	Pointed interproximal papilla Scalloped gingival margin Often shows marginal groove	Blunted, swollen papilla Loss of papilla Flattened scallop pattern Gingival swelling masks marginal groove
	Adaptation	Flat ("knife-edged") margin Tightly adapted to teeth	**Edematous**/Swollen ("rolled") margin Easily deflectable
	Other	Commonly has orange-peel texture ("stippling")	Smooth and shiny gingival margin May have **fistula/sinus tracts** Margin may be friable
Clinical measurements/ signs of periodontal disease	Probing depth	Low (1–3 mm usually)	High (>4 mm) Probing may be painful
	Gingival bleeding	None or insignificant	Present (at least 10% of sites)
	Clinical attachment	Intact (ideally 0 mm) Sulcus feels firm and tight	Loss of attachment (>0 mm, especially if interproximally)
	Tooth mobility	None (or little for mandibular incisors; small teeth; petite individuals)	May be easily detectable
	Recession	Ideally none	Common
	Amount of gingiva	Greater than probing depths	May be less than probing depth
	Furcation	Ideally none	Common
	Plaque	None to low	Clearly detectable
	Calculus	None to low	Clearly detectable
Radiographs		No bone loss	May have bone loss
Medical history		Typically healthy	Often has medical condition
Dental history		Usually has regular preventive care; frequent oral hygiene	Typically sporadic dental care and oral hygiene
Age		Typically younger	Typically older

state is called "healthy, but reduced periodontium," and has the following characteristics:
- Low probing depths.
- Little (< 10% of sites) or no bleeding on probing.
- Clinical attachment levels greater than zero/presence of radiographic bone loss.
- Gingival recession may be present.
- Tooth mobility may be present.
- Often, has a history of past periodontal treatment.
- Likely needs continued periodontal preventive care to prevent disease recurrence.

"Periodontal health" can also be achieved in **edentulous** areas of the jaw as there is no tooth-soft tissue interface where periodontal disease can develop. Here, the residual gingiva, away from any teeth, will appear healthy and there is no disease activity other than slow ridge resorption from lack of use.

1.4 Anatomy, Histology, and Clinical Relevance

The anatomy and histology of periodontal tissues are important for diagnosis and disease development as shown here.

1.4.1 Relationship between Clinical Landmarks and Tissue Histology

Gingival landmarks are related to unique histologic features of each gingival area (see ▶ Fig. 1.3):
- **Marginal gingiva** or free gingiva consists of keratinized stratified squamous epithelium resting on a small area of connective tissue apical to it. There is no fiber attachment to the underlying tooth. This makes the free gingiva flexible, and allows the insertion of a periodontal probe. Since this area is closest to the tooth surface, this area will display the earliest signs of periodontal inflammation. In healthy tissues, the marginal groove usually corresponds to the level of the periodontal sulcus.

- **Attached gingiva** consists of a thick layer of stratified squamous keratinized epithelium that usually lack residual cell nuclei in the most superficial layer (orthokeratinized). On the hard palate, and occasionally in gingiva, the superficial layer may retain greatly reduced cell nuclei (parakeratinized). The epithelium is firmly attached to underlying dense connective tissue with interlocking tissue fingers (rete pegs), and the underlying dense connective tissue is firmly attached to the periosteum of alveolar bone and teeth through gingival fibers. In a **thin biotype**, the gingiva is thin, translucent, relatively smooth, and has long and thin, friable dental papillae. In a **thick biotype**, the gingiva is very thick and heavily stippled with a dense, fibrous connective tissue core, and has short, stubby interdental papillae.
- **Palatal gingiva** is similar to the attached gingiva found on facial surfaces, but may also contain minor salivary glands and islands of adipose tissue, loose connective tissue, nerves and blood vessels, in addition to dense connective tissue. The epithelium and dense connective tissue of the hard palate also tend to be thicker and denser than their facial gingiva counterpart, which makes the palatal gingiva lighter in color than facial gingiva, and makes it more difficult to reflect palatal gingiva during surgery.
- **Mucosa** is a soft, flexible tissue that covers most of the oral cavity and allows jaw, lip, and tongue movement. It consists of a relatively thin nonkeratinized squamous stratified epithelium that has shallow rete pegs and rests on a deep bed of loose connective tissue. Clinically, since the epithelium is thinner and so it is more transparent. This tissue appears darker than gingiva and contains numerous small surface blood vessels that are clearly visible.
- **Interdental papilla** consists of smooth, keratinized-stratified squamous epithelium, and dense connective tissue near the interproximal alveolar bone. For anterior teeth, the interdental papilla usually is pyramid-shaped, whereas, for posterior teeth, it is saddle-shaped around the contact point. The depression around the contact point is called a **col** (see ▶ Fig. 1.4). Periodontal disease usually starts

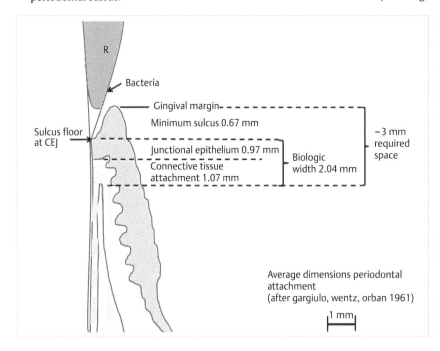

Fig. 1.4 Average dimensions of the dentogingival junction in periodontal health. R = Restoration. For most patients, a space of at least 3 mm between a restoration and alveolar bone is needed in order to prevent chronic inflammation, attachment loss, bone loss, and gingival recession.

R

Bacteria

Gingival margin

Minimum sulcus 0.67 mm

Sulcus floor at CEJ

Junctional epithelium 0.97 mm

Connective tissue attachment 1.07 mm

Biologic width 2.04 mm

~3 mm required space

Average dimensions periodontal attachment (after gargiulo, wentz, orban 1961)

1 mm

interproximally, and this tissue usually suffers the worst destruction during periodontal disease.
- **Sulcular epithelium** is the tissue facing toward the tooth within the sulcus, and consists usually of a thin layer of stratified squamous epithelium. In the absence of periodontal inflammation, it lacks rete pegs. In response to periodontal diseases, this tissue proliferates and forms a rough surface as seen in (▶ Fig. 1.3d), and it develops rete pegs.
- **Junctional epithelium** is the epithelium adjacent to the root surface at the base of the sulcus. Unlike sulcular epithelium and attached epithelium containing several distinct cell layers (basal, spinous, granular, and keratinized), junctional epithelium only contains the basal layer and a suprabasal layer that does not keratinize. If it is healthy, it forms a tight barrier against bacteria or periodontal probing and therefore it is responsible for low periodontal probing depths during periodontal health.

1.4.2 Dentogingival Junction and Biologic Width

The connective tissue and junctional epithelium attached to the tooth along with the sulcular epithelium facing the tooth are part of the dentogingival junction. The area of epithelium and connective tissue attachment to the tooth is also defined as "supracrestal attached tissue" in the newest (2018) periodontal disease classification scheme. For every patient and tooth location, there is a minimum width of this supracrestal attached tissue, which most commonly is still referred to as "biologic width". The average biologic width is about 2 mm, and a minimal sulcus is about 1-mm deep (▶ Fig. 1.4). The biologic width can vary between patients and sites depending on a patient's biotype, history of periodontal diseases, and other local factors, such as the presence of restorations.[1] The biologic width is important for several reasons:
- *For restorative purposes*: If a restoration is placed closer to the alveolar bone than the biologic width, it will likely trigger inflammation, bone loss, and gingival recession at this site. In order to prevent bone loss and gingival recession, a restoration should never extend closer than 1 mm toward the sulcus floor. If a restoration needs to be extended beyond this limit, a "clinical crown lengthening" procedure

can re-establish the biologic width surgically. In this procedure, a surgeon will typically remove bone around a tooth so that there is sufficient space for the gingiva to attach to the tooth apical to the restorative margin.
- *For periodontal diagnosis*: This allows for predicting if attachment loss is present. On average, if the radiographic distance between cemento-enamel junction (CEJ) and crestal bone is less than 2 mm, then there is likely no attachment loss.
- *For implant therapy*: This allows estimating bucco-lingual bone width for implant placement prior to diagnostic imaging. On average, gingival tissue is 2-mm thick. One can estimate the width of the underlying bone from the ridge width by subtracting 2 × 2 mm from the clinically visible ridge width, and then predict if there is sufficient bone for implant placement.

1.4.3 Epithelial Attachment to Underlying Tissues

The dentogingival junction contains the junctional epithelium that is attached to the tooth. Junctional epithelium is unique as it attaches to both teeth and connective tissue and therefore it has two genuine basement membranes. Epithelial cells attach to these basement membranes with hemidesmosomes, which are protein platforms on an area of thickened, cholesterol-stiffened cell membrane that is then anchored to the cytokeratin skeleton of the cell (▶ Fig. 1.5). This platform consists typically of five common proteins:
- 230 kD bullous pemphigoid antigen (BPAG1) and plectin, which anchor the inside of the hemidesmosome to cell's cytoskeleton.
- 180 kD bullous pemphigoid antigen (BPAG2) and type XVII collagen (COL17A1) that make up the transmembrane portion of the hemidesmosome.
- Integrins such as the alpha 6 beta 4 integrin-specific to junctional and sulcular epithelium, which attaches the hemidesmosome to the basement membrane.

The basement membrane consists of many proteins, but key proteins include the following:
- Laminin is a cross-shaped, high molecular weight molecule that is a binding target for integrins of hemidesmosomes. In turn, laminins are anchored by other proteins such as collagen

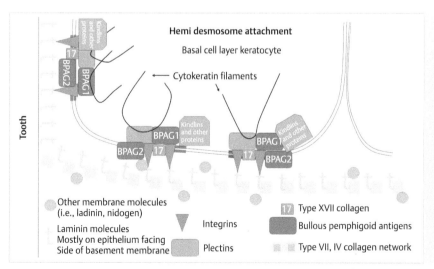

Fig. 1.5 A simplified diagram of the hemidesmosome attachment of the basal cell layer keratinocytes in the junctional epithelium. Keep in mind that even though the bullous pemphigoid antigens, type XVII collagen and integrins are the major cell membrane-supported components of the hemidesmosome, many other proteins such as the kindlins may be bound to the desmosome for regulation of integrin binding activity and stabilization of the protein complex. If any of these molecules is defective, or if autoimmune disease targets any of these proteins, epithelial attachment to underlying tissues will be impaired and serious blistering skin diseases are the consequence.

Hemi desmosome attachment

Basal cell layer keratocyte

Cytokeratin filaments

Tooth

Other membrane molecules (i.e., ladinin, nidogen)

Laminin molecules
Mostly on epithelium facing
Side of basement membrane

Integrins

Plectins

Type XVII collagen

Bullous pemphigoid antigens

Type VII, IV collagen network

type IV and VII chains and integrin, nidogen, and perlecan molecules.
- Collagen type IV and VII chains, which form the dense protein mat backbone of the basement membrane (▶ Fig. 1.5).
- Ladinin, nidogen, and perlecan cross-link various integrins, collagens, and laminins to form a secure attachment within the membrane and the underlying connective tissue fibers. Basement membranes can also contain growth factors and other molecules that control growth and differentiation of attached cells.

The attachment between epithelial cells is similar, as it involves desmosomes. Desmosomes are similar in structure and function to hemidesmosomes, but contain different proteins that are responsible for attachment to adjacent epithelial cells and not basement membranes (▶ Fig. 1.6):
- Plakoglobin and plakophilin form the internal part of the desmosome, and bind desmoplakin that anchors the desmosome to the cells' internal cytoskeleton.
- E-cadherin or carcinombryonic antigen-related cell adhesion molecule 1 (CEACAM-1) creates the transmembrane protein platform of the desmosome. In attached gingiva, the platform primarily consists of E-cadherin, whereas CEACAM-1 is the primary desmosome platform protein in sulcular and junctional epithelium.
- Desmogleins connect the desmosome platform of one cell to that of another by binding desmocollin in a Velcro-like attachment.

1.5 Clinical Significance of Cellular Attachment

The significance of these molecules becomes apparent in any autoimmune disease that targets these molecules. For example, in pemphigus vulgaris, autoantibodies target desmoglein, preventing desmosome attachment and leading to blister formation within the epithelium. In mucous membrane pemphigoid, autoantibodies may target the bullous pemphigoid antigen, laminins, or integrins, causing the epithelium to separate from the underlying connective tissue. Any condition that interferes with these molecules leads to the clinical appearance of "desquamative gingivitis," where there is significant inflammation and ulceration of the gingiva.

Cellular attachment is also important for the development of periodontal disease. Cells in the junctional epithelial layer are only loosely connected with few desmosomes, and the occasional gap junction. Therefore, periodontal bacteria, capable of initiating periodontal disease, can penetrate the junctional epithelium with relative ease. As the bacteria invade the epithelium, neutrophils will be attracted and migrate through the junctional and sulcular epithelium aided by the expression of CEACAM-1 molecules. The resulting inflammation further loosens the junctional epithelium, and, clinically, this becomes apparent as increased probing depth as a periodontal probe can easily penetrate through diseased junctional epithelium. The loose organization of junctional epithelium also allows for tissue liquid to seep through, creating a steady stream of gingival crevicular fluid through the sulcus.

1.5.1 Connective Tissue Attachment

The dentogingival junction also contains connective tissue that attaches gingiva to teeth and underlying bone. As part of normal connective tissue function, fibroblasts produce connective tissue matrix and continually produce, ingest, or degrade mostly type I and type III collagen in response to mechanical forces. Meanwhile, cementoblasts slowly deposit cementoid matrix on root surfaces nearby and osteoblasts deposit osteoid matrix on nearby alveolar bone, with the major protein component of both matrixes being type I and type III collagen as well. Collagen fibers from surrounding tissues may become entrapped in the growing osteoid and cementoid matrices, which then calcify and partially trap these collagen fibers. These fibers are known as Sharpey's fibers and they anchor teeth, connective tissue, and alveolar bone together. Periodontal fibroblasts tend to remodel collagen fibers into discrete parallel bundles to resist mechanical forces on a given tooth. These fiber bundles are divided into the dentoalveolar group or periodontal ligament fibers within the tooth socket and the gingival fiber group outside of the tooth socket. The dentoalveolar group consists of (▶ Fig. 1.7a) the following:
- *Crestal alveolar fibers*: A small group of fibers connecting the coronal third of the tooth root to the alveolar crest, and they resist both occlusal and lateral forces.
- *Horizontal fibers*: A relatively small group of fibers connecting the middle and coronal third of a tooth to the sides of a tooth socket. They resist the lateral movement of teeth.

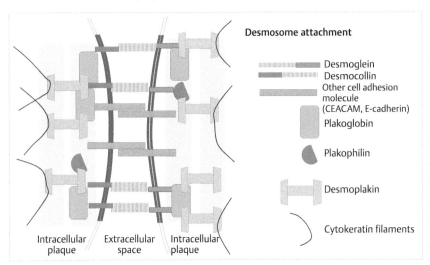

Desmosome attachment

- Desmoglein
- Desmocollin
- Other cell adhesion molecule (CEACAM, E-cadherin)
- Plakoglobin
- Plakophilin
- Desmoplakin
- Cytokeratin filaments

Intracellular plaque   Extracellular space   Intracellular plaque

Fig. 1.6 The major components of the most common attachment within oral epithelium, the desmosome. The importance of these attachment proteins is demonstrated by autoimmune and genetic defects that target these proteins, which tend to be severe skin blistering diseases and other life-threatening diseases.

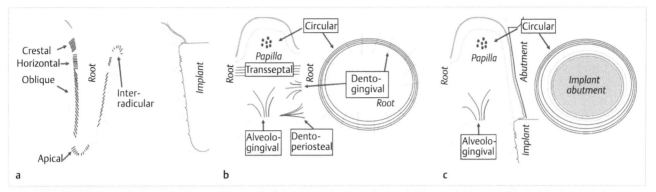

Fig. 1.7 Fiber attachment to teeth and implants. (**a**) Periodontal ligament fiber groups attaching to teeth. Dental implants generally are in direct contact with bone, and lack periodontal ligament. (**b**) Gingival fiber groups around teeth. (**c**) Generally, no gingival fibers attach to implants. The gingiva around implants is supported by the circular and alveologingival group.

- *Oblique fibers:* The majority of fibers that connect the apical and middle third of a tooth root to the side of a tooth socket. They are the primary fibers resisting apical tooth movement while chewing.
- *Apical fibers*: A small group of fibers connecting the root tips to the base of the tooth socket, and preventing the tooth from getting pulled out of the socket if sticky food is chewed.
- *Interradicular fibers:* These are only found on multirooted teeth, and connect the interdental septum with the furcation area. Like apical group fibers, they resist occlusal movement.

The gingival fibers consist of (▶ Fig. 1.7b) the following:
- **Transseptal fibers** connect tooth roots in a mesial-distal direction coronal to the interdental septa and maintain interproximal contacts. These fibers may be responsible for orthodontic relapse.
- **Alveologingival fibers** connect the gingiva with the underlying alveolar bone, and prevent the movement of attached gingiva.
- **Dentogingival fibers** connect the coronal most part of the tooth root to the overlying gingiva.
- **Dentoperiosteal fibers** connect the coronal most part of the tooth root to the facial/lingual periosteum, and add to the resistance against lateral tooth movement.
- **Circular fibers** are the only fibers that do not insert into either bone or tooth root. They encircle a tooth in the marginal gingiva and ensure the tight adaptation of marginal gingiva to a tooth crown or implant-supported crown. These fibers are also the only notable fiber group that forms in the soft tissue around dental implants (▶ Fig. 1.7c).

1.5.2 Cells, Vessels, and Nerves

The connective tissue of periodontal ligament and gingiva is a typical dense irregular connective tissue. Their cellular content and clinical significance are as follows:
- **Fibroblasts** are the most common cells, and produce the connective tissue matrix, which is mostly type I and type III collagen. Periodontal ligament fibroblasts are specially adapted for producing and maintaining periodontal ligament fibers. Abnormal collagen production or breakdown leads to gingival enlargements as seen in hereditary gingival fibromatosis and some forms of gingival enlargement. Genetic conditions resulting in defective or deficient matrix protein predispose subjects to severe periodontal disease or premature tooth loss.

- Various immune cells, such as neutrophils, dendritic cells, T-cells, and plasma cells are found in the connective tissue apical to the junctional and sulcular epithelium. While their numbers are sparse in periodontal health, plaque buildup will lead to a rapid increase in neutrophil numbers initially followed by large numbers of plasma cells in areas of chronic inflammation. Neutrophils can be a significant source of collagenases contributing to the loss of collagen fibers and attachment loss in periodontal disease. B-cells and plasma cells can be a significant source of RANK ligand, which favors bone loss seen in severe periodontal disease. T-cells produce various inflammatory cytokines, which may perpetuate chronic inflammation and tissue damage.
- **Melanocytes** within the basal cell layer of the gingiva may provide racial pigmentation.
- **Epithelial cell rests of Malassez** are remnants of Hertwig's root sheath and may give rise to lateral periodontal cysts or abscesses.
- Nerve fibers from terminal branches of the trigeminal nerve allow for the detailed sensing of chewing, food texture, and temperature. Ruffini endings are the primary tactile sensors in periodontal ligament. Gingiva also contains Merkel cells that can detect touch. Pain is sensed by naked, argyrophilic nerve fiber endings embedded in gingiva and periodontal ligament. Alveolar bone itself contains few nerve fibers, which often permit periodontal surgery or implant surgery with infiltration anesthesia.
- Various strongly interconnected blood vessels provide a rich blood supply. Generally, blood flows from the vestibule and apical areas to the coronal and interproximal aspect of the alveolar ridge, and from distal to mesial. The periodontal ligament is nourished from many small blood vessels that reach out from the center, cancellous portion of the alveolar bone through the cribriform plate into the tooth socket. Gingiva receives blood from blood vessels branching out from the cancellous portion of the bone through the cortical compact bone into the gingiva, and from blood vessels within the connective tissue portion of the gingiva, arising from larger blood vessels deep under the vestibular mucosa (▶ Fig. 1.8).

The periodontal blood supply has several clinical implications. Since blood vessels in the gingiva and periodontal ligament are small, bleeding from periodontal procedures most likely is caused by cut capillaries and stoppable with firm, sustained

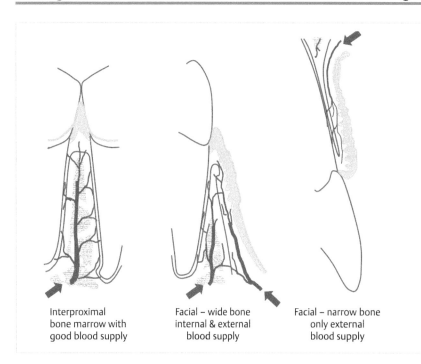

Fig. 1.8 Blood flow of gingiva, alveolar bone, and periodontal ligament follows an apical to coronal and distal to mesial pattern. Periodontal ligament is well nourished through capillaries and blood vessels arising from the bone marrow of interseptal and apical bone. Facial bone is nourished from both internal sources and from the overlying gingiva if the facial bone is thick. Thin facial bone is nourished mostly through the overlying gingival tissue, which can present surgical problems and pose a risk for bone loss and gingival recession.

Interproximal bone marrow with good blood supply

Facial – wide bone internal & external blood supply

Facial – narrow bone only external blood supply

pressure. Since blood supply arises from the vestibule, surgical incisions for periodontal surgery are usually made as coronal as possible to avoid tissue necrosis after surgery. The blood supply also explains why paper-thin facial bone can exist around anterior teeth since it is nourished through the gingival blood supply. However, if the overlaying gingiva is reflected during surgery, this paper-thin bone loses its blood supply and likely resorbs during healing, which causes bone loss and soft tissue recession.

1.6 Contribution of Microbes to Periodontal Disease

Common periodontal diseases are microbial infections. A common goal of periodontal therapy is to reduce microbial contaminants on tooth surfaces that are in contact with periodontal tissues.

1.6.1 Plaque, Calculus, and Oral Hygiene

In clinical practice, microbial contamination is assumed if tooth surface deposits are found. The surface accretions are named as follows:
- **Acquired pellicle** is a thin, translucent, slightly gray, or brown film of proteins that immediately forms over the enamel surface after polishing once saliva contacts the tooth. Acquired pellicle does not contain bacteria and usually is not visible clinically.
- Tooth staining is a thin, nonproteinaceous, brown, or black surface film caused by the deposition of colored organic molecules from tobacco, coffee, tea, mouth rinses, or other strongly colored foods.
- Bacterial staining is an uncommon patchy red, orange, green, black, or brown surface stain created by bacterial colonies.

- Food debris consists of freshly impacted food particles with few bacteria, and can be rinsed off.
- **Material alba** is an unstructured, loose, white, granular film consisting of salivary proteins, cell debris, bacteria, and degranulated neutrophils. Unlike plaque, material alba can be rinsed off.
- **Dental plaque** is an organized, dense, sticky, and white or off-white biofilm containing mostly rods, cocci, and filamentous bacteria (▶Fig. 1.9). It cannot be rinsed off, but oral hygiene methods can eliminate it. Besides water, plaque contains about 11% weight in inorganic material, 11% protein, 6% carbohydrates, and minor amounts of lipids and other substances.
- **Dental calculus** is a darkly colored, mineralized, hard plaque that consists 70 to 90% of calcium phosphate salts (▶Fig. 1.10). Calcium hydroxyapatite and octacalcium phosphate are most commonly found in mature calculus, whereas magnesium whitlockite and brushite are found in immature calculus. Oral hygiene methods cannot remove calculus, and calculus tends to form near salivary gland orifices. Calculus can form within 24 hours, and formation rate depends on local salivary flow rate, calcium ion levels, local pH, plaque accumulation, and the presence of urea or ammonia-producing bacteria.[2] If calculus forms in a periodontal pocket, it is usually a hard, dense, and rough root surface deposit, which is colored brown, black, or green from pigmented bacteria or hemoglobin breakdown.

Of these accretions, only plaque and calculus near the gingival margin and within pockets are related to periodontal disease. The rate of plaque and calculus accumulation depends on many factors such as:
- *Softness and stickiness of food*: Enhances microbial growth as it prolongs nutrient availability.
- *Sucrose content of food*: Enhances the growth of mutans type streptococci that produce a sticky glucan matrix using glucosyltransferase enzyme.

- Calcium content of food and saliva enhances the mineralization of plaque into calculus.
- Alkalinity of foods and saliva enhances the mineralization of plaque into calculus.
- Saliva protein content enhances pellicle and calculus formation.
- Salivary flow enhances calculus formation by supplying additional calcium ions.
- Soft tissue movement and occlusion prevent plaque accumulation.
- Shedding rate of epithelial cells influences the rate of material alba formation.
- Frequency and effectiveness of oral hygiene methods that remove plaque.
- Frequency and effectiveness of professional tooth cleaning that removes surface deposits.
- Local anatomic and restorative factors such as malpositioned teeth, root concavities, enamel defects, bulky restorations, and orthodontic appliances create niches for plaque growth.

The combination of these factors determines if a patient accumulates calculus quickly, or where in the oral cavity plaque and calculus accumulate. In general, patients can effectively brush facial tooth surfaces, resulting in little plaque, calculus, and periodontal disease on facial surfaces. In contrast, patients

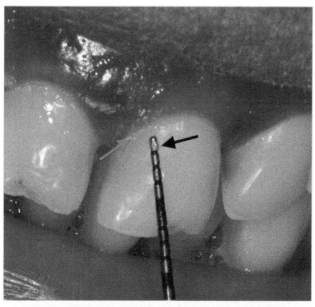

Fig. 1.9 Plaque near the gingival margin (*red arrow*) and collecting as off-white, sticky material on the tip of a periodontal probe (*black arrow*).

usually find interproximal oral hygiene difficult to achieve, resulting in interproximal areas having higher plaque levels. In addition, plaque at these sites is able to mature, and is more likely to contain a disease-causing microbial community. Consequently, periodontal disease usually begins interproximally, and the worst damage is seen here. While plaque can mineralize into calculus interproximally, the largest amounts of supragingival calculus are usually seen near the opening of salivary ducts (parotid gland-buccal of maxillary 1st molars; Wharton's duct-lingual of mandibular incisors) as saliva flow and calcium content are highest here.

1.6.2 Models of Periodontal Disease—One Does not Fit All

Dentists have grappled with understanding and classifying periodontal diseases as the source of tooth loss and gingival inflammation for more than a century. Various disease models have been proposed that apply to some periodontal diseases and explain some aspects of periodontal disease:

- *General plaque hypothesis*: The amount of plaque or bacteria correlates to inflammation and periodontal disease severity. This model applies best to plaque-associated gingivitis in young, healthy patients. In experimental gingivitis, healthy subjects stop oral hygiene after having their teeth cleaned professionally. Within days, the number and diversity of bacteria increase toward a more gram-negative, anaerobic flora of spirochetes, rods, filamentous bacteria, and motile bacteria. Within 7–10 days, this is followed by significant inflammation. Resumption of oral hygiene reduces bacterial counts and diversity, and restores gingival health (▶ Fig. 1.11).
- *Specific plaque hypothesis*: Specific bacteria cause periodontal disease similar to medical infectious disease. This applies best to rare periodontal diseases caused by agents of systemic disease such as Neisseria, Treponema pallidum, Mycobacteria bacteria, Candida, and other fungal or viral infections. It also applies to some cases of severe periodontitis exhibiting a molar/incisor pattern associated with leukotoxic strains of *Aggregatibacter actinomycetemcomitans* bacteria. With any of these perio-dontal diseases, disease activity ceases once these organisms are eliminated with appropriate antimicrobial therapy.
- *Plaque ecology*: Environmental changes favor growth of disease-causing bacteria. This was originally developed to explain caries development but it also applies to periodontal disease. For example, creation of an overhanging restoration creates a niche for plaque retention, allowing growth of disease-causing bacteria that need a protected environment.

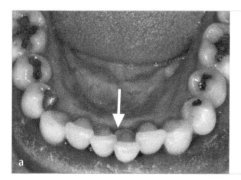
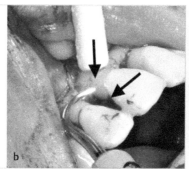

Fig. 1.10 Calculus types. (a) Typical off-white, hard supragingival calculus building up on lingual surfaces of crowded mandibular incisors, filling the interproximal space (*white arrow*). (b) Typical black subgingival calculus discovered during periodontal surgery (*black arrows*).

- *Dysbiosis*: An existing microbial community associated with health undergoes changes in microbial composition that then promote disease development. In periodontitis, it is thought that the addition of various key microbial species to dental plaque is the initiator of disease development. Some of these key specises such as *Porphyromonas gingivalis* can manipulate the local immune system to maintain persistent chronic inflammation. This chronic state of inflammation produces constant tissue damage, which then allows these key species and many other organisms to feed on tissue by-products.[3]
- *An integrated model*: Periodontal microbes interact with the local immune system to cause inflammation. Long-term inflammation interferes with normal cell functioning in periodontal tissues that leads to clinically observable signs and symptoms of periodontal disease. The general degree and speed at which periodontal disease happens are influenced by the overall systemic and genetic health of a patient, with conditions diminishing immunity and soft tissue function leading to more severe disease. Local differences in periodontal destructions are caused by local factors that either favor plaque retention or present some form of chronic trauma (▶ Fig. 1.12).
- *Burst model*: Periodontal disease activity happens in repeated short episodes of active disease. For each individual patient, disease experience will differ at any given point of time (▶ Fig. 1.13). This applies to most cases and stresses the importance of frequent follow-up with patients who have periodontal disease as this will increase the chance of observing and stopping active disease.

1.6.3 Establishment of a Periodontal Disease-causing Microbial Community

Development of plaque-associated periodontal diseases hinges on the development of a microbial community that triggers chronic and deep inflammation in periodontal tissues. Clinically, the amount of visible plaque often corresponds to gingival inflammation, but not to probing depth, attachment loss, or bone loss. Plaque formation generally proceeds as follows:

- *Acquired pellicle formation*: Salivary proteins, such as acidic proline-rich proteins, coat a tooth as soon as it erupts into the oral cavity, or as soon as saliva contacts a polished tooth surface.
- *Growth of early colonizers*: Mostly gram-positive, aerobic coccoid bacteria including oral viridans streptococci, such as *Streptococcus mitis* and *S. salivarius,* form sparse colonies on the acquired pellicle within 24 hours. Other streptococcal species, such *S. oralis, S. mutans, S. anginosus, S. gordonii,* and some *Actinomyces* species, grow and displace earlier colonists.
- *Growth of intermediate colonizers*: After several days of plaque formation, additional bacteria, mostly gram-positive, facultative anaerobic rods, such as *Actinomyces naeslundii,* attach to the early colonizers, forming a more complex biofilm on the tooth surface.
- *Growth of late colonizers*: As the biofilm matures and thickens after 1 week, pockets of low-oxygen environment develop where anaerobic rods and fusiform bacteria, such as *Fusobacterium nucleatum,* can grow. *F. nucleatum* and

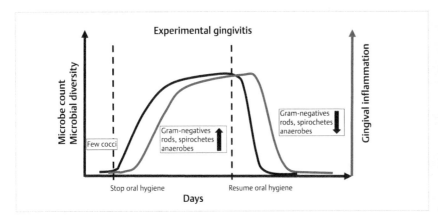

Fig. 1.11 Experimental gingivitis model. Cessation of oral hygiene leads to plaque accumulation on previously cleaned teeth. As plaque accumulates, bacterial counts, diversity, gram-negatives, rods, spirochetes increase. This is followed by gingival inflammation, resulting in significant gingivitis 7–10 days after oral hygiene cessation. Restoration of oral hygiene restores the original state of gingival health.

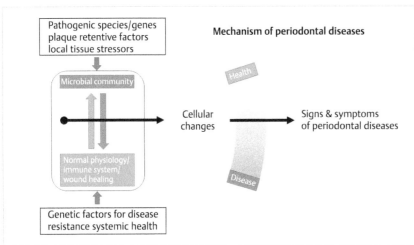

Fig. 1.12 Periodontal diseases produce clinical signs and symptoms depending on the competing forces between the disease-causing microbial community and the periodontal tissues immune system and wound healing capacity to restore periodontal health. If the balance tips toward consistent, continuous cell damage, signs and symptoms appear and the clinical impression of a particular periodontal disease becomes apparent. This interplay is influenced by many factors, such as the presence of more **virulent pathogenic** species or gene products from different microorganisms, plaque-retentive factors, and local tissue stressors, such as occlusal trauma, genetic factors, and systemic conditions.

similar bacteria are important in that they can bind to many other bacteria and produce metabolites that aid the growth of early and late colonizers. Bacteria, such as *F. nucleatum,* also produce tissue-damaging factors, such as porins, which enhances local inflammation that releases tissue amino acids required for bacterial growth. It is at this stage, where gingival inflammation becomes clinically apparent.

- *Infection with periodontal pathogens*: Gram-negative, anaerobic bacteria associated with severe periodontal disease, such as *P. gingivalis, Tannerella forsythia, Treponema denticola* (Hertwig's), and other oral spirochetes, become established, attaching to other bacteria and using metabolic products of other bacteria. For example, *P. gingivalis* attaches to fimbria and aggregation factor produced by *A. naeslundii* and develops a synergistic metabolic relationship with *T. forsythia.*

Early colonizers are associated with periodontal health. They may even be protective to some degree, as they compete with other bacteria for nutrients, produce hydrogen peroxide that prevents growth of many gram-negative bacteria, and release **biocins**, which are antimicrobial proteins that kill other bacteria. Many of these bacteria also release acidic metabolic by-products, which contributes to dental caries on susceptible tooth surfaces, if a consistently low local pH can be maintained by these bacteria.

Late colonizers are associated with gingival inflammation and risk of developing attachment loss or bone loss, and the so-called "red complex" bacteria, including *P. gingivalis, T. forsythia,* and *T. denticola,* are associated with deep probing depth and attachment loss. However, even in sites with severe periodontal disease, these bacteria make up only about 3% of all bacterial DNA content in the site. The continued presence of early and intermediate colonizers mutually benefits the bacteria within the biofilm as various members of the biofilm use each other for attachment as described in the **Kolenbrander model** of dental plaque,[4] and the bacteria utilize each other's metabolic by-products to satisfy their nutritional needs (▶ Fig. 1.14).

Various other bacterial species called "novel putative periodontal pathogens," even viruses and enteric amoebas, have been associated with severe chronic periodontal diseases as well. Besides "red complex" bacteria, late colonizers may also include other microorganisms that are associated with either atypical periodontal diseases related to immunosuppression and genetic disorders, or aggressive periodontal diseases that affect young, healthy patients. The later colonizer *A. actinomycetemcomitans* serotype b is associated with aggressive periodontal disease in young patients.

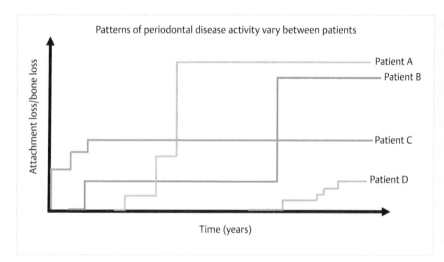

Fig. 1.13 Different patients will experience different disease activity over time, and disease activity will come in quick bursts of tissue destruction that likely occur between dental appointments.

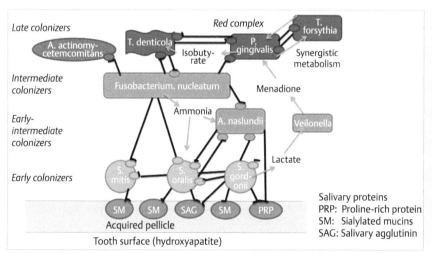

Fig. 1.14 In dental plaque, intermediate and late colonizers adhere to each other and utilize waste products as metabolites (*blue*). (Simplified Kolenbrander model with added metabolic pathways.)

1.6.4 Red Complex Bacteria Contribution to Periodontal Disease Development

Unlike many medical infections, red complex bacteria make up only a small fraction of the entire biofilm. The reason that these few bacteria can induce disease is that they provide mechanisms to prevent a successful immune response and allow the entire microbial community to persist and continually stimulate the immune system for more ineffective responses. Here are some key organisms that demonstrate multiple virulence factors, which contribute to the development of destructive periodontal disease:

- *P. gingivalis* is a black-pigmented, anaerobic rod that thrives off tissue breakdown products caused by inflammation. The following factors aid its ability to cause periodontal disease:
  - Major and minor fimbriae attach to other bacteria, tooth surfaces, and human cells.[5]
  - *Gingipains*: Lysine and arginine proteases that digest tissue and immune proteins.
  - Ability to invade epithelial and endothelial cells for the evasion of immune cells.
  - Noxious volatile organic compounds induce tissue damage and cause halitosis
  - Atypical **Lipid A** component of lipopolysaccharide triggers ineffective immune response.
  - Outer membrane vesicles trigger inflammation and impair cell function at a distance.
- *T. denticola* is one of many gram-negative, anaerobic oral spirochetes associated with severe periodontitis, necrotizing periodontal disease, and abscesses. It produces:
  - Major sheath protein binds to human proteins and *F. nucleatum*; it also impairs neutrophil migration and macrophage function.
  - Cystalysin protein lyses red blood cells, which are a food source for oral spirochetes.
  - Dentilisin, a prolyl-phenylalanine-specific protease, digests tissue matrix, and immune proteins. It also allows it to bind to *P. gingivalis* and *T. forsythia*.

- *T. forsythia* is a gram-negative anaerobe rod requiring amino acids for growth. It lives in metabolic synergy with the other red complex bacteria, and produces:
  - Sheath protein BspA, which allows attachment to epithelial cells, *F. nucleatum,* and stimulates destructive immune responses.
  - Several proteases, karilysin, mirolysin, and mirolase that breaks down tissue matrix and complement.
- *A. actinomycetemcomitans* is not a member of the red complex and is commonly found in small numbers in the oral cavity as harmless commensalist.
  - Some strains, however, produce leukotoxin, a pore-forming toxin that destroys neutrophils. These strains are associated with localized severe periodontitis exhibiting a molar/incisor pattern that causes rapid bone and tooth loss in young patients. Production of this toxin is in part regulated by a quorum sensing system using Lux proteins.
  - Some strains (serotype b) produce lipopolysaccharides that are more effective in inducing inflammatory responses and are associated with severe periodontal disease.

While these are some of the best known periodontal disease-causing bacteria, it is important to realize that many other bacteria and microbes may be involved in periodontal disease, and some of these have not yet been identified or studied. It is also likely that not a single species cause disease, but it is the total sum of bacteria and expressed genes of all microbes that cause disease.

1.6.5 Effect of Plaque Retentive Local Factors on Periodontal Disease

While poor oral hygiene typically leads to higher levels of plaque everywhere, in most patients, periodontal disease affects teeth unequally, with incisors typically having the least amount of periodontal disease, and molars having the most amount of tissue destruction. Differences in periodontal disease experience between teeth are most likely due to local factors that protect plaque from removal during oral hygiene and professional tooth cleaning as shown in ▶ Table 1.2.

Table 1.2 Factors that favor plaque retention and maturation

Anatomical	Restorative	Periodontal
Furcation entrances	Overhanging margins	Deep pockets
Root projections	Open margins	Calculus deposits
Enamel pearls and projections	Poor interproximal contacts	Bulky gingiva
Enamel defects	Subgingival restorative margins	Localized gingival recession
Dentin ridges and concavities	Caries	Sensitive gingiva/tissue
Aberrant cusps	Bulky restorations	Lack of keratinized gingiva
Dental invaginations	Undercontoured restorations	Tooth mobility
Tipped/crowded teeth	Pontics	
Partially impacted 3rd molars	Cantilevers	
Unevenly erupted teeth	Extracoronal attachments	
Shallow/tight vestibule	Splints	
	Rough restorative materials	
	Removable partial dentures	
	Orthodontic appliances	
	Exposed implant surface	
	Deeply placed implant platform	
	Loose restorative components	
	Restorative flash	
	Extruded cement	
	Sensitive teeth	

Most of these factors directly protect an area of plaque from removal. Some of these factors, such as tooth mobility, make plaque removal less efficient, whereas lack of keratinized gingiva may cause local tissue to be sensitive and provide a deterrent against a patient's hygiene efforts. Regardless of the mechanism, these factors allow long-term retention of plaque, which allows plaque to mature and become a niche for possible infection with periodontal pathogens. Presence of these factors at a given site often explains local differences in periodontal disease activity and tissue damage.

1.7 Host Defense Mechanisms and Periodontal Disease

As microbes try to colonize the periodontal sulcus and extract as many nutrients as possible from the surrounding tissue and oral cavity, the human body attempts to restrict this colonization. Although this is successful for mild periodontal diseases, this backfires in the periodontitis-type periodontal diseases where an ineffective immune response contributes significantly to the clinical appearance of periodontal destruction.

1.7.1 Innate Immunity: Protection Against Periodontal Infection

For many individuals, mature plaque may develop after several months, but destructive periodontal disease takes decades to develop. This may happen as the individual never contracts virulent late colonizers, and also because of innate immunity that keeps the microbial community confined to the sulcus through these mechanisms:

- *Physical barrier*: Gingival epithelial cells are generally tightly connected with many desmosomes and isolated gap junctions, further bound to a basement membrane made of a dense network of collagens and other proteins. The exception to this is the junctional epithelium, where epithelial cells are only loosely connected.
- *Constant epithelial shedding*: Basal cells of these epithelia proliferate constantly, renewing the epithelium and shedding individual cells along with any attached bacteria into the oral cavity.
- *Gingival crevicular fluid*: Tissue fluid leaks through the basement membrane and epithelium as there are no tight junctions in the junctional epithelium, resulting in a constant flow from the base of the sulcus into the oral cavity, which helps to flush out microbes from the sulcus. Inflammation increases this flow, which may help limit further inflammation.
- Antimicrobial peptides and proteins are produced by epithelial cells, neutrophils, and salivary glands. These can function in several ways:
  - Decoy attachment molecules, which prevent bacterial adhesion molecules from attaching properly to tissues.
  - Chelator molecules that reduce the availability of key nutrients, such as iron.
  - Protease inhibitors that block the action of gingipains and other tissue-degrading enzymes produced by bacteria.
  - Peroxidases, such as myeloperoxidase, that promote oxidative damage to bacteria.
  - Cationic peptides, such as LL-37, formed from degraded cathelicidin that disrupts bacterial cell walls.
  - Antimicrobial proteins, such as lysozyme, that enzymatically digest cell walls of gram-positive bacteria,[6] and beta-defensins, which form pores in microbial membranes.

Clinical relevance: Genetic defects affecting these proteins result in severe periodontal disease. For example, in Papillon-Lefèvre syndrome, there is a defect in the cathepsin C gene, which encodes a protein that then fails to activate protease-3, which in turn fails to produce functional cathelicidin, and patients affected by this syndrome then develop severe bacterial infections including periodontal disease.

- **Neutrophils** are found normally in small numbers near the dentogingival junction, and are recruited by epithelial and fibroblasts cells that emit chemokines after exposure to periodontal bacteria. Neutrophils are very efficient in killing periodontal bacteria, and are the reason why destructive periodontal disease usually develops very slowly.

The general mechanism on how epithelial cells, fibroblasts, and neutrophils can detect and fight of periodontal bacteria is made possible by the presence of many bacterial molecules associated with normal microbial function and not found in human cells. These are called "pathogen-associated molecular patterns" and are detected with various receptors as shown in ▶ Table 1.3.

Binding of microbial molecules to these pattern-recognition receptors activates signaling cascades within the cell. Commonly, these are pathways, such as the nuclear factor kappa of activated B-cells (NFκB), mitogen-activated protein kinase, and the stress-activated protein kinase/Jun amino-terminal kinase pathways, which lead to expression of many genes related to immune activation.[7]

In epithelial cells and fibroblasts, this usually leads to expression of chemokines (i.e., Interleukin-8 or CXL-8, macrophage inflammatory protein [MIP-1α] and growth-related oncogene

Table 1.3 Molecular patterns associated with microbes and cellular receptors

Molecular pattern (PAMP) (and oral organism that possesses it)	Receptor (pattern-recognition receptor)
Cell wall fragments (as in oral bacteria, yeast)	TLR2
Flagellin (as in motile bacteria, i.e., spirochetes)	TLR5
Formylated methionine (fMLP) (any oral bacteria)	fMLP receptor
Intracellular bacteria (i.e., intracellular *P. gingivalis* bacteria)	NOD-1, NOD-2
Lipopolysaccharide, lipooligosaccharide, lipid A (gram-negative bacteria)	CD14 together with TLR4
Lipopeptides (bacteria)	TLR2 with TLR6 or TLR1
Mannose-containing branched carbohydrates (oral yeasts such as Candida species)	Various scavenger receptors
Unmethylated CpG pattern nucleotides (any microbe)	TLR9
Viral RNA/DNA fragments (i.e., herpes, cytomegaloviruses in sulcus)	Various TLRs (TLR3,7,8)

Abbreviations: CD, cluster of differentiation; CpG, cytosine-purine-guanosine; NOD, nucleotide-binding oligomerization domain-containing (protein); TLR, toll-like receptor.

family chemokines) that attract immune cells like neutrophils. These same cells will also release cytokines (i.e., Interleukin-1, 6, Tumor-necrosis factor alpha) that activate immune cells.

In neutrophils, binding of bacterial proteins to pattern-recognition receptors, in the presence of cytokines, leads to full activation of neutrophils. This results in:

- Transfer of granules filled with antibacterial substances, such as cathelicidin, lysozyme, and myeloperoxidase, to the cell membrane.
- Granule release.
- Release of matrix metalloproteinases that aid movement of neutrophils through the connective tissue epithelium into the sulcus, and also removes periodontal tissue fibers.
- Engulf microbes.
- Burst and release a web of DNA that entraps and kills more bacteria.
- Production of various chemokines and cytokines recruiting and activating more immune cells.

Clinical significance: Genetic defects in these pattern-recognition receptor/activation cascade/chemokine homing systems at a minimum result in a high risk of life-threatening bacterial infections and severe destructive periodontal disease early in life. Although there is some genetic redundancy that protects against fatal immune defects from the loss of one receptor or signaling molecule, there are several examples where mutations lead to severe periodontal disease:

- *Chediak-Higashi syndrome*: A mutation in a protein-regulating vesicle transport causes neutrophils to be unable to release their antimicrobial granules, thus resulting in recurrent severe bacterial infections and periodontal disease.
- *Leukocyte adhesion deficiency syndromes (LAD-1, LAD-2; lazy neutrophil syndrome)*: Neutrophils lack functional receptors that allow them to leave blood vessels at the site nearest to infection, resulting in generalized severe destructive periodontal disease early in life and risk of life-threatening infections.
- *Congenital neutropenia, cyclic neutropenia, agranulocytosis, Kostmann syndrome, Fanconi anemia, aplastic anemia,* and *chemotherapy*: Lack of neutrophils causes severe periodontal disease and life-threatening bacterial infections.

Although neutrophils are largely protective against periodontal disease as shown by these conditions, overly activated neutrophils can produce excessive tissue damage as the antimicrobial molecules released by them can also damage surrounding normal periodontal tissue. The normal function of neutrophils and the innate immunity, in general, limits the damaging effect of microbes in the periodontal sulcus, and helps achieve a steady state between tissue damage and wound healing that is limited to the immediate tissues surrounding the sulcus (▶ Fig. 1.15).

1.7.2 Adaptive Immunity and Chronic Periodontal Disease

It is still unclear what causes the progression from gingivitis to periodontitis, and when this happens, as the majority of adults apparently never progress from gingivitis to periodontitis. The presence of red complex bacteria, such as *P. gingivalis,* is not sufficient by itself to cause destructive periodontal disease. One key for the transition from mild gingival inflammation to destructive periodontal disease may be the adaptive immune system. While neutrophils are important in keeping periodontal disease in check, the majority of immune cells found in gingiva of patients with clinically recognizable gingivitis are lymphocytes and plasma cells. Although these cells are concerned with antibody production, these cells produce ineffective IgG2 antibodies that do not control periodontal disease. As periodontal microbes are not cleared from the sulcus, the following cells may be involved in tissue destruction:

- *Dendritic cells and macrophages*: Recognize invading microbes, engulf, and process them to small peptides that they present on their cell surface in major histocompatibility complex receptors. These cells migrate to local lymph nodes and present these peptide-filled receptors to lymphocytes. If they encounter a lymphocyte that recognizes the peptide, they release a variety of cytokines that stimulate the lymphocyte to proliferate and differentiate into a functional B or T-cell.
- *CD4+ T-cells/T helper (Th) cells*: Depending on the macrophage or dendritic cell's released cytokine profile, it will drive the development of naïve Th-cells into different T-cell subsets:
  - *Th1* promotes cell death in cells infected with intracellular parasites such as viruses or intracellular bacteria.
  - *Th2* stimulates the production of antibodies by B-cells differentiating into plasma cells. Generally, this is protective against bacterial and viral infections as antibodies

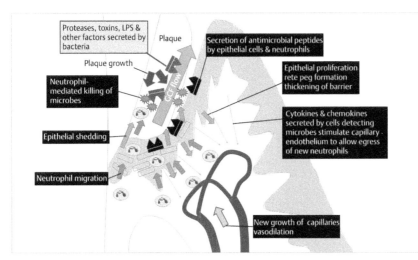

Fig. 1.15 Even though bacteria can become established in the sulcus, inflammation stays localized the junctional and sulcular epithelium as the epithelium, neutrophils, and supportive connective tissues counteract microbial growth and virulence factors. The epithelium serves as physical barrier and proliferates in response to bacteria, which leads to increased thickness and development of rete pegs. Proliferation also leads to increased epithelial shedding, which also helps to eliminate attached bacteria, along with a stream of gingival crevicular fluid that ejects loose microbes. Epithelial cells secrete antimicrobial peptides and messenger molecules that lead to recruitment and replenishment of neutrophils, which also limit microbial growth.

neutralize these microbes. This is effective against *A. actinomycetemcomitans* and it usually keeps damages localized to few teeth, but fails against *P. gingivalis* and allows continued tissue loss in periodontitis.
- ○ Treg cells are a set of diverse Th cells that limit inflammation and promote wound healing.
- ○ Th9 cells promote survival of Treg cells.
- ○ Th17 cells promote strong, and maybe excessive neutrophil responses to bacterial infection, which leads to tissue damage.
- **B-cells**, some of which differentiate into plasma cells that produce antibodies.

The presence of an adaptive immune response is important in limiting periodontal infections, as lack of T-cells in DiGeorge and Wiskott-Aldrich syndromes leads to severe periodontal disease. Severe periodontal disease is also a typical sign of AIDS caused by uncontrolled long-term HIV infection. On the other hand, cells in adaptive immunity may play a significant role in periodontal disease:
- Periodontal tissues affected by periodontitis contain large numbers of Th17 cells.
- Th17 cells promote activation of neutrophils, which release matrix metalloproteinase that degrade collagen fibers in periodontal tissues. This loss of collagen fibers may favor attachment loss.
- In tissues affected by periodontitis, a significant amount of RANK ligand is produced by:
  - ○ Th17 cells.
  - ○ B-cells.
- RANK ligand induces the development and activation of osteoclasts, which remove bone. In periodontitis, more RANK ligand is produced than osteoprotegerin (OPG), which is a decoy receptor for RANK ligand and prevents bone loss. Consequently, bone metabolism is skewed toward continued bone loss[8,9] (▶ Fig. 1.16).

1.7.3 Mechanisms Leading to Gingival Erythema and Bleeding

The earliest sign of periodontal disease is gingival erythema. The color of the gingival margin depends on:
- Hemoglobin (red) in red blood cells within gingival capillaries. Inflammation leads to the production of vasoepithelial growth factor (VEGF), which causes an increase in capillaries. Inflammation also leads to widened capillaries, and both are responsible for increased gingival redness.
- Oxygenation of hemoglobin (dark red color, if deoxygenated). A decrease in blood flow leads to darker, more "cyanotic" appearance of the gingiva in severe inflammation.
- Translucency of keratinized epithelial cells. The increased thickness of gingival epithelium blocks some of the red color of underlying tissue, resulting in the pale pink appearance of gingiva.
- Presence of melanocytes (brown-black). This is responsible for racial pigmentation.
- Presence of colored substances in the gingiva. This is uncommon, but leads to discolored gingiva if amalgam or metal fragments become imbedded in gingiva, or to marginal discoloration in the presence of environmental heavy metal exposure.

Many inflammatory mediators, such as prostaglandin E2 and proteolytic enzymes released by tissues and bacteria, weaken or damage blood vessel walls, causing an increased flow of plasma into the tissue, leading to gingival edema or swelling and generally more fragile blood vessels in the gingiva. Inflammation also weakens the basement membrane and desmosomal attachment of epithelial cells, causing junctional epithelium to detach or ulcerate in response to periodontal disease. Insertion of a periodontal probe into an inflamed pocket can easily penetrate the junctional epithelium and rupture capillaries in the area, leading to the clinical sign of gingival bleeding on probing.

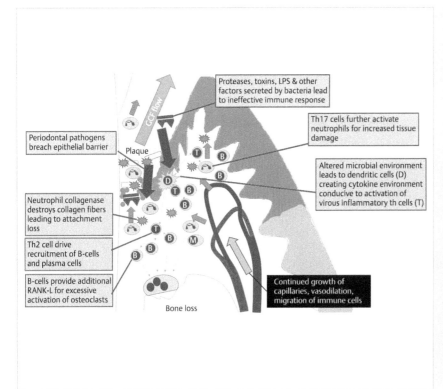

Periodontal pathogens breach epithelial barrier

Plaque

GCF flow

Proteases, toxins, LPS & other factors secreted by bacteria lead to ineffective immune response

Th17 cells further activate neutrophils for increased tissue damage

Altered microbial environment leads to dendritic cells (D) creating cytokine environment conducive to activation of virous inflammatory th cells (T)

Neutrophil collagenase destroys collagen fibers leading to attachment loss

Th2 cell drive recruitment of B-cells and plasma cells

B-cells provide additional RANK-L for excessive activation of osteoclasts

Bone loss

Continued growth of capillaries, vasodilation, migration of immune cells

Fig. 1.16 In periodontitis, the balance between immune defense and microbial growth breaks down as the microbial community changes and some microbes either are able to invade tissues or evade the immune system with various virulence factors. While the previous protective mechanisms, such as neutrophil migration, bacterial killing, epithelial functions, and crevicular fluid flow, continue, they are no longer effective. This happens as the changed bacterial environment also triggers a changed cytokine environment produced by dendritic cells (D) and other antigen presenting cells that now stimulate development of various inflammatory T-helper cells (T). For example, Th17 cells are generated that further activate neutrophils, and these overactive neutrophils produce greater tissue damage. For example, the increased amount of neutrophil collagenase aids further destruction of collagen fibers, leading to attachment loss. Also, Th2 cells recruit and activate B-cells and plasma cells (both labeled B) that produce ineffective antibody, and produce RANK-ligand, which in concert with inflammatory mediators tips the RANK-L/OPG balance to favor osteoclast activation and bone loss.

1.7.4 Mechanism Leading to Pocketing and Attachment Loss

The probing depth is a measure of soft tissue height relative to the sulcus/pocket floor and is determined by:

- A relatively fixed epithelial thickness of about 1 mm. This thickness is created by the differentiation process of epithelial cells, and is limited by nutrient diffusion.
- A variable connective tissue thickness that can change depending on the cell content, matrix content, and liquid content of the tissue. Since periodontal inflammation leads to an increased influx of immune cells while at the same time producing fluid inflow from leaky capillaries as described above, it leads to an increase of connective tissue thickness and swelling of the marginal gingiva as a whole. Other conditions such as medications (e.g., calcium channel blockers, phenytoin, and cyclosporine) or genetic conditions (i.e., hereditary gingival fibromatosis) that stimulate either proliferation of fibroblasts or increased deposition of connective tissue matrix produce the same effect. The now inflated marginal gingiva is taller compared to the apical connective tissue attachment, thus resulting in a deeper pocket as the gingival margin moves more coronal in relation to the tooth.
- The degree to which the periodontal probe penetrates the junctional epithelium. If healthy, the sulcular epithelium is tightly packed, and a periodontal probe does not penetrate it with light pressure. If diseased, the epithelium is weakened by proteolytic enzymes and a periodontal probe can penetrate it, which leads to greater probing depths.

The base of a pocket can migrate apically in response to attachment loss, which reflects the loss of collagen fibers attached to the root surface. Collagen fiber alterations, as a result of gingival inflammation, develop early in the disease process, starting around blood vessels before clinical signs of gingival erythema develop, and affecting most collagen fibers in established gingivitis. Even though there is loss of collagen fibers in gingivitis, it likely is not enough to be clinically noticeable. Instead, there may be a balance between collagen loss and production as fibroblasts continually produce collagen, and protease inhibitors, such as tissue inhibitors of matrix metalloproteinases prevent excessive collagen breakdown.

However, the balance may eventually tip toward excessive collagen destruction, and there is a gradual loss of collagen attachment to the tooth as the added proteolytic insult from immune cells and bacteria overwhelms the regenerative capacity of fibroblasts in maintaining tissue attachment. While this may not be noticeable clinically as histologic attachment loss always precedes clinical attachment loss, enough tissue attachment is lost to allow for a periodontal probe to sink past the CEJ for clinical detection of attachment loss.

1.7.5 Mechanism Leading to Bone Loss

Bone constantly remodels in response to mechanical forces as osteoblasts deposit bone and osteoclasts remove bone. This also applies to the alveolar bone that houses teeth, as chewing slightly forces teeth into the tooth socket and apply tensile force on the alveolar bone on the side of the socket through the oblique fibers. The constant remodeling process of the alveolar bone allows maintenance of supportive bone for normal function, and supports tooth position changes that are necessary because of tooth attrition. The primary mechanism that regulates and balances bone resorption and deposition is the balance between "receptor activated nuclear factor kappa B" ligand, or RANK-L molecule, and OPG. If RANK ligand (a.k.a., TNSF11, TRANCE, OPGL, or ODF) binds to the RANK receptor, it triggers a signaling cascade that leads to expression of NFκB-controlled genes, which ultimately lead to bone resorption. OPG is a protein that sequesters RANK ligand. In a bone, osteoblasts produce roughly equal amounts of OPG and RANK ligand, thus allowing for the limited stimulation of osteoclasts and keeping a balance between bone resorption and bone deposition. In destructive periodontal diseases, B-cells and Th17 cells produce additional RANK ligand, which then tips the balance toward bone loss.[10]

In addition to increased levels of receptor activator of nuclear factor kappa-B ligand (RANKL) leading to osteoclast activation, many inflammatory cytokines produced during periodontal inflammation, such as Interleukin-6, Interleukin-1, and Tumor necrosis factor alpha, which are produced by macrophages and neutrophils reacting to periodontal bacteria, can substitute for RANKL and activate osteoclasts to begin bone formation. Likewise, bacterial products, such as *P. gingivalis* and lipopolysaccharide, can directly induce osteoclast activation.[11]

1.7.6 Mechanism Leading to Mobility and Tooth Loss

Teeth are secured to the tooth socket through periodontal and gingival fibers. Except for teeth with severe bone and attachment loss, most of the tooth support is provided by periodontal fibers. Periodontitis gradually destroys attachment fibers, and bone loss from periodontal disease reduces the alveolar bone height, which then increases mechanical stress on the remaining periodontal fibers. The increased stress on the fibers may lead to lasting mechanical damage, and overpower the ability of fibroblasts to compensate the increased mechanical demand by adding collagen fibers. The resulting loss of fibers eventually leads to tooth mobility.

There is no specific attachment level or percentage of bone loss where a tooth develops mobility or where a tooth will be lost since root surface area, anatomy, and bone density play a role in developing tooth mobility and tooth loss. In general, it seems that the chance for tooth loss dramatically increases after about 8 mm or 60% attachment loss (based on average root length).

1.7.7 Effect of Genetic Factors on Periodontal Disease

For most patients at a given time, the immune response balances the damaging effect of a disease-causing microbial community, and this immune response itself features multiple balancing forces, such as the right amount of protective neutrophil activity, the right amount of T-helper cell set activation, and the RANK ligand/ OPG balance. Any disturbance of this system leads to an increased likelihood of severe periodontal

infection as shown by the numerous genetic conditions that result in some type of immune defect such as:
- Trisomy 21 (general immune defects).
- Papillon-Lefevre (neutrophil defect).
- Congenital agranulocytosis (lack of neutrophils).
- Lazy leukocyte syndrome (neutrophil defect).
- Chediak Higashi (neutrophil defect).
- Cohen syndrome (lack of neutrophils).
- Congenital neutropenia (lack of neutrophils).
- Zimmerman-Laband (lack of neutrophils).
- Glycogen storage disease type I (generalized immune defects).
- Klinefelter syndrome (generalized immune defects).

Or, connective tissue function defect such as:
- Ehlers-Danlos (collagen assembly defect).
- Marfan syndrome (collagen assembly defect).
- Hypophosphatasia (bone metabolism defect).

However, even in individuals not affected by a specific genetic disorder, periodontal disease has a marked genetic component. This genetic component is the cumulative effect of various subtle polymorphisms, or genetic variations of promoters and other regulatory genes that control the production of immune proteins and connective tissue function.

An example of this is the IL-1 genotype, which leads to higher levels of Interleukin 1 (IL-1) in response to infections. Interleukin 1 has many functions, but in the context of periodontal disease, it is associated with inflammation and bone destruction. Clinically, the presence of IL-1 genotype can be tested with a commercial kit. However, this test is only significant in smokers, where a positive test result corresponds to a higher risk of periodontal disease.[12]

Generally, the presence of a specific polymorphism is associated with a weak, and likely clinically insignificant risk of enhanced periodontal disease. It is possible that a collection of polymorphisms may be associated with clinically significant risk, but since there is no commercially available test for polymorphisms other than for the IL-1 genotype, genetic testing is generally not useful yet.

1.7.8 Effect of Medical Factors on Periodontal Disease

Generally, periodontal disease can be enhanced by medical conditions that promote inflammation. Likewise, periodontal disease can influence medical conditions by contributing to systemic inflammation, either through release of inflammatory mediators or through seeding circulating blood with bacteria (▶Fig. 1.17).

The contribution to systemic inflammation can be significant as the surface area of inflamed periodontium can approach up to 39 cm² in size. This large amount of inflamed tissue releases significant, measurable amounts of inflammatory mediators into the systemic circulation. These can then exacerbate inflammation somewhere else, such as in arthritic joints or cardiovascular disease, contribute to undesired tissue reactions, such as insulin resistance or preterm labor. The list of conditions associated with or interacting with periodontitis keeps growing, including conditions, such as diabetes mellitus, atherosclerosis, cardiovascular disease, stroke, obesity, certain types of pneumonia, rheumatoid arthritis, birth complications, kidney disease, oral cancer, and erectile dysfunction.

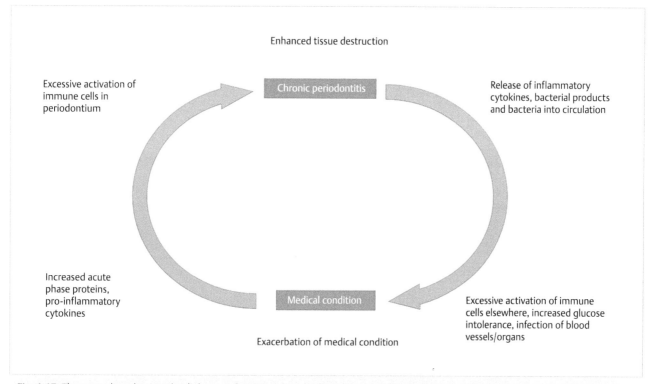

Fig. 1.17 The general mechanism that links periodontitis and medical conditions is inflammation.

1.7.9 Periodontitis, Diabetes Mellitus, and Obesity

The relationship between diabetes mellitus, obesity, and periodontitis exemplifies the circular relationship described in the previous paragraph (▶Fig. 1.18):

- Inflamed periodontal tissues release inflammatory cytokines such as TNF-alpha and IL-6 into blood. Excess adipose tissue also releases these mediators.
- These circulate to other organs.
- TNF-alpha and IL-6 promote an acute phase response and counteract the effect of insulin.
- This results in increased blood glucose, lipids, fibrinogen, and other acute phase proteins.
- Increased blood glucose producing **advanced glycation end products** (AGEs). Increased blood lipids also lead to higher levels of oxidized blood lipids.
- AGEs, oxidized blood lipids, acute phase proteins enhance the activation of immune cells.
- Enhanced activation of immune cells in periodontal tissues adds to tissue damage.

This relationship produces a 3-fold increase in severe periodontitis in those with HbA1c levels greater than 9, and reduces treatment success. However, periodontal treatment decreases inflammation, and improves HbA1c levels by about 0.3 to 0.5%[13] in type II diabetes.

1.7.10 Atherosclerosis, Heart Attacks, and Strokes

Atherosclerosis is caused by injury to the smooth endothelial lining of blood vessels, which then produces an area on the blood vessel wall where leukocytes and platelets can accumulate, and further damage the endothelium in an attempt to repair the original injury. This leads to the eventual narrowing of blood vessels, risking thrombosis, which can trigger tissue infarct conditions, such as strokes and heart attacks, depending on the organ involved. The most medically relevant risk factors for atherosclerosis are sedentary lifestyle, obesity, high blood lipid levels, tobacco use, and diabetes mellitus. Periodontitis poses a minor but statistically significant risk as individuals with moderate to severe periodontitis have about 1.2-fold increase in strokes or heart attacks compared to other individuals. There also is a direct link between periodontitis and atherosclerosis as periodontal bacteria, such as *P. gingivalis,* can be found in atheromas, trigger atheromas in animal models, and can cause endothelial injury through local immune cell activation within the atheromas.

1.7.11 Birth Complications

Preterm births, where birth happens before 37 weeks of pregnancy, are a major public health concern. Preterm newborns tend to be underweight, have immature, nonfunctional organs,

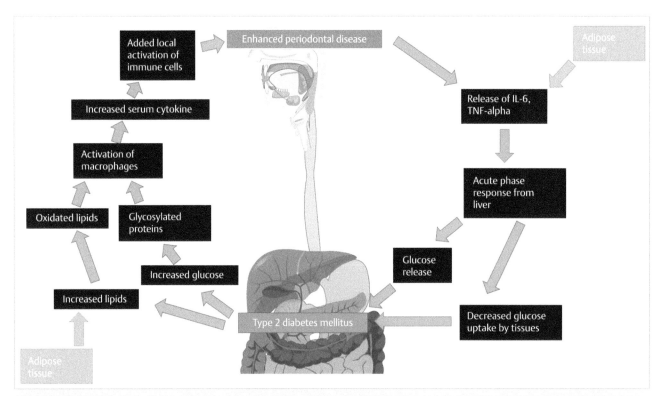

Fig. 1.18 Type II diabetes mellitus results in both increased plasma glucose and lipid levels, which lead to increased oxidative stress and generalized activation of macrophages in the circulation which are attempting to remove damaged proteins. This leads to a general increase in cytokine levels in serum, which contributes to local activation of immune cells in periodontal disease, leading to over activation and excessive tissue damage. Cytokines, such as IL-6 and TNFα, trigger an acute phase response from the liver. Part of this response is an increased level of glucose release from the liver, and decreased uptake by tissues. This in turn contributes to insulin resistance.

and often need weeks of intensive medical and caregiving support to survive. Preterm newborns are less likely to survive infancy and have a higher risk of developing neurologic and developmental conditions. The most medically relevant risk factors are lack of prenatal care, stress, domestic violence, previous preterm labor, uterine abnormalities, preeclampsia, tobacco use, poor overall health, or systemic infections. Periodontal inflammation poses a lesser, but still significant risk as it is consistently associated with preterm birth, low birth weight, and stillbirths. This may happen as a result of blood-borne invasive periodontal bacteria infecting the uterus, or caused by inflammatory mediators (i.e., prostaglandin E2) produced by periodontal inflamed tissues triggering labor in a susceptible uterus. It is unclear, however at this time, if periodontal treatment during pregnancy can reduce birth complications.

1.7.12 Pneumonia

Pneumonia is a severe lung infection that can be fatal for hospitalized, institutionalized, or older individuals. Death rates for patients in intensive care units who contract pneumonia while connected to a ventilator approach 40%. Medically relevant risk factors include serious illness, loss of consciousness, malnutrition, and length of hospital stay. Periodontitis and poor oral hygiene are a minor, but significant risk factor for both hospital-acquired and community-acquired pneumonia. The mechanism is thought to involve either aspiration of oral bacteria from plaque-covered teeth, aspiration of bacterial enzymes that either damage lung epithelium, or prevent clearance of aspirated bacteria or inflammatory mediators from the oral cavity that makes lung epithelium more susceptible to bacterial infection. Oral hygiene or repeated application of antiseptic mouthwash-soaked sponges significantly reduces the incidence of pneumonia in a hospital setting or nursing home.

1.7.13 Other Medical Conditions

The list of medical conditions affected by periodontitis is growing as more association studies show small, but significant statistical associations with various medical conditions. These include conditions as diverse as some types of oral cancer, hypertension, osteoporosis, and erectile dysfunction. Likely more clinically relevant, since periodontal treatment may help to improve these conditions are chronic kidney disease and rheumatoid arthritis.

In chronic kidney disease, the loss of functional nephrons leads to impaired excretory kidney function as measured through the glomerular filtration rate, which leads to a higher risk of cardiovascular disease and death. Major risk factors for kidney disease are developmental kidney abnormalities, increasing age, chronic exposure to kidney toxins, and systemic conditions, such as obesity and type II diabetes mellitus. Patients with chronic kidney disease have a higher risk of severe periodontitis, and periodontal treatment may aid in improving kidney function, presumably by reducing systemic inflammation that contributes to kidney damage.

Similarly, rheumatoid arthritis is associated with more severe periodontal disease. Inflammatory mediators from the oral cavity presumably enhance inflammation elsewhere, leading to destruction of joint surfaces. Periodontal treatment has a small, but significant beneficial effect in these conditions. In rheumatoid arthritis, it will reduce systemic markers of inflammation and lead to slight overall improvement of joint function.

1.7.14 Aging

Bone loss and attachment loss become more widespread and severe with age. Although aging does not cause periodontal disease, the number of chronic medical conditions, such as type II diabetes mellitus, increases with increasing age, leading to a higher risk for periodontal disease. According to the free radical theory, continued oxidative stress through the production of oxidative molecules, during normal metabolism and immune function, leads to cumulative molecular and tissue damage. Eventually, this can no longer be fully compensated, leading to signs of aging. In the oral cavity, this leads to thinner, more fragile oral tissues that are more prone to injury, decreased regenerative potential and slower wound healing.

1.7.15 Tobacco Use

Tobacco use leads to many harmful health effects including a more than 5-fold worse risk of severe periodontitis. Periodontal therapy including implant therapy is less likely to succeed in smokers compared to nonsmokers. The effect of tobacco on the periodontal microflora seems minor, although some studies show an increase in *P. gingivalis* and *A. actinomycetemcomitans*. Various molecules liberated by smoking adversely affect immunity and wound healing. For example, nicotine is a potent vasoconstrictor, leading to decreased blood flow in gingival tissues. Reactive molecules found in tobacco smoke, such as carbon monoxide, acrolein, and aldehyde, directly damage tissues leading to a more fibrotic gingiva that is less prone to gingival bleeding in the presence of periodontal inflammation. Tobacco use also alters the cytokine environment in periodontium, and diminishes the production of protease inhibitors, which normally protect against proteases released by bacteria and immune cells, thus leading to greater tissue damage.

1.8 Wound Healing

Periodontal therapy is critically dependent on wound healing. Whereas the main goal of periodontal therapy is to restore periodontal health, periodontal procedures only remove tissue irritants and set the stage for wound healing, which then may produce periodontal health if healing is successful.

1.8.1 Phases of Wound Healing

There are four phases, discussed below, of wound healing, which may happen concurrently in different parts of a surgical wound.

Hemostasis

The first step in healing is bleeding. Surgical or injury from bacteria or immune cells breaches a capillary wall, which brings blood in direct contact with connective tissue that contains factors that either activate platelets or initiate coagulation. Arterioles also constrict as the result of tissue damage, slowing blood flow and allowing efficient coagulation. Clinically, this leads to reduced bleeding about 5 to 10 minutes after the initial flap elevation in periodontal surgery. Since bleeding from any invasive periodontal treatment is most likely from capillary beds, applying firm pressure on bleeding periodontal tissues effectively stops bleeding after 5 to 10 minutes. Coagulation forming a waterproof blood clot is usually complete after 24 hours.

Defects in the coagulation cascade, either created by anticoagulants or genetic conditions, may result in prolonged bleeding. Coagulation will happen eventually, but produces large, fluid-filled clots that delay healing. Clinically, this effect is typically insignificant for patients who receive periodontal surgery and take Aspirin or other nonsteroidal anti-inflammatory drugs (NSAIDs). Prolonged bleeding may be observed with patients taking oral antiplatelet agents (i.e., Clopidogrel) and anticoagulants (i.e., Coumadin and Rivaroxaban), but these medications typically should not be discontinued for routine periodontal surgery. Prolonged bleeding is likely with untreated moderate-severe von Willebrand disease or Hemophilia, and periodontal surgery for these patients requires collaboration with a hematology team for the administration of replacement factor prior and after surgery.

Inflammation

Almost concurrent with coagulation, and peaking 12 to 24 hours after injury, inflammation develops. This usually clears bacteria and damaged cells from the wound, and allows normal wound healing progression. If a wound becomes infected, it will delay healing as inflammation will disrupt the deposition of extracellular matrix and prevent normal function of connective tissue cells. For periodontal surgery, postoperative infections usually become apparent in the first few days after surgery. Since increasing pain severity is an early sign of postoperative infection and inflammatory pain usually is worst the day after surgery, it is useful to check on a patient 1 to 2 days after a periodontal surgery with a follow-up phone call.

Diabetes mellitus delays wound healing as the deposition of glucose-modified proteins triggers enhanced and prolonged inflammation, and clinically this may result in delayed wound closure and incomplete bone regeneration after regenerative surgeries and bone grafting.

Granulation

Once the wound is free of bacteria, these cells will attempt to migrate into and over the wound.
- Keratinocytes from the surrounding wound edges migrate over the wound surface at a rate of 0.5 to 1.0 mm per day, primarily driven by epidermal growth factor secreted by salivary glands. These cells are the fastest moving cells in a wound, and usually reach exposed root surfaces first.
- Fibroblast migrate into the wound, primarily driven by transforming growth factor beta released by anti-inflammatory T-regulatory cells, and platelet-derived growth factors (PDGF) released by platelets. PDGF and platelet concentrates can be used clinically to speed up soft tissue healing, and favor bone growth. Fibroblasts also secrete tissue plasminogen activator that begins an enzyme cascade resulting in dissolution of the blood clot.
- Endothelial cells from surrounding capillaries grow in response to the hypoxia in the center of the blood clot, and by VEGF produced by fibroblasts. Nerve growth factor and insulin-like growth factors promote growth and differentiation of fibroblasts and endothelial cells.
- Osteoblasts are the slowest migrating cells and need a stable wound environment devoid of motion for growth. For this reason, it takes time to regenerate bone, and it is usually more difficult to regenerate hard tissue versus soft tissue. Clinically, some bone morphogenetic proteins can be used to stimulate bone formation.

Granulation tissue is typically dark red as it contains many capillaries, and fragile. Tobacco use most likely interferes with wound healing as it limits blood flow, which reduces the speed at which precursor cells arrive, and through direct toxic effects on the developing and maturing cells in the area.

Maturation

Periodontal soft tissue usually matures within 6 to 8 weeks, producing typical pink gingiva as blood vessels reduce in number and epithelium achieves its normal thickness. Within the connective tissue of the maturing wound, the fibroblast number reduces and the original collagen fiber network consolidates, producing some wound contraction.

Within a grafted extraction socket or periodontal defect, stromal cells from the surrounding alveolar bone marrow infiltrate the area, possibly attracted by bone morphogenetic proteins released by some graft materials. Stromal cells differentiate into osteoblast and begin depositing bone matrix, which happens within 8 weeks. By about 3 months, bone matrix is sufficiently mineralized to be detected radiographically, and within 1 year, it will have completely remodeled.

1.8.2 Regeneration versus Repair

Wound healing is an adaptive survival strategy that aims to prevent exsanguination and microbial infection. There are two types of wound healing:
- *Repair*: After wound healing, new tissue has different make-up as the original tissue, and may be smaller in size or less functional. For humans, this is the typical mode of wound healing.
- *Regeneration*: After wound healing, new tissue has the same make-up and characteristics as the original tissue. For periodontal therapy, this is the ideal, but rarely achieved outcome.

After periodontal therapy, regeneration and repair produce different outcomes (▶ Fig. 1.19):
- *Formation of a long junctional epithelium*: As epithelial cells migrate fastest, they reach the instrumented root surface first and grow along the root surface until encountering periodontal ligament, forming a thin, but long layer of epithelial cells tightly packed against the root surface in absence of inflammation. Clinically, this will appear as healthy gingiva with reduced probing depth, but in the presence of plaque, the epithelium will detach and the pockets recur. This is the typical outcome of effective scaling and root planing.
- *Gingival recession*: Gingiva heals into a compact, thin soft tissue layer overlying alveolar bone with a normal-sized junctional epithelium. Clinically, this is seen as the loss of root coverage (gingival recession) and reduced probing depth. This is the typical and desired outcome of traditional pocket reduction surgery (i.e., gingivectomy, gingival flap surgery, and osseous surgery).

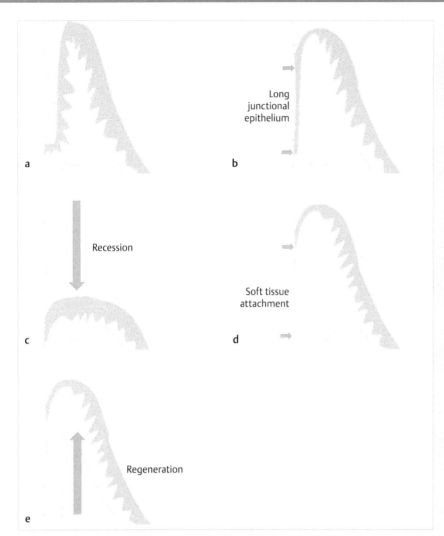

Fig. 1.19 There are four outcomes of healing after periodontal therapy. **(a)** With destructive periodontal disease, direct and indirect damage from the bacteria infection creates a deep pocket, attachment and bone loss. **(b)** After professional removal of plaque and calculus deposits, the root surface is clean, but epithelium contacts the root surface and migrates apically to form a long junctional epithelium. Clinically, this will appear as much reduced pocketing and gained attachment, but this can be lost quickly if the epithelium detaches from the root surface in response to new periodontal infection. **(c)** Traditional pocket-reduction surgeries usually create gingival recession as the tissue is healthy, but much reduced. **(d)** Sometimes, healing allows soft tissue to reattach to the root surface with occasional islands of epithelial tissue. **(e)** The most desired outcome is periodontal regeneration that rebuilds lost bone, cementum, periodontal ligament, and gingival fiber attachment. While partial regeneration is common, full regeneration is rare and difficult to achieve.

- *Soft tissue attachment*: Fibroblasts reach the root surface and collagen fibers become entrapped in developing cementum, producing a soft tissue attachment. There is no bone formation and there may be clusters of epithelial cells on the root surface. Clinically, this appears as thick, healthy gingiva with reduced probing depth, but no radiographic bone gain. This is a desired outcome of root coverage procedures.
- *True regeneration:* The original tissue structure featuring soft tissue and bone is restored in its entirety. Most likely, regenerative surgery produces a mix of regenerated tissue, soft tissue attachment, long junctional epithelium and recession. True regeneration can only be determined histology from a block section of the regenerated tissue.

1.8.3 Unique Aspects of Tissue Healing around Dental Implants

As dental implants are surgically implanted into bone, wound healing produces unique features:
- A direct bone-titanium interface. There is no intervening soft tissue analogous to periodontal ligament around implants. This has several important clinical consequences:
  - Once an implant is completely integrated into bone, it must experience complete bone loss around the implant to display mobility. A mobile implant is a failed implant.
  - Unlike teeth, there is little concern about the ratio between the length of the implant and the supported restoration. A short implant can support a large crown.
  - Unlike teeth, conventional orthodontic treatment cannot move implants. Implants do not respond to facial growth in the same way as teeth.
  - The lack of periodontal ligament space with embedded immune cells and blood vessels may contribute to the difficulty in treating infections around implants.
  - Unlike teeth, implants cannot maintain a thin buccal layer of bone as there is no blood supply and no mechanical stimulation from a periodontal ligament.
  - It is difficult to create a tight interproximal contact between implant-supported restorations as typical restorative methods such as interproximal wedges cannot separate implants.
- No gingival attachment (although some newer implant systems may produce attachment). Instead, gingival epithelial cells form a tight cuff around the implant platform and along the abutment while gingival circular fibers maintain close contact.
  - Plaque-induced inflammation around implants quickly results in deep pocketing and risks bone loss around the implant.
  - Usually, there is some degree of initial bone loss of up to 2 mm around the implant platform to accommodate this long junctional epithelium.

1.8.4 Clinical Implication: Postoperative Instructions

Wound healing has very practical applications in describing postoperative instructions for patients who received surgery (see ▶ Video 1.1):
- The most important instruction is "Do not spit, rinse, brush teeth, floss, suck liquid through a straw; look at the surgery area by stretching the mouth, or allow your tongue to feel the surgery area for the first 24 hours. Do not try to remove the stitches on your own." This is important for wound stability as the blood clot is fragile for the first 24 hours and could easily dislodged, thus delaying wound healing. Suturing helps to stabilize the wound and speeds up healing.
- "Bleeding will stop within the first 24 hours. Apply pressure with wet gauze to stop bleeding if you notice bleeding." Make use of the fact that cross-linking fibrin happens in the first 24 hours, and that pressure will both slow blood flow and stabilize the blood clot, while gauze provides a foreign surface that triggers clotting.
- "Manage pain by applying ice on and off" and "take [your NSAID of choice] for pain as needed." Ice controls swelling and provides mild anesthesia, whereas NSAIDs control swelling and prostaglandin-related pain.
- "We will call you tomorrow to see how you are doing, and we want to check the site about 1 week from today." Infections and postoperative complications arise most likely in the first few days, and the procedure will be most likely successful if there are no complications within the first week.

1.8.5 Clinical Implication: Wait Times after Surgery for Dental Procedures

Wound healing also dictates how long one must wait for a specific surgical outcome:
- *Soft tissue healing*: It usually completes in 6 to 8 weeks. The tissue is mature enough by this time to permit impression taking and restoration after pocket reduction surgery, crown-lengthening surgery, or second-stage implant surgery. For anterior sites, it may be advisable to wait 3 months or more to ensure that the gingival margin is stable and will not expose the crown margin.
- *Hard tissue healing*: It usually completes in 3 to 12 months depending on the amount of bone formation needed and tolerance for continued bone remodeling. Usually, the wait times are as follows:
  - *3 months*: Restoration after crown lengthening/osseous surgery for anterior maxillary teeth; second-stage procedure after uncomplicated implant placement that achieved 30 Ncm insertion torque (which may also be immediately restored at time of placement); implant placement after uncomplicated extraction/ridge preservation.
  - *6 months*: Implant placement after complex ridge preservation or ridge augmentation procedures; second-stage procedure for implants placed either with bone graft/sinus lift procedure, or implants that failed to achieve 30 Ncm insertion torque.
  - *8–12 months*: Implant placement after sinus augmentation procedures; second-stage procedure for implants placed at the time of sinus augmentation procedure.
  - *12 months*: Stable, long-term result of regeneration and root coverage procedures can be measured at this time.

1.9 Developmental Influences

While the onset of periodontal disease symptoms happens long after tooth development for most patients, events that take place during tooth development may shape a patient's periodontal disease experience decades later.

1.9.1 Tooth Development

The beginnings of human tooth development may be traced back to the development of neural crest cells during the neurula stage in a 4-week old human embryo:
- *Week 4*: Tube-shaped embryo curls into a C-shape due to the rapid growth of the anterior end of the neural tube, which is destined to become the brain. As it grows, it curls over the portion of the embryo containing the developing heart, forming a fold that is destined to become the face and neck.
- *Week 5*: Tissue bulges appear in this region, forming the mandibular pharyngeal arch, maxillary processes, and median nasal and lateral nasal processes. Other pharyngeal arches form a tube that becomes the esophageal tract, oropharynx, and other parts of the neck and middle ear. From within this tube, a small tissue swelling at the base of the mandibular process grows anteriorly. This swelling forms the tongue as cells from the 2nd, 3rd pharyngeal arches and neck muscles migrate there.
- *Week 6*: Maxillary and median nasal processes fuse to form the maxilla and hard palate, whereas the mandibular processes form the floor of the mouth over the next 3 weeks. Neural crest cells migrate to the tissues overlying the future jaw bones and mix with the existing mesodermal tissues to form ectomesenchyme. The ectomesenchyme forms a band of denser epithelial tissue called dental lamina. According to the field theory, concentration gradients of different proteins such as the homeobox proteins, wingless, and sonic hedgehog family proteins and growth factors such as hepatic growth factor, bone morphogenetic proteins, fibroblast growth factor, and direct ectomesenchymal cells, to form different types of tissues and tooth types. Alternatively, according to the clone theory, number of teeth, type, and position may also be determined by the number of cell divisions as the dental lamina grows posteriorly. Other neural crest cells mix with ectodermal placode cells to form the trigeminal ganglion neurons, whose axons form the future trigeminal nerves.
- *Week 7*: Mandibular jaw bone begins to form near the mental foramen, and wraps around the decaying **Meckel's cartilage**, which was the previous supporting element of the mandibular arch. Bone also begins to form in the h week near the nasal capsule and spreads posteriorly from there to form the maxilla.
- *Week 8–9*: The dental lamina thickens further and forms tissue ingrowths called dental buds at every site destined to have a tooth. These dental buds grow toward the developing jaw bone, and eventually enlarge to form first cap- and then bell-like structures, which are called enamel organs and destined to become the enamel portion of teeth. As these dental lamina cells develop bell-like structures, they entrap mesenchymal cells, which will form eventually the pulp and dentin portion of teeth. This area surrounded by the enamel organ is called the dental

papilla. The cells in the center of the enamel organ at the tip of the dental papilla differentiate further, become denser, and form preameloblasts. These preameloblasts form a structure called the enamel knot, and this structure determines the future tooth shape. The preameloblasts also induce the adjacent dental papilla cells to differentiate into odontoblast, which then further stimulate the preameloblasts to become ameloblasts and deposit enamel. Once enamel is deposited, the odontoblasts begin to secrete dentin matrix, which then mineralizes into dentin. As this process begins at the cusp tips of developing teeth, the edges of the enamel organ continue to elongate with a layer of inner enamel epithelium cells destined to become ameloblasts, an intervening layer of stellate reticulum and an outer layer of outer enamel epithelium. This process continues along the sides of the tooth until the tooth crown is complete.

- *Week 12–16*: Teeth begin to mineralize and this process continues until the crown of the deciduous teeth are complete. The same process begins later for the permanent dentition from tooth buds.

1.9.2 Root Development and Tooth Eruption

As the enamel organ grows and extends away from the cusp tips, there comes a point where the outer and inner enamel epithelia fuse without intervening stellate reticulum. This point becomes the CEJ as the inner enamel epithelium, from this point on, fails to produce ameloblasts. Instead, it continues to induce osteoblasts, forming the root of the teeth. From this point on forward, it is called Hertwig's root sheath.

The root sheath continues to elongate, and differences in cell growth determine the direction of the root growth. In addition, local differences in cell growth of the root sheath lead to tissue tongues that grow toward the opposing side of the root sheath, creating furcation entrances and separating roots. If growth is interrupted, resulting in a hole within the root sheath, it produces an accessory foramen in the root. Ultimately, the growth of the root sheath tapers off, and it constricts toward the root apex of each root.

As the root grows, alveolar bone develops around it and axon fibers become trapped in the dental papilla, forming the pulpal nerve network. As root formation ends, Hertwig's root sheath breaks up and largely disappears. As the root sheath dissipates, cells from the mesenchyme surrounding the root become in contact with dentin, which triggers these mesenchymal cells to differentiate into cementoblasts. These cementoblasts deposit cementum on the root surface, and during this process, collagen fibers produced by nearby developing fibroblasts become entrapped into the tooth surface. Simultaneously, as bone formation begins near the tooth, collagen fibers become entrapped in bone forming bundle bone. The collagen fibers entrapped in both cementum and bone are called Sharpey's fibers and form the periodontal ligament.

As the tooth root develops and becomes surrounded by bone, root growth pushes the crown toward the oral cavity. As the tooth is pushed toward the oral cavity, the epithelial strand of the tooth bud along with the enamel organ is pushed against the epithelium of the oral cavity. In time, the outer enamel epithelium fuses with the oral epithelium, forming a channel through which the tooth erupts. Once the tooth erupts, the inner enamel epithelium degenerates to a reduced enamel epithelium that forms a thin film over the erupting crown, and is subsequently shed when the tooth is exposed in the oral cavity.

1.9.3 Clinical Implications for Periodontal Treatment

Any disturbance in tooth development will affect the formation, shape, and position of each tooth. Disruption of the enamel bud through disease or environmental factors usually results in the lack of tooth formation.

Root Anatomy and Surface Defects

On a smaller scale, abnormalities in root sheath growth produce aberrant root anatomy, such as additional roots, excessively curved or thin roots, dilacerated roots, or ridges and grooves on the root surface. Enamel pearls develop if there is a local zone of inner enamel epithelium that maintains the ability to form ameloblasts. Cervical enamel projections form if there is the tongue of inner enamel epithelium that maintains enamel formation capacity while surrounding cells stop producing enamel.

Depending on how far mesenchymal cells migrate toward the CEJ and how far the root sheath breaks up determine the shape and size of the CEJ. If cement production is exuberant, it may cover part of the enamel as well. Contrary, if the root sheath persists near the CEJ, no cementum will be produced there, producing a CEJ prone to root sensitivity.

Potential for Cyst Formation

The root sheath disintegrates almost completely, but may leave some remnant clusters of epithelial cells. These clusters, the cell rests of Malassez, can sometimes become active and form a growing ball of epithelial cells that then can become fluid filled, leading to lateral periodontal cysts. It also is speculated that these cysts may become infected during periodontal disease, and form periodontal abscesses occasionally.

Altered Passive Eruption

As the root grows, it pushes teeth toward the oral cavity in a process called active eruption. This process causes gingival epithelium and outer enamel epithelium to fuse, forming a channel through which the tooth erupts. Once the tooth erupts, the extraneous epithelial cells produced by this process die off through apoptosis, thus reducing the amount of gingiva covering the tooth in a process called passive eruption.

If apoptosis is insufficient in reducing the amount of excess gingival cells, the tooth will remain covered partially with gingiva resulting in short teeth and a gummy smile. Likewise, there may be excessive bone formation past the CEJ, preventing complete tooth eruption. In either case, it will appear that a tooth has not fully erupted, which is called "altered passive eruption."

Use of Enamel Matrix Derivatives and Growth Factors

As tooth development leads to the growth of cementum, periodontal ligament fibers, and bone, clinicians have, for long, attempted to trigger elements of tooth development with the addition of various growth factors to periodontal therapy. The most well-known example is the use of enamel matrix derivatives (Emdogain), which is derived of porcine tooth buds and said to stimulate periodontal regeneration by recapitulating tooth development. There is also interest in using various molecules that are involved in tooth development such as fibroblast growth factor and bone morphogenetic proteins in stimulating development of new tissue.

1.10 Essential Takeaways

- Periodontal disease is a common entity. When normal periodontium is subjected to bacterial insults and modified by the host's immune system, disease results.
- Plaque biofilm is a structured community of various bacterial species. Early microbial colonizers facilitate the arrival for late, anaerobic, gram-negative colonizers, such as the "red complex" (*P. gingivalis*, *T. forsythia*, and *T. denticola*), which trigger disease.
- Innate host defenses, such as the physical barrier wall in the gingiva, shedding of bacteria attached epithelial cells, sulcular flushing with crevicular flow, antimicrobial peptide and protein production, are initiated and modified by the various types and numbers of microorganisms in the plaque community.
- Neutrophils and T-cells play a role in wound healing and trigger destructive periodontal disease by altering the host innate immune response.
- Periodontal disease is characterized by gingival erythema, swelling, and tooth mobility from attachment, and bone loss.
- Genetic conditions influence and modify the severity of disease.
- Inflammation appears to be the primary link to medical conditions.
- Wound healing consists of coagulation, inflammation, granulation, and maturation. Bacterial clearance is critical in each phase for healing to occur.
- Regeneration is the desired goal, but repair is often the result after surgery.
- Postop healing and integration of implants occur without a periodontal ligament and are therefore unique relative to natural teeth.
- Root anatomy is determined during tooth development, and some regenerative procedures aim to recapitulate steps in tooth development.

1.11 Review Questions

Consider the following case for the practice questions below:

A 25-year old dental student is examined by another dental student during a clinical teaching session simulating an initial comprehensive exam. Neither one is aware of any pain or other symptoms of dental disease. They both are healthy, have no known allergies, and receive regular dental care. They are also very serious about oral hygiene, brush three times a day using a powered toothbrush, and floss regularly. The patient's oral appearance is shown in ▶ Fig. 1.20 and a panoramic radiograph is shown in ▶ Fig. 1.21.

7	8	9	10	11	Tooth	22	23	24	25	26
323	212	322	212	213	PD (facial)	212	212	212	212	213
					BOP (facial)					
323	323	323	323	323	PD (lingual)	323	323	323	323	323
					BOP (lingual)					
0	0	0		0	Highest CAL	0	0	0	0	0
					Furcation (lingual)					
					Furcation (buccal)					
0	0	0	0	0	Tooth mobility	0	0	0	0	0

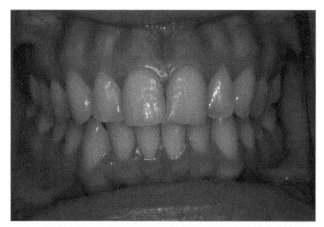

Fig. 1.20 Clinical view of facial gingiva.

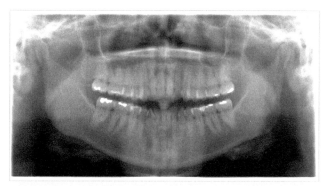

Fig. 1.21 Panoramic radiograph.

Learning Objective: Recognize normal anatomy of healthy periodontal tissue.

1. Evaluate the following statements, regarding this patient's incisors and canines.
   Statement 1: Periodontal chart measurements suggest periodontal health.
   Statement 2: Clinical appearance and measurements suggest the need for further evaluation with periapical radiographs.
   A. Both statements are true
   B. Both statements are false
   C. The first statement is true, the second is false
   D. The first statement is false, the second is true

2. This dental student is seen several years later in a private dental office. The presentation is essentially unchanged, but overzealous tooth brushing induced some tooth abrasions on the facial surface of the canines and premolars (teeth nos. 5, 6, 11, 12). This also resulted in 2 to 3 mm gingival recession and an attachment level of 2 mm at the same location. Probing depths are still 1 to 3 mm, there is no bleeding on probing, and clinical attachment level is still zero at all teeth other than the affected canine and premolars. The patient's periodontal condition is best described as:
   A. Periodontal health
   B. Healthy, but reduced periodontium
   C. Diseased periodontium
   D. Cannot say/not enough information

3. Now a dentist in her 40s, she cracked tooth no. 12 while eating a sandwich during a dental conference and a former classmate is helping her out with repairing this tooth with an onlay restoration. While periodontal health has not changed since the initial exam, the lingual cusp fractured to about 1 mm below the distolingual gingival margin. Probing depths in this area are 2 to 3 mm, and the sulcus is still 1 mm below the fracture. The radiographic bone level is 2 mm below the CEJ. There is no pulp exposure and endodontic tests produce normal findings. Which of the following statements about this case is correct?
   A. The restoration will violate biologic width
   B. The biologic width is larger than normal
   C. The dentogingival junction is 3-mm wide
   D. Crown lengthening is not needed

4. Around age 50, this student develops an autoimmune disease, where a serum test reveals antibodies against desmoglein. In periodontal tissues, this will result in:
   A. Intraepithelial blister formation
   B. Potential for rapid attachment loss
   C. Severe bacterial infections
   D. Mucosal detachment from underlying tissue

Learning Objective: Describe the contribution of microbes to the periodontal disease process.

5. Prior to the onset of the autoimmune disease, this individual had consistently low plaque scores and no signs of periodontal disease. A sample of the microbial flora on tooth no. 9 facial surface would reveal predominantly:
   A. Actinomyces species
   B. Fusobacterium species
   C. Streptococcal species
   D. Staphylococcal species

6. The facial gingival margin of no. 9 became ulcerated and sensitive to brushing and she stopped brushing this area for 1 week. Relative to other bacterial types, which bacterial type decreases?
   A. Gram-positive
   B. Anaerobes
   C. Rods
   D. Motile

Learning Objective: Describe cellular and molecular events that lead to clinical signs and symptoms of periodontal disease.

7. To treat the autoimmune disease, a physician prescribes corticosteroid therapy and orders a complete blood count with differential as part of monitoring therapy progress. The physician notes a steep reduction of leukocytes, especially neutrophils, to 0.5×10^9/L (normal 2.5–7.5×10^9/L). This produces a _____ risk of bacterial infection, which _____ with attachment loss.
   A. Low, correlates
   B. Low, is unrelated
   C. High, correlates
   D. High, is unrelated

8. The physician adjusted the dose of corticosteroids to a lower level that allows rebound of neutrophil numbers to normal levels, but eliminates the autoantibody. At age 55, periodontal charting is essentially unchanged, with only minor attachment loss at canines and first premolars, low probing depths, and few isolated areas of gingival bleeding during professional tooth cleaning. Evaluate the following statements.
   Statement 1: The gingival bleeding was caused by periodontal disease.
   Statement 2: This individual likely has genetic factors that are protective against periodontal disease.
   A. Both statements are true
   B. Both statements are false
   C. The first statement is true, the second is false
   D. The first statement is false, the second is true

9. Given the trend in this case, you would expect increasing age to:
   A. Increase risk for periodontal disease
   B. Lead to thinner and more fragile oral tissue
   C. Increase risk for pneumonia from oral microbes
   D. Lead to deeper pocketing

Learning Objective: Describe how periodontal tissue recovers from injury caused by bacteria or tissue trauma.

10. At age 65, tooth no. 12 fractures, and it is not restorable. She sees her nephew who has been practicing dentistry

for 2 years, and has the tooth removed. At the end of the procedure, she is instructed to bite down on a piece of gauze. Why?
A. Provide mechanical stimulation to fibroblasts
B. Keep bacteria from contaminating the site
C. Widening the tooth socket so as to counteract wound contraction
D. Aid hemostasis and coagulation

11. Several months later, a dental implant is placed in this area and restored. The maxillary sinus is close to the site, thus an 8-mm short implant is placed that supports a 10-mm tall restoration. Evaluate the following statement/ reasoning pair.
Statement 1: The poor implant to crown ratio is a concern.
Statement 2: Since there is no fiber attachment to the implant.
A. Both the statement and the reason are correct and related
B. Both the statement and the reason are correct but NOT related
C. The statement is correct, but the reason is NOT
D. The statement is NOT correct, but the reason is correct
E. NEITHER the statement NOR the reason is correct

Learning Objective: Describe how tooth development influences periodontal disease and treatment.

12. When tooth no. 12 was removed, it became evident that it had a mesial and a distal root. This happened because …
A. Each cusp developed its own root sheath
B. Different areas of the root sheath grew at different speeds
C. Cells underwent apoptosis in two areas of the root diaphragm
D. Odontoblasts paused dentin deposition in the tooth center

13. Evaluate the following statements:
Statement 1: Addition of enamel matrix proteins to an implant site will aid bone growth around the implant at the no. 12 site.
Statement 2: If sinus surgery was considered for the no. 12 site, the addition of bone morphogenetic protein is likely to induce bone growth.
A. Both statements are true
B. Both statements are false
C. The first statement is true, the second is false
D. The first statement is false, the second is true

1.12 Answers

1. **C.** Statement 1 is correct, because the reported probing depths are very low (1–3 mm), there is no bleeding on probing, tooth mobility, or attachment loss. If bleeding was present, it would indicate at least the presence of gingival inflammation, and if attachment loss was present, it would indicate the presence of periodontitis. Statement 2 is incorrect, as it seems unlikely that the patient has any

bone loss in this area requiring further evaluation with a periapical radiograph. There is no visible sign of gingival recession, or measured attachment loss, or deep probing depth suggesting bone loss inducing periodontal disease, and there is no suggestion in this case that the patient has any endodontic infection or other conditions. In an apparently healthy patient presenting for an initial comprehensive exam as shown in this case, the only radiographs one would order other than a panoramic radiograph are bitewing radiographs that evaluate posterior teeth for interproximal caries.

2. **B.** This choice is correct as there is attachment loss, but no evidence of current periodontal disease. Unlike in the original presentation, there is now evidence of attachment loss, which makes choice **A** incorrect. However, low probing depths, absence of bleeding, and no other sign or symptom of disease indicate absence of periodontal disease (**C**).

3. **D.** Crown lengthening is not needed, as the restoration does not violate biologic width. **A** is incorrect as the sulcus is still 1-mm apical to the fracture line, which will be where the restorative margin will be located. As such, a minimal sulcus is maintained and the dentogingival junction not invaded. **B** is incorrect, as the biologic width implied by the radiograph is 2 mm, and there is no evidence of a thick biotype. **C** is incorrect, as a 3-mm wide dentogingival junction is much thicker than normal and would likely produce wider distance from the alveolar crest to the CEJ.

4. **A.** Desmoglein is found in desmosomes connecting epithelial cells to each other, and antibodies will prevent proper desmosome function. This will cause separation of epithelial cells within the epithelium, leading to intraepithelial blister formation (**A**). Desmoglein is not a typical component of hemidesmosomes, which attach cells to the underlying basement membrane, and this attachment is not affected by this type of autoantibody (**D**). Rapid attachment loss (**B**) is typical for conditions affecting immunity or collagen function, and not connected to desmoglein. Severe bacterial infections (**C**) typically suggest a neutrophil defect, and not related to desmoglein.

5. **C.** A clean facial, supragingival tooth surface usually contains only a few isolated oral streptococci. Actinomyces species follow if plaque is allowed to accumulate, but not on a clean surface. Fusobacteria is a sign of mature plaque, which is not possible in this case with low plaque levels. Staphylococci are not commonly found in the oral cavity.

6. **A.** When oral hygiene ceases, the number of bacteria increases along with increased gram-negatives, anaerobes, motiles, and rods. Consequently, the number of gram-positives decreases relative to other bacteria.

7. **C.** This level of neutrophils suggests moderate-severe neutropenia, which puts this patient at high risk of bacterial infections, including periodontal disease that leads to attachment loss.

8. **D.** Statement 1 is likely incorrect as the case description suggests continued periodontal health, and isolated bleeding was most likely caused by instrumentation trauma

during the tooth cleaning. Statement 2 is likely correct as there is still no sign of significant periodontal disease despite the history of neutropenia and mature age.

9. **B.** Choice **A** is incorrect, as age by itself does not cause attachment loss or periodontal disease. **C** is likely incorrect as this patient does not have periodontal disease and likely maintains good oral hygiene, which eliminates a source of microbes that could cause pneumonia. **D** is incorrect, as pocketing does not necessarily increase with increasing age (as it could be treated).

10. **D.** The instruction of biting down on a piece of gauze aids hemostasis by applying pressure on a bleeding extraction socket, and it provides a foreign surface that induces coagulation. Mechanical stimulation of fibroblasts may happen during granulation, which is long after the patient removes the gauze. Gauze is too porous to prevent entry of bacteria to the extraction socket. The extraction socket should be left alone, and not "widened" after tooth removal.

11. **D.** The statement is not correct as the implant-to-crown ratio does not play the same role as crown-to-root ratio in teeth. The reason by itself is correct as there is no periodontal ligament or fiber attachment to implants. As a statement/reasoning pair, this combination does not make sense for implants as the reason for the concern about crown-to-root ratio in natural teeth is the amount of fiber attachment.

12. **B.** Furcation entrances and separate roots are formed when parts of the root sheath grow faster than other parts, which then leads to invaginations in the root sheath that can fuse and form a furcation entrance. **A** is incorrect as this forms separate teeth. **C** creates accessory foramina. **D** leads to dentin defects.

13. **D.** Enamel matrix derivatives are said to recapitulate tooth development and aid regeneration of lost periodontal attachment. Bone morphogenetic proteins are capable of inducing bone. Therefore, the first statement is incorrect, but the second statement is correct.

1.13 Evidence-based Activities

- Search the internet for photographs of the oral cavity and identify landmarks. Decide if the photographs show healthy or diseased periodontal tissues and explain why?
- Pick a microbe and search for virulence factors using the PubMed or EMBase Databases. Debate in class if your bacterium is more responsible than others when causing dental disease.
- Pick a virulence factor, such as *P. gingivalis* LPS, and map a molecular pathway that leads from *P. gingivalis* LPS

binding to a pattern-recognition receptor all the way to clinically observable changes in tissue using scientific studies and reviews found in the PubMed or EMBASE databases.

- Go to the University of Texas Health Science Center School of Dentistry at San Antonio's library of critically appraised topics (CAT) at https://cats.uthscsa.edu/ and search for a review on the link between cancer and periodontal disease. Read any CAT you can find, and debate if the conclusion is still correct based on current literature.
- Create a CAT on the merit of periodontal treatment for preventing heart disease (or any other topic for which a CAT is not available) following the outline provided by Sauve S., et al. in "The critically appraised topic: a practical approach to learning critical appraisal" (Ann R Coll Physicians Surg Can 1995; 28:396–398).

References

[1] Schmidt JC, Sahrmann P, Weiger R, Schmidlin PR, Walter C. Biologic width dimensions—a systematic review. J Clin Periodontol 2013;40(5):493–504

[2] Jin Y, Yip HK. Supragingival calculus: formation and control. Crit Rev Oral Biol Med 2002;13(5):426–441

[3] Hajishengallis G, Lamont RJ. Beyond the red complex and into more complexity: the polymicrobial synergy and dysbiosis (PSD) model of periodontal disease etiology. Mol Oral Microbiol 2012;27(6):409–419

[4] Kolenbrander PE, Palmer RJ Jr, Rickard AH, Jakubovics NS, Chalmers NI, Diaz PI. Bacterial interactions and successions during plaque development. Periodontol 2000 2006;42:47–79

[5] Mysak J, Podzimek S, Sommerova P, et al. Porphyromonas gingivalis: major periodontopathic pathogen overview. J Immunol Res 2014:476068

[6] Bechinger B, Gorr SU. Antimicrobial Peptides: Mechanisms of Action and Resistance. J Dent Res 2016

[7] Ding PH, Wang CY, Darveau RP, Jin LJ. Nuclear factor-κB and p38 mitogen-activated protein kinase signaling pathways are critically involved in Porphyromonas gingivalis lipopolysaccharide induction of lipopolysaccharide-binding protein expression in human oral keratinocytes. Mol Oral Microbiol 2013;28(2):129–141

[8] Raphael I, Nalawade S, Eagar TN, Forsthuber TG. T cell subsets and their signature cytokines in autoimmune and inflammatory diseases. Cytokine 2015;74(1):5–17

[9] Moutsopoulos NM, Kling HM, Angelov N, et al. Porphyromonas gingivalis promotes Th17 inducing pathways in chronic periodontitis. J Autoimmun 2012;39(4):294–303

[10] Belibasakis GN, Bostanci N. The RANKL-OPG system in clinical periodontology. J Clin Periodontol 2012;39(3):239–248

[11] Scheres N, de Vries TJ, Brunner J, Crielaard W, Laine ML, Everts V. Diverse effects of Porphyromonas gingivalis on human osteoclast formation. Microb Pathog 2011;51(3):149–155

[12] Huynh-Ba G, Lang NP, Tonetti MS, Salvi GE. The association of the composite IL-1 genotype with periodontitis progression and/or treatment outcomes: a systematic review. J Clin Periodontol 2007;34(4):305–317

[13] Engebretson S, Kocher T. Evidence that periodontal treatment improves diabetes outcomes: a systematic review and meta-analysis. J Periodontol 2013;84(4, Suppl):S153–S169

2 Gathering Periodontal Data

Abstract

The most important aspect of periodontal treatment is a thorough patient evaluation as without it, neither comprehensive diagnosis nor treatment planning is possible. Patient evaluation must investigate the systemic background of the patient's periodontal condition and look for local factors that influence the disease. The systemic background can be investigated through an attentive review of the medical history and past treatment. Detail-oriented extraoral and intraoral examinations can reveal various local factors that contribute to a patients' periodontal disease. In some cases, additional endodontic, radiographic, microbiologic, histologic, and genetic tests may need to be used to investigate unusual disease.

Keywords: history, measurements, radiographs, problem list

2.1 Learning Objectives

- Assess the systemic context of a patient's periodontal condition.
- Evaluate a patient's clinical periodontal condition for current status and local contributing factors.
- Use radiographic imaging and adjunctive tests to corroborate periodontal findings and uncover contributing factors.
- Prepare a problem list that leads to an etiology-based treatment plan.

2.2 Case

A 56-year old Caucasian female presented with pain from several teeth and wants to "take better care of her teeth." She states that the pain is mild and tolerable but fluctuates in intensity and never goes away completely. The pain comes from several teeth in the mouth, which makes it hard for her to point out the worst offending tooth. She noticed that it usually is triggered by eating cold or sweet foods, such as chilled soda, and it diminishes after a while when she does not eat. She did not seek care for the toothache elsewhere and tried avoiding seeing a dentist because of concerns about treatment costs. She denies having any anxiety about treatment. She has not seen a dentist since 5 years ago, where she received sporadic dental care. She uses a soft manual brush for about a minute twice a day to brush her teeth with a scrubbing technique, uses floss once a day, and uses a generic antiplaque mouth rinse once daily.

She does see a physician regularly, who prescribed 100-mg Losartan, 50-mg Levothyroxine, and 100-mg Gabapentin for her to take once daily, and takes these medications to treat her hypertension, hypothyroidism, and nerve pain in her hip. She denies having any other conditions; taking any supplements, recreational drugs, or using tobacco.

Extraoral exam reveals no findings other than a mild popping sound in the left temporomandibular joint (TMJ) halfway during mouth opening and closing. Intraorally, tissues appear normal other than marginal gingival erythema, and a small amount of purulent discharge next to no. 19 in an area of deeply erythematous marginal gingiva. Wear facets are present on most teeth and there are abfractions on the canine and first premolar facial surfaces, which also were the sites of facial gingival recession. A heavy centric occlusal contact was noted between no. 19 and no. 14, with no. 14 slightly supraerupted and no. 19 slightly submerged compared to teeth nos. 18 and 15. The patient is in Angle Class I with a deep overbite and shallow overjet.

The periodontal exam reveals several areas with slightly increased pocketing to about 5 mm around some molars, and a deep, wide 9-mm pocket on the facial side of no. 19. At this site, probing caused some discomfort to the patient, and when the probe was withdrawn, several drops of purulent discharge began to seep from the pocket entrance. This site was also coincident with the marginal erythema noted earlier, and the roof of the furcation could be felt about halfway under the tooth.

Radiographic examination showed mild generalized radiographic bone loss that correlated with the clinically observed mild generalized clinical attachment loss. There was a well-defined periapical radiolucency at tooth no. 14, and recurrent caries on the mesial surface of no. 15. There also was an area of reduced density within the furcation area of no. 19, and somewhat irregularly shaped crestal bone in all molar areas. Several crowns displayed open margins, especially on teeth nos. 3, 14, and 31. Tooth no. 29 had significant recurrent caries on the distal side of the tooth. Several of the patient's direct restorations had a degraded radiographic appearance with either poorly defined interproximal contacts, rough surfaces, restorative material overhangs, or a thick bonding agent-composite fill interface.

The patient was asked again to identify the area with the most severe pain, and the patient pointed to the upper left side. Closer inspection of these teeth revealed that the crown on no. 14 was slightly loose. The patient reported that the crown and associated root canal was completed more than 10 years ago. The patient did not remember any problems experienced during and after treatment back then. Pulp testing was performed on teeth nos. 13, 14, and 15, with an ice pellet. Tooth no. 13 produced a normal short-lived episode of pain when cold was applied and tooth no. 15 a slightly more pronounced, but still short-lived episode of pain. Unexpectedly, tooth no. 14 produced pronounced and lingering pain when cold was applied to the tooth, and it replicated the patient's pain complaint most closely. None of the three teeth produced pain on palpation or percussion.

Clinical appearance (▶Fig. 2.1) and radiographs (▶Fig. 2.2) are as shown in these figures.

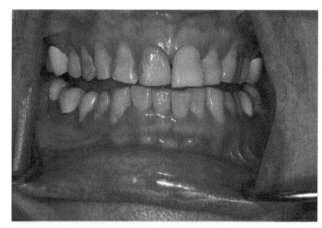

Fig. 2.1 Clinical presentation.

Fig. 2.2 Case X-ray series.

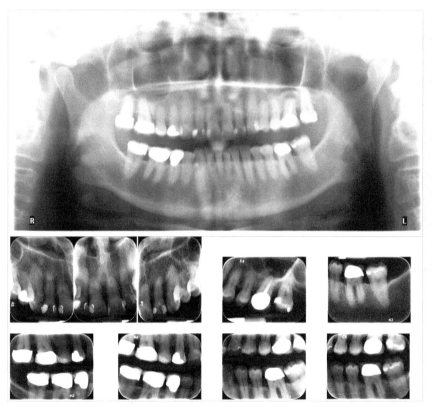

Findings in the periodontal chart are as follows:

Maxilla facial		1	2	3	4	5	6	7	8	9	10	11	12	13	14	15	16
	PD		425	425	423	223	222	212	212	212	213	213	313	314	213	513	
	BOP					1								1				
	CAL		3	3	1	1		1	1	1	1	3	1	2	3		
	GR		1										2		1	2	
	MGJ		323	434	434	434	434	434	545	545	544	422	423	433	433	434	
	Furc																
	PLQ		0	0	1	1	0	0	2	2	1	1	1	1	1	2	
Maxilla lingual	PD		424	523	212	313	311	212	211	312	212	212	212	212	424	513	
	BOP		1			1										11	
	CAL			2												2	
	GR		1	2											1		
	Furc																
	Mobil										1				2		
	PLQ		0	2	0	0	0	0	0	0	0	0	0	1	0	2	

Mandible lingual		32	31	30	29	28	27	26	25	24	23	22	21	20	19	18	17
	PD		213	514	313	222	223	212	212	213	312	212	223	313	521	333	
	BOP		1 1	1													
	CAL		1									2	3	2		2	
	GR		1														
	MGJ		323	222	212	223	212	212	212	212	222	223	333	334	334	444	
	Furc														2		
	PLQ		2	1	1	1	1	1	1	1	1	1	1	1	2	0	
Mandible facial	PD		213	412	212	212	213	413	213	313	313	313	313	224	593	324	
	BOP			1												1	
	CAL			1	2	2	1				1	1			9		
	GR		1	1	2	1	1							1	1		
	MGJ		223	212	222	323	000	655	554	555	655	433	000	101	222	122	
	Furc														2		
	Mobil																
	PLQ		1	1	1	2	2	2	2	1	1	1	1	1	2	1	

Abbreviations: BOP, bleeding on probing (1), suppuration (2); CAL, clinical attachment level; Furc, furcation involvement (Glickman class); GR, gingival recession; MGJ, position of mucogingival junction from margin; Mobil, tooth mobility (Miller grade); PD, probing depths; PLQ, plaque level (0 = none, 5 = heavy).

What can be learned from this case?

Unlike the patient case presented in Chapter 1, this patient presents with definite signs of periodontal disease, such as pocketing, bleeding and suppuration on probing, gingival recession, furcation involvement, and bone loss. Moreover, this patient presents with tooth pain.

Pain should always be addressed first. One way to diagnose oral pain is to consider the possible sources and rule them out based on clinical findings.

- Nonodontogenic pain is unlikely. There is no history of neurologic conditions (referred pain, headaches, migraines, and neuralgias) or signs and symptoms of aggressive tumors (swelling and unexpected weight loss). The examination did not reveal signs of significant TMJ conditions, such as a displaced disk or arthritis (no pain on palpation and normal exam/radiographic findings).
- Pain from occlusion is unlikely as there is no pain during percussion or occlusion
- In tooth no. 19 suppuration and deep pocket indicate periodontal infection and severe inflammation, which cause discomfort during probing.
- Teeth nos. 3 and 31 have open margins, and tooth no. 15 has recurrent caries. These teeth may produce sharp, short-lived pain when air is blown over the exposed margins or caries but have otherwise normal pulp vitality test results. Since the patient experiences pain after eating sweets, recurrent caries at no. 15 is a more likely source of pain.
- Tooth no. 14 is likely the main source of the patient's pain as testing replicated symptoms. Although periapical radiolucency suggests previous root canal treatment, intense pain during pulp vitality testing suggests irreversibly damaged pulp tissue. Given the radiographic presentation, it seems likely that root canal treatment failed or canals were missed during root canal treatment.

Acute infections have the second highest priority in treatment, and purulence at no. 19 suggests active infection. Here, a severe periodontal disease resulted in an isolated area of large bone loss that can be visualized when changing contrast and brightness on the digital radiograph, or with adjusting voltage and exposure time for several repeated conventional radiographs of no. 19 (▶ Fig. 2.3).

Isolated areas of bone loss should trigger a search for local factors enhancing periodontal disease. In this case, the local factor is the furcation involvement and the unique occlusal relationship between no. 14 and no. 19 in this case. Tooth no. 14 protrudes slightly in relation no. 15, and no. 19 is slightly submerged in relation to no. 18. Both teeth have wear facets and there is a heavy occlusal contract at maximum intercuspation and in excursive movement. Chronic excessive occlusal force from this heavy contact may have led to increased attachment loss and bone loss in response to the already occurring periodontal infection near the furcation entrance. For no. 14, the heavy occlusal force may have contributed to the cemental breakdown under the crown, which lead to the crown loosening and bacterial reinfection of the root canals.

The 5-mm pockets seen around the molars with isolated bleeding on probing are also linked to local factors: subgingival, open margin at the interproximal space between teeth nos. 2 and 3; open margin, open contact, and rough surface at the interproximal space between nos. 14 and 15; recurrent caries at no. 29; and bulky contour of no. 30.

The patient's general level of periodontal disease activity is mild and typical for her age and dental history, since plaque

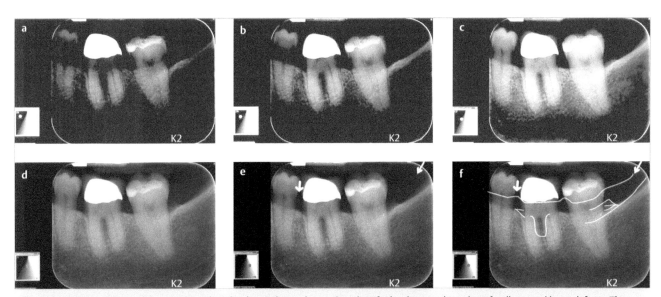

Fig. 2.3 Changing density and contrast on digital radiographs can be used to identify the shape and number of walls around bone defects. The process is as follows: (a) Adjust contrast so that it shows the maximum of bone structure, and lower brightness so that only the most radiodense objects such as dentin, enamel, external oblique ridge, and restorations remain. (b) Increase brightness until the densest parts of crestal bone appear. This will also outline the apical base on any bone defects. (c) Increase brightness further until faint parts of the alveolar crests appear, showing any walls of bony defects such as the bone spur distal to tooth no. 18 and the shallow vertical defect between this bone spur and the external oblique ridge. Notice also the faint line outlining the likely facial bone loss around the furcation of no. 19. (d, e) Increase brightness even more to show the faint gingival shadow (as shown in **e** with the *arrows*), which provided an estimate of tissue thickness. (f) Gingival shadow and bone defects outlined. Note the U-shaped area of bone loss at the furcation of tooth no. 19, the shallow 1-wall defect mesial of no. 19, and the shallow, but complex multi-wall defect at the distal of tooth no. 18 created in part by the overlying external oblique ridge. Thickened soft tissue overlies this multi-wall defect as seen by the thick tissue shadow (*white line, arrows*).

levels are low and there are no major systemic contributing factors at this time.

The abfractions and facial gingival recession seen in this case are most likely related to occlusal trauma and are linked to the wear facets of those teeth. While not indicated in the patient's dental history, the presence of wear facets and abfractions suggests that the patient bruxes her teeth and this possibility must be considered during the treatment.

Finally, the low amount of keratinized gingiva abbreviated as "MGJ" in the chart since it marks the position of the mucogingival junction (MGJ) relative to the gingival margin and lack of it at the canines are associated with a shallow lingual vestibule and numerous frenum attachments on the facial side of the mandibular ridge. This lack of MGJ may make brushing mandibular teeth more difficult, and may have contributed to periodontal disease activity at some point in the past. Currently, however, plaque levels are low, and the lack of MGJ may not be a significant factor in this patient.

2.3 Assessing the Systemic Context of a Patient's Periodontal Condition

2.3.1 Chief Complaint and the History of Present Illness

One of the most important aspects of a patient interview (see ▶ Video 2.1) in preparation for a comprehensive periodontal exam is to let the patient voice their concerns and treatment goals. Allowing the patient explaining their symptoms and probing the patient's concerns with the right type of skilled open-ended questioning often provide important clues for fast diagnosis. For efficiency, patient assessment should start with an open-ended question like "What brings you here today?" The answer, the "chief complaint" (CC), should be recorded verbatim, and usually presents the patient's most pressing concern. This should be followed up with open-ended, but directed questions to find out details about the patient's CC, which are collectively known as "history of present illness." Whereas most patients seeking care at a general practice will present with concerns unrelated to periodontal disease, a small proportion of patients will present either because they feel they need a "cleaning" or actually have symptoms of periodontal disease.

CCs related to periodontal conditions usually fall in the following categories, and should be investigated with the following questions:

- *"Want cleaning"/ "want check-up for gums:"* What makes you feel you need a cleaning/exam? Any concerns about the gums? When were the last cleaning/exam?
- *Referrals/ "was sent here:"* Who referred patient? Why? What treatment was done prior to the current visit?
- *"Loose teeth"/tooth mobility/shifting of teeth*: What teeth are loose/have shifted? How bad? How does it affect eating, drinking, speaking, and swallowing? When noticed? Any gum problems before?
- *Pain*: How severe? (use a visual analog scale) Where? How does it feel like? When does it happen? When first noticed? Is it changing in any way since it first started? What

makes it worse triggers it? What makes it better? How do you manage your pain? How does it affect you? Have you already seen someone else about the pain?
- *Gingival bleeding/swelling*: Where? What triggers it? How severe? When did the patient notice it for the first time? What makes it better? Had previous treatment for it?
- *Gingival recession*: Where? When first noticed? Noticed any changes recently? Had previous treatment for it?
  - ○ The following questions checking possible contributing factors for gingival recession: ever been told you had gum disease? How do you clean your teeth? Have you had braces? Do you use smokeless tobacco? Have piercings? Grind or clench teeth?

The patient's responses are often relevant for diagnosis as the symptoms usually correspond to clinical findings or certain periodontal diseases. If the CC is about:
- Wanting a "cleaning" or "check-up," then there will likely be significant calculus and plaque accretions. This may also indicate difficulty to commit to regular periodontal care.
- Being "sent here" or "referred here," usually this implies deep pockets, severe attachment loss/bone loss, mobile teeth, or extensive subgingival calculus deposits.

If the CC mirrors any of the following symptoms of periodontal disease, such as:
- "Loose teeth," it is most likely related to tooth mobility caused by severe attachment and bone loss. These patients may also report that teeth have "drifted" or "shifted" recently, and these patients may have some difficulty with eating or speaking as teeth no longer occlude properly, or the tooth mobility causes pain. In our experience, a CC of "loose teeth" most likely is associated with generalized severe periodontitis, or with combined periodontal endodontic lesions (more of this in Chapter 3). Much less common, but important to remember is that tooth mobility can also be caused by occlusal trauma, abnormal root anatomy (short tooth roots, root resorption, orthodontics-associated root resorption, and microdontia), rare genetic syndromes, and rare malignancies such as Langerhans' cell histiocytosis.
- "Bleeding gums," it usually indicates severe gingival inflammation. Gingival bleeding may be noticed by patients after brushing, flossing, or eating solid foods. Rare, but important to remember is that spontaneous gingival bleeding can also occur in patients with necrotizing periodontal diseases, severe coagulation defects, platelet disorders, and acute myeloid leukemia.
- Pain, it usually indicates severe disease if the pain originates from the periodontal tissues. While periodontal disease in most of the patients causes little to no pain, severe inflammation in the periodontal tissues can produce a constant, "dull," "sore," and maybe "itching" type of pain. Often, patients with gingival pain report that scratching or brushing the gingiva vigorously relieves pain. Chewing may aggravate the pain. Sharp pain is either related to occlusion (pain occurs or gets worse during chewing) or a pulpal condition (replicable with cold or other types of stimulation).
- "Receding gums" or "long teeth," it is related to gingival recession either caused by severe periodontal disease or other factors that cause isolated areas facial or lingual recession. Patients may also complain about the appearance of brown or yellow root surfaces, exposure of metal crown

margins, spaces appearing between the teeth, or the "gums receding." If there is a generalized loss of gingiva, with the loss of interproximal tissues, then the patient most likely has a form of periodontitis. If the recession is limited to a few teeth, local factors as explored with the questions above are more likely the cause of recession.

2.3.2 Medical History

A thorough medical history and review of systems are essential for safe patient care and are useful for the identification of risk factors linked to periodontal disease or treatment complications. For these reasons, it is important to obtain the following information.

Physician Contact Information

For patients with complex medical histories, it is often necessary to collaborate with a patient's primary physician and medical specialists. Therefore, the names, phone numbers, and fax numbers of a patient's primary physician and medical specialists should be recorded and verified either prior to the exam or before the patient leaves after the initial visit.

Medications

The most important aspect of the medical history is the list of medications as these are indicative of significant medical conditions and may interfere with periodontal treatment.[1] Supplements and recreational drugs should be considered as "medications" for their potential to interact with dental anesthesia and periodontal disease. Medications should be checked against a database (i.e., Lexicomp, Physician Desk Reference) and their typical use, mechanism of action, potential for drug interaction, and oral side effects researched. The following types of medications are relevant for periodontal treatment:

- *Amphetamines* are associated with gingival enlargement.
- *Antidepressants (tricyclics and monoamine oxidase inhibitors)* have severe hypertension risk with epinephrine.[2]
- *Anti-HIV medications* can have oral side effects such as xerostomia and gingiva discolorations. Anti-HIV medications tend to have renal toxicity, and NSAIDs should be avoided.
- *Anticoagulants* pose bleeding risks during invasive procedures.[3] Consult with a physician to lower bleeding risk or achieve an international normalized ratio (INR) target of less than 2.5 prior to surgery.
- *Antiplatelet agents* may pose bleeding risks during invasive procedures. Usually, bleeding risk is not significant, and medication should not be discontinued.[4]
- *Beta-blockers and nonselective* may produce orthostatic hypotension. Epinephrine may increase blood pressure while lowering pulse.
- *Bisphosphonates* use may pose a risk for osteonecrosis (0.1 to 4% for users of oral bisphosphonates, 10% after IV bisphosphonate administration) after periodontal surgery, scaling and root planing, or even the presence of periodontal disease.[5]
- *Calcium channel blockers* are associated with gingival enlargement (<10% of users).
- *Calcium supplements* interfere with tetracyclines (i.e., doxycycline).

- *Corticosteroids* lead to infection and adrenal crisis risk. Consult with the physician and consider doubling corticosteroid dose on the day of the procedure, along with antibiotic prophylaxis.
- *Cyclosporine* lead togingival enlargement (up to 60% with cyclosporine; less with sirolimus and tacrolimus) and postoperative infection risk. Consider antibiotic prophylaxis.
- *Deferiprone* (an iron chelator) may cause neutropenia and sever periodontal disease.
- *Digoxin* leads to severe hypertension risk with epinephrine.
- *Dilantin/phenytoin* results in gingival enlargement (40% of users).
- *Estrogen replacement/birth control* results in enhanced gingival inflammation. It may be associated with pyogenic granuloma.
- *Methotrexate and immunosuppressive medications* lead to postoperative infection risk. Consider antibiotic prophylaxis.
- *Minocycline* can cause gingival discoloration.
- *NSAIDs* lead to occasional bleeding risk. They are associated with lichenoid lesions and renal toxicity.
- *Phenobarbital* is infrequently associated with gingival overgrowth.
- *Supplements such as garlic, gingko, ginger, chamomile, vitamin E, and large doses (several grams) of fish oil supplements* may pose a bleeding risk.
- *Thyroid hormone replacement* (i.e., Synthroid) may cause possible hypertension risk with epinephrine. It is occasionally associated with bleeding risk from acquired von Willebrand disease.
- *Valproic acid* is infrequently associated with gingiva overgrowth.
- *Xerostomic medications:* There are over 400 medications that are associated with xerostomia, which is associated with both increased caries and periodontal disease risk.

Medical History/Review of Systems

Medical conditions are of interest for periodontal treatment since they either present a treatment risk or interact with periodontal disease. Consequently, periodontal assessment requires a thorough medical history and review of systems.

Generally, medical conditions present the following five types of concerns for periodontal treatment:

- *Need for antibiotic prophylaxis for periodontal exams:* Bacteremia caused by periodontal probing may pose a risk of serious infection for patients with some medical conditions, typically conditions linked to bacterial endocarditis[6] or the presence of implanted medical devices such as total joint replacements,[7] catheters, ports, stents, and vena cava filters. Usually, this requires consultation with the patient's physician, and a dose of antibiotics (2-g amoxicillin or 600-mg clindamycin) may need to be prescribed 1 hour before the periodontal exam.
- *Need for antibiotics to prevent postoperative infections after invasive treatments:* Periodontal procedures such as scaling and surgery introduce bacteria into oral tissues and cause bacteremia. This creates a risk of postoperative infections for patients with weakened immune responses, in addition to patients with implanted medical devices or at risk for

bacterial endocarditis. Generally, consultation with the patient's physician can assist in judging the risk of infection and prescription of antibiotics either for the procedure or afterward should be considered.

- *Risk of medical emergencies during dental procedures:* Periodontal procedures may be lengthy, stressful, and uncomfortable for patients and often require the administration of local anesthesia. This increases the risk of medical emergencies occurring during treatment. For patient's safety, it is important to identify conditions that pose a risk for medical emergencies, and be prepared to address these emergencies if they arise.[8]

- *Treatment modifications needed:* For some medical conditions, adjusting the way treatment is delivered may improve patient comfort or lessen the risk of medical emergencies.
- *Periodontal-systemic relationships:* Some medical conditions influence periodontal disease and vice versa. These may exacerbate periodontal disease or lessen the chance of treatment success. Periodontal disease treatment may also aid in improving medical conditions, and knowledge of these relationships can motivate some patients for periodontal treatment.

The medical conditions that are a concern for periodontal treatment are listed in (▶Table 2.1a-b).

Table 2.1 (a) Medical conditions affecting periodontal treatment (part 1)

Condition	AE	AT	Medical emergency risk
AIDS	X	X	
Anemia, severe		?	Hypoxia with sedatives
Angina			Myocardial infarct (especially, if unstable angina)
Anxiety			Anxiety attack may mimic myocardial infarct
Asthma			Asthma attack, patient should bring inhaler
Atherosclerosis			Myocardial infarct, stoke
Endocarditis, past	X	X	
Bleeding disorder	?	?	Internal/joint bleed, prolonged bleeding from surgery
Bronchitis, COPD			Hypoxia with sedatives
Cancer		?	
Cardiac dysrhythmia			Cardiac arrest, stroke (depends on dysrhythmia)
CHF			Heart failure, hypoxia
Dementia			Stroke (if dementia caused by previous stroke)
Diabetes mellitus		X	Hypoglycemia (especially, Type 1)
Epilepsy			Seizure
GERD/reflux			May mimic myocardial infarct
Hypertension			Myocardial Infarct, stroke (long-term risk)
Hypothyroidism			Hypertensive crisis triggered by epinephrine (unlikely)
Leukemia/lymphoma	?	X	
Liver cirrhosis		?	Bleeding risk, adverse drug reactions
Medical implants	?	?	
Myocardial infarct	?		(new) Myocardial infarct
Obesity			Myocardial infarct, stroke (long-term risk)
Organ transplant	X	X	
Osteoporosis, severe			Bone/hip fracture
Pacemaker	?	?	Cardiac arrhythmia (if pacemaker malfunctions)
Pregnancy			Hypotension, preterm labor (unlikely)
Prosthetic heart valve	X	X	
Renal disease	?	?	Adverse drug reaction
Rheumatoid arthritis		?	
Sickle cell disease		X	Sickle crisis
Stroke			(new) Stroke
Total joint replacement	X	X	

Abbreviations: AE, need for antibiotic prophylaxis for exam; AT, need for antibiotic prophylaxis for treatment; CHF, congestive heart failure; COPD, chronic obstructive pulmonary disease; X, likely need; ?, may need or consult with treating physician.

Table 2.1 **(b)** Medical conditions affecting periodontal treatment (part 2)

Condition	Treatment modification	Perio-systemic relationship
AIDS	Refer to physician prior to PT	Severe, unusual PD
Anemia, severe	Monitor SpO_2, supply O_2 antibiotics for aplastic anemia	Oral signs of anemia, severe periodontal disease risk with aplastic anemia
Angina	Conservative treatment	
Anxiety	Consider anxiolytic	
Atherosclerosis	Avoid neck palpitation, possible bleeding risk	PT ↓ 0.7 mg/L CRP, ↓ 0.2 mmol/L Trig and cholesterol, ↓ 0.4% HbA1c
Bleeding disorder	Consult with hematologist Focus on disease prevention	
Bronchitis, COPD	Monitor SpO_2, supply O_2,	1.3 × more likely with CP
Cancer	Consult with oncologist; PT depends on treatment stage	Oral metastasis risk, long-term effects
Congestive heart failure	Monitor ECG, vitals; supply O_2	More likely to have CP
Dementia	Conservative treatment, ensure informed consent	Tooth loss associated with dementia
Diabetes mellitus, severe	Conservative treatment, short AM appointments	2–3 × more likely CP, PT ↓ 0.3–0.4% HbA1c
GERD/reflux	Avoid recline	
Hypertension	Short appointments, caution with epinephrine	1.5 × more likely with CP
Hypothyroidism	Caution with epinephrine	
Leukemia/lymphoma	Consult hem/oncologist; PT depends on treatment stage	Risk of severe periodontal disease
Liver cirrhosis	Lower medication dosing	
Medical implants	Consult with surgeon who placed device	
Myocardial infarct	Delay PT after recent MI short, PM appointments	1.2–1.5 × odds of myocardial infarct with CP
Obesity	Short appointments	1.3–1.8 × odds of CP
Organ transplant	Consult with medical specialist	Severe PD risk
Osteoporosis, severe	Prevent falls	Worsens CP; CP increases hip fracture risk
Pacemaker	Avoid electrosurgery, magnetostrictive ultrasonics	
Pregnancy	Avoid teratogens, radiation (1st trimester), NSAIDs (3rd), recline	Enhances gingival inflammation; PD may increase risk of birth complications
Prostate enlargement	Avoid opioids	
Psychiatric conditions	Conservative PT	
Renal disease	Avoid NSAIDs; lower medication dosing	PT improves GFR
Rheumatoid arthritis	Conservative PT, prevent disease	1.1 × more likely CP; PT improves DAS28
Sickle cell disease	Monitor SpO_2, supply O_2 caution with $epinephrine_2$	
Stroke	Avoid PT after recent stroke, conservative PT; simplify oral hygiene; consent issue	1.2–2 × odds with CP
Tuberculosis, active	Delay PT until treated	

Abbreviations: CP, chronic periodontitis (as reported in prior to 2018); PD, periodontal disease; PT, periodontal treatment.
"Conservative PT": Disease prevention; Surgical PT leans toward extractions, resective surgery.

For patients with severe medical conditions, it is usually better to provide treatments in short appointments, and patients tend to tolerate dental procedures better in the morning, unless they have cardiovascular conditions. Supplemental oxygen supplied through a nasal cannula is often beneficial for patients with anemia, respiratory conditions, and cardiovascular conditions. Although epinephrine is a useful vasoconstrictor for periodontal surgery, it may cause discomfort or trigger medical emergencies in patients with sickle cell disease, severe cardiovascular disease, or thyroid conditions.

For patients with cancers including leukemia and lymphoma, periodontal treatment depends on the stage of cancer treatment. Prior to cancer treatment, the focus needs to be on rapid oral disease elimination with the removal of any diseased teeth or teeth that are at risk for disease. During cancer treatment, dental treatment should focus on preventing infections and managing oral side effects of cancer therapy. After cancer treatment, treatment should continue on disease prevention, and monitor any oral signs of cancer recurrence.

Information that Needs to Be Gathered

For conditions that impact periodontal therapy, it is useful to obtain more information from a patient and a patient's physician to gauge the severity of the medical condition. For conditions that impact periodontal disease, this information will aid in gauging the impact of a patient's medical condition (▶ Table 2.2).

Table 2.2 Additional information that should be obtained for conditions affecting periodontal treatment

Condition	Factors to gauge impact	Major impact expected
AIDS, HIV	CD4+ count, HIV viral load	CD4+ <200, high virus titer
Anemia, severe	Type of anemia, current effect of anemia on living CBC lab results	Fanconi, Diamond-Blackfan, thalassemia major/intermedia low hemoglobin, RBC count
Angina	When does it occur (stable, unstable)	Spontaneous (unstable angina)
Anxiety	When does it occur, how severe	Dental-related; severe panic attacks
Atherosclerosis	How was it diagnosed, where, what medications	If it affects head and neck arteries
Bleeding disorder	• What type • INR/PT for anticoagulant therapy • Factor level for Hemophilia, vWD • Current problems caused by condition	Moderate-severe hemophilia/vWD; INR > 3.5 Large bruises with no impact; joint disease
Bronchitis, COPD	How severe; impact on living?	Needs supplemental oxygen
Cancer	Where, what type, what stage, how treated?	Current cancer, chemo/radiation therapy
Congestive heart failure	How severe; impact on living?	Cannot recline; needs supplemental oxygen; ejection fraction <70%
Dementia	How severe? Dependence on caregiver	Needs assisted living
Diabetes mellitus, severe	What type? Severity? Effect on living? Glucose levels, HbA1c	Evidence organ damage; Glucose > 150 mg/dL; HbA1c > 9
GERD/reflux	How severe? How far able to recline?	Cannot recline
Hypertension	How severe? Effects of blood pressure?	Headache, blurry vision
Hypothyroidism	How severe?	
Leukemia/lymphoma	What type? What stage? Effect of cancer so far?	Advanced stage, aggressive or incurable type of cancer. Symptoms of disease progression
Liver cirrhosis	How severe? Needs liver transplant?	Signs and symptoms of liver failure
Medical implants	What type? Need antibiotic for dental treatment?	
Myocardial infarct	When? How severe? What was done?	Less than 6 months ago
Obesity	How diagnosed? Underlying medical condition? BMI/Weight/Height?	Thyroid/genetic cause BMI > 40
Organ transplant	What organ? Success? Impact on living?	
Osteoporosis, severe	How diagnosed? What bones affected? Had fractures? T-score	Previous hip, vertebra fracture T-score < –2.5
Pacemaker	When placed? Why? Previous problems with dental treatment?	Dental equipment caused pacemaker to malfunction
Pregnancy	How far along? Current comfort level sitting, laying on back, getting up?	1st, 3rd trimester. Has difficulty getting up, reclining
Psychiatric conditions	Impact on living? Dependence on care taker	
Renal disease	How severe? Need for dialysis/transplant? GFR	Receives dialysis/on wait list GFR < 30
Rheumatoid arthritis	What joint affected? How severe?	Hand, TMJ joint affected
Sickle cell disease	Previous sickle crisis? Impact on living?	Crisis in dental office; receives blood transfusion
Stroke	How severe? Impact on living?	Not coherent. Needs caregiver
Tuberculosis	When diagnosed? Was symptomatic?	Has active, productive cough

Abbreviations: BMI, body mass index; GFR, glomerular filtration rate; INR/PT, international normalized ratio/prothrombin time; TMJ, temporomandibular joint; vWD, von Willebrand factor deficiency.

Recreational Drugs Associated with Periodontal Disease

Recreational drugs can have a variety of effects on the oral cavity, and a thorough medical history should include questions on recreational drugs (▶Table 2.3).

Genetic Conditions Associated with Severe Periodontal Disease

A number of specific genetic conditions are associated with severe periodontal disease (▶Table 2.4).

Table 2.3 Recreational drugs relevant for periodontal disease

Drug	Information needed	Significance	Periodontal impact
Alcohol	What beverage? How much? How often?	Oral cancer risk; risk of liver cirrhosis, malnutrition, neurologic conditions, social problems if excessive	Linear dose relationship alcohol-CP
Cocaine, crystalline/powder	How used? How often?	Dental erosion; risk of tissue necrosis where applied. Cocaine users tend to also use tobacco, marijuana, or alcohol	Unknown effect
Crack cocaine/free base	How often?	Oral blisters and burns from extreme heat of smoked crack cocaine. Crack cocaine uses ten to also smoke tobacco, marijuana	More severe PD
Marijuana/cannabis	How consumed? How much per day? For how many years? When?	Smoked marihuana may have similar oral cancer risk to tobacco. Some marijuana users may also experiment with other recreational drugs	Increased periodontal disease similar to tobacco
Tobacco	What type? How much per day? For how many years? When? How used?	Heavy smoker 1 pack/day; Pack of cigarettes/day times year relates to cancer, stroke, COPD risk	5–20 × more likely CP; PT less successful

Table 2.4 Genetic conditions associated with severe periodontal disease

Condition	Typical features	Cause of periodontal disease
Chediak-Higashi	Oculocutaneous albinism, coagulation deficiency, ataxia, and seizures	LYST gene defect leads to defect in lysosome function, which interferes with immune cell function
Cohen syndrome	Developmental delay, microcephaly, myopia, retinal dystrophy, thick hair and eyebrows, long eyelashes, unusual shaped eyes, short philtrum, prominent nos. 8 and 9	Unknown
Congenital agranulocytosis/Kostmann syndrome	Recurrent infections and anemia	Defective expression of Bcl-2 gene leads to excess apoptosis of myeloid progenitor cells
Congenital neutropenia	Recurrent infections, osteoporosis, and leukemia risk	Various mutations (i.e., ELANE gene) lead to premature death of developing neutrophils in bone marrow
Ehlers-Danlos, periodontal type/type VIII	Joint hypermobility, skin hypermobility, tissue fragility; and lack of attached gingiva	C1R, C1S gene defects leads to defective complement pathway
Glycogen storage disease type I/von Gierke disease	Hypoglycemia, lactic acidosis, hyperuricemia, hyperlipidemia, thin arms, legs; short stature; and risk of osteoporosis, kidney disease, and adenomas	Neutropenia through unknown mechanism
Hypophosphatasia	Ricketts; early loss of teeth; and abnormal tooth development	ALPL gene defect leads to abnormal bone/teeth mineralization
Klinefelter syndrome	Low testosterone, delayed puberty, gynecomastia, reduced facial hair, and infertility	Unknown
Leukocyte adhesion deficiency	Delayed loss of umbilical cord and severe bacterial/fungal infections	Defective beta2 integrin prevents migration of leukocytes toward infection
Marfan syndrome	Vision problems (dislocated lens, early glaucoma); defective heart valves, sunken/protruding chest; tall stature; and risk of aortic dissection	Defective fibrillin leads to overgrowth and instability of tissues
Papillon-Lefévre	Palmoplantar keratosis, severe periodontitis	Defective cathepsin C gene leads to ineffective killing of bacteria
Trisomy 21/Down syndrome	Intellectual disability, characteristic facial appearance, hypotonia, risk of celiac disease, heart disease, and hypothyroidism	Unknown
Zimmerman-Laband	Gingival overgrowth, narrow facial appearance, overgrowth of tongue, and long/slender fingers	Unknown

Autoimmune Conditions Associated with Severe Periodontal Disease

Autoimmune conditions affecting soft tissues can produce the clinical signs of "desquamative gingivitis," where vesicle formation and epithelial sloughing produces ulcerations. Typically, this can be caused by the following autoimmune conditions, and these conditions are described in many oral pathology textbooks:[9]

- Pemphigus vulgaris.
- Mucous membrane pemphigoid.
- Lichen planus/lichenoid reactions.
- Erythema multiforma.
- Lupus erythematosus.
- Linear IgA disease.
- Chronic ulcerative stomatitis.

For any of these conditions, consultation and referral to a medical specialist is essential for resolution of oral disease.

Demographic Factors

Demographic factors generally have limited relevance for diagnosis and treatment, but are useful in assessing the overall risk of periodontal disease. When assessing a patient or describing a case, the following demographic factors should be considered:

- *Social environment*: Generally, this is encapsulated by the employment status of an adult patient, and caregiving for children and special needs patients. Low socioeconomic status correlates with poorer overall and oral health, including periodontal disease.[10]
- *Age*: Damage caused by periodontal disease accumulates with age.[11] Patients with significant periodontal disease at a young age have a high risk of continued periodontal disease and tooth loss. Typically, anything more than mild radiographic bone loss is not seen under age 40.
- *Gender*: Males usually have more significant periodontal disease compared to females with similar overall health.
- *Ethnicity/race/geographic origin*: Periodontal disease experience varies across different populations and in different countries. In the United States, Hispanics have the highest level of periodontitis, followed by non-Hispanic blacks, Asian Americans, and non-Hispanic whites.

Dental History

While the lack of preventive dental care is not predictive for periodontitis, the dental history provides clues on a patient's oral hygiene habits, past compliance with treatment, and the likelihood of treatment success. The following questions pertaining to oral hygiene and previous dental treatment need to be answered:

- *Oral hygiene*: How are teeth brushed? How often? How is the space between teeth cleaned? How often? What toothbrush, paste, floss, and mouthwash is used?
- *Previous dental treatment*: Information about the previous dentist: how often seen for dental treatment? What was done? What was planned? What was the reason for leaving? Problems with previous dental treatment? Received previous periodontal treatment? By a specialist?

2.4 Evaluating the Current State of the Periodontal Condition

The periodontal condition always should be evaluated at any examination visit. While a detailed oral exam of a new patient may take 1 hour for complicated cases in the hands of an experienced provider, the collection of periodontal data, such as probing depth and bleeding on probing, can often be done in less than 15 minutes.

Typically, a periodontal exam requires a mirror, caries explorer, periodontal probe, gauze, articulating paper, and an articulating forceps. A furcation probe (i.e., Nabers probe) aids furcation detection. For the radiographic examination of a new patient or for a patient experiencing new disease, an X-ray holder kit (i.e., Rinn [R] kit) and radiographic sensors or film for taking radiographs are needed. If there are signs of root canal infections, such as bone loss around the apex of teeth, tooth pain or fistula tracts, endodontic ice, pulp testers, paper point, and gutta-percha points are needed.

2.4.1 General Head, Neck, Oral Mucosal, and Hard Tissue Exam

A general assessment of the head, neck, and oral cavity should be performed as part of a periodontal exam. While this can be brief, here are rare, but important findings that should be checked.

Head and Neck Exam

The head and neck evaluation should be brief. It relies on careful observation, which checks for signs of significant medical conditions affecting oral health (see ▶Video 2.2):

- Patient gait, ability to walk and communicate:
  - *Impaired*: Stroke or other severe neurologic conditions (i.e., Parkinson).
- Hands:
  - Upturned fingernails: Severe anemia.
  - Dark discoloration of nail bed: Medications or environmental toxins (i.e., heavy metals).
  - Pinpoint bruises in nail bed, large bruises: Bleeding disorders or anticoagulant therapy.
  - Swollen joints: Arthritis or gout.
- Face:
  - Drooping/loss of muscle tone on one side of face: Previous or ongoing stroke.
  - Facial asymmetry: May correlate with temporomandibular joint disorders (TMD).
  - Localized swollen, red tissue: Usually, the sign of tissue infection.
  - Localized swollen, gradually enlarging tissue: Can be a sign of neoplasm.
  - Enlarged temporalis and masseter muscle: Often a sign of bruxism.
  - Abnormal skin color: Pale lips, mucosa—anemia. Chronically flushed skin may indicate various conditions from severe hypertension to emphysema to polycythemia vera.
  - Spider veins/telangiectasia, solar elastosis: Cancer risk.
  - Ulcerations: If not healing, may present squamous and basal cell carcinomas.

○ Moles of unusual size or irregular, ill-defined borders: Possible melanoma.
○ Areas of numbness: Trigeminal nerve damage.
• *Lymph nodes* should be palpated at regular intervals. Palpation will reveal either:
○ *Nothing:* This is the most common outcome. Healthy nodes are barely felt with pressure.
○ *Swollen, warm, tender, doughy lymph nodes:* Indicative of a local infection.
○ *Firm, large "lump" that may be fixed to surrounding tissue:* Rare. Sign of cancer.
• *Thyroid:* Should be palpated: enlargement or abnormal shape may be a sign of thyroid neoplasm.
• *TMJ:* Should be palpated during opening and closing. Look for:
○ *Pain:* Sign of disk displacement. Periodontal procedures may aggravate pain.
○ *Clicks and popping sounds at different positions:* Suggest disk displacement.
○ *Clicks at the same position:* Common sign of anatomical irregularity on joint surface.

Oral Mucosa Exam

Periodontal disease is associated with increased risk for oral cancer, and an oral mucosal screening for cancer should be performed at every exam (see ▶ Video 2.3). This consists of the following two components:
• *Oral inspection for color changes and ulceration in the following areas:* The upper and lower lip, corners of the mouth; labial and buccal vestibules; lingual vestibule; floor of the mouth; ventral side of the tongue; lateral borders of the tongue; dorsum of the tongue; hard palate; soft palate; pharyngeal arches and faucillar pillars; and oropharynx, maxillary tuberosity, and the retromolar pad.
• *Palpation of salivary glands:* This should be done with two hands, one intraorally and one extraorally, to feel for soft salivary glands and check for the production of saliva from the submandibular, lingual, and parotid glands.

The presence of any oral piercings should be noted as they are associated with gingival recession.

Hard Tissue Exam

Many local factors that enhance the severity of periodontal disease at a given tooth can be noticed during the hard tissue exam (see ▶ Video 2.4). Teeth should be examined clinically and with diagnostic radiographs to evaluate the presence of the following factors:
• *Caries* creates rough, plaque-retentive surfaces favoring periodontal disease. Caries either feels like a sticky surface with a sharp caries explorer, or feels rough and concave. Interproximal caries is readily seen on radiographs as a dark shadow near the contact point.
• *Calculus* can be felt as a rough patch, wedge, or ledge that sticks out of the tooth surface. If severe, it can be seen as a radiopaque spike on the root surface.
• *Open contacts* cause food impaction and are associated with increased pocketing and bone loss. Floss readily passes through the contact, and there may be a radiographic gap.
• *Open margins* at or below the gingival margin are associated with increased bleeding on probing and pocketing. A sharp

explorer will stick to the same area when run across the restoration margin in apically and coronally.
• *Overhanging restorations* are associated with increased periodontal disease, and often can be seen radiographically. This will feel as a "step out" when an explorer is dragged over the restorative margin, as a sharp explorer will only stick to the margin in one direction, but not the other.
• *Rough restorative surfaces and broken restorations* contribute to plaque retention and increasing probing depth, and are felt as rough surface with an explorer.
• *Subgingival margins* attract more plaque and are associated with increased gingival inflammation.
• *Overcontoured or bulky restorations* may lead to worsened plaque accumulation conceptually, but a study suggests this effect is very slight.
• *Furcation entrances*[12] are difficult to treat periodontally and diminish long-term survival.
• *Crowding and associated fixed orthodontic appliances* interfere with oral hygiene.
• *Rotation/tipping* interferes with oral hygiene.
• *Enamel ridges and projections* interfere with scaling and root planing.
• *Root surface concavities* interfere with scaling and root planing. Maxillary first premolars have deep interproximal root concavities that are notoriously difficult to treat periodontally.
• *Enamel pearls* are most likely found on first and second maxillary molars between the distobuccal and palatal root, and associated with deep pocketing in molars.
• *Partially erupted teeth/partially impacted* 3rd *molars* may produce a pocketing. Removal of 3rd molars may leave residual pockets.

Occlusal Evaluation

Occlusal factors may play a large role in periodontal disease in some patients, but it is unclear if they play a major role,[13] or a minor role for the average patient. Generally, the following factors should be assessed:
• *Angle Class:* Severe Angle Class II and Class III are more likely associated with gingival recession.
• *Overjet and overbite:* If severe, associated with increased bone loss.
• *Vertical dimension at rest:* Closed vertical dimension is associated with bruxism. To evaluate, have the patient swallow or pretend to say the letter N silently for a few seconds. Both maneuvers will leave the patient's mandible in a resting position, and the posterior teeth should clearly not contact the opposing arch.
• *Signs of parafunctional habits:*
○ *Severe attrition:* Suggests bruxism.
○ *Tooth or restoration fractures:* More likely seen with clenching than bruxism.
○ *Thickened, festooned gingival margins:* Bruxism or clenching.
○ *Generalized tooth mobility:* Bruxism or clenching.
○ *Generalized widened periodontal ligament in the absence of systemic disease.*
○ *Crenellation marks on the tongue:* Suggest clenching.
○ *Lack of fingernails and chipped anterior teeth:* Suggest nail biting.

- A distinct area of excessive wear the size and shape of a pipe stem for pipe chewers.
- *Occlusal interference contacts:* Associated with worse probing depths over several years, and may be associated with angular bone defects. Evaluate by drying teeth, and having patient tap teeth together with occlusal paper. Occlusal contacts should be evenly spread out among posterior teeth with no heavy marks. Excursive movements should disclose posterior teeth smoothly, with gliding contacts limited to canines.
- *Signs of occlusal trauma:* Occlusal trauma is most likely associated with enhanced periodontal disease severity. Signs of occlusal trauma include the following:
  - *Fremitus* is associated with gingival clefting and recession. Fremitus can be determined readily in the maxilla by placing a finger lightly on the facial surface of the maxillary teeth, having the patient tap their teeth together, and feeling for tooth movement upon occlusal contact.
  - Excessive occlusal wear and large wear facets.
  - Tooth mobility in the absence of major bone loss.
  - Tooth/restorative fractures.
  - Funnel-shaped or widened periodontal ligament on radiographs.
  - Vertical bone defects in the absence of anatomical or restorative factors.
  - Abfractions that correlate with interference contacts.
  - Pain on occlusion.

2.4.2 Periodontal Assessment

Patient safety: A periodontal exam may pose a significant infection risk for immunocompromised patients, patients with implanted medical devices, or patients at high risk for infective endocarditis. In these cases, consult with the patient's physician, and consider using prophylactic antibiotics 1 hour prior to the exam.

Whereas the evaluation of the head, neck, oral mucosa, and hard tissue checks for systemic and local factors affecting periodontal treatment, the evaluation of periodontal tissues provides the basis for diagnosis of periodontal disease and treatment need. This part of the evaluation process checks the following:

General Gingival Appearance

- *Method*: Visual inspection of the mucosa and gingiva on buccal and lingual aspects of both maxilla and mandibular areas, including edentulous areas (see ▶ Fig. 2.4, for examples of gingival appearance).
- *What to evaluate?*
  - Color:
    - *General color*: Pale pink, coral pink, tan, or brown/black pigmented.
    - *Patches of color changes*: Lighter pink, yellow, white, brown/black/blue patches.
    - *Translucency of gingiva:* Is the tissue thin and translucent, or thick and opaque?
    - *Areas of erythema.*
    - *Location of erythema:* Papillary, marginal, or diffuse.
    - *Severity of erythema:* Mild, severe (beefy-red), or cyanotic.
  - Texture:
    - *Surface texture*: Stippled or smooth?
    - *Degree of surface texture:* Rough, granular, or smooth?
  - Shape:
    - *Size of gingival scallop*: Tall or low papilla heights relative facial/lingual margin?
    - *Thickness of gingival margin:* Knife-edged or rolled?
    - *Depth of vestibular mucosa:* Deep or shallow?
    - *Gingival Recession:* Present or absent?
  - Presence of unusual characteristics:
    - McCall's Festoons? Associated with occlusal trauma.
    - Stillman's clefts? Associated with underlying bone dehiscence.
    - Purulent discharge? Presence of a fistula? Associated with local infections.
    - Localized swellings/growths? Local infections, reactive, or neoplastic growths.
    - Visible surface blood vessels in the gingiva? Associated with gingival bleeding.

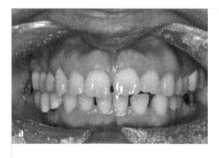
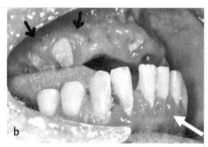
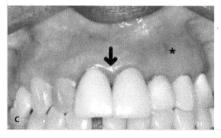
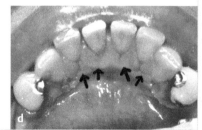

Fig. 2.4 (a) Normal pink stippled scalloped gingiva and dark pink mucosa in a patient with thick gingival biotype. (b) Festooned gingiva (*black arrows*) around maxillary root tips and severely inflamed cyanotic swollen spongy papilla around mandibular teeth (*white arrow*). (c) Papillary erythema and edema (*arrow*) and fistula tract (*star*). (d) Stillman's clefts, most likely created as a result of abscess formation close to the gingival margin (*arrows*).

- Significance:
  - Areas with erythematous, smooth, and rolled margins likely to have deep pocketing; areas of pink, stippled, and knife-edged gingiva likely to have shallow pocketing.
  - Fistulas and purulent discharge should be followed with pulp vitality testing of nearby teeth.
  - Thick, opaque tissue with low scallop indicates a thick biotype. Thin, translucent tissue with high scallop indicates a thin biotype.

Pocketing/Probing Depths

- Method (see ▶ Fig. 2.5, ▶ Video 2.5)
  - Technique:
    - Insert probe gently at distal line angle, following the long axis of the tooth root, until rubber band-like resistance is found. If probe encounters hard surface, move probe sideways or toward tissue until it drops further into sulcus. Note the position of gingival margin along with probe marking, and note the nearest exposed probe mark. This marks the local probing depth.
    - Walk probe into distal contact point, angling it up to about 45 degrees relative to tooth, and feeling for any drop in sulcus surface. Memorize deepest probing depth.
    - Walk probe back to facial/lingual surface and to mesial line angle; angle it parallel to root surface. Find the deepest insertion point and memorize probing depth here.
    - Walk probe into mesial contact point, angling it up to 45 degrees relative to tooth and feeling for any drops. Memorize the deepest depth and record these three depths.
    - While checking probing depths, assess: (1) firmness of sulcus floor. It should feel just like touching a rubber band; (2) roughness of the root surface. Clean surfaces feel smooth; (3) presence of pain with light probing force; (4) bleeding after probing.
  - For consistency:
    - Same type of periodontal probe should be used for all exams.
    - Consistent, gentle pressure should be used (about 25 grams). Higher pressure is acceptable but it causes patient discomfort.
  - For efficiency:
    - A consistent measurement pattern should be used for all exams.
    - Probing depths should be read and recorded in triplets (i.e., 3–2–3).
    - Measurement pattern should match the pattern set by HER software, if used.
    - Keyboard shortcuts and data entry devices (i.e., DentalRat, voice recognition) are useful.
- Special circumstances:
  - *Calculus impedes probing*: Remove excess calculus ultrasonic scaler or hand scaler until the ultrasonic tip reaches the rubbery bottom of the sulci. This can be billed as "debridement."
  - *Buccal surfaces of 2nd or 3rd molars*: Insert a mouth mirror into the buccal vestibule next to the molars with the back end of the mirror facing the cheek mucosa, and ask the patient to move the lower jaw away from the teeth to be measured.
  - *Lingual surfaces of incisors:* Use headrest to tilt patient's head back and chin up. Use a mirror only if necessary.
  - *Implants*: Use a plastic periodontal probe if available to find probing depths. If the peri-implant tissue appears pink and healthy, use minimal force.

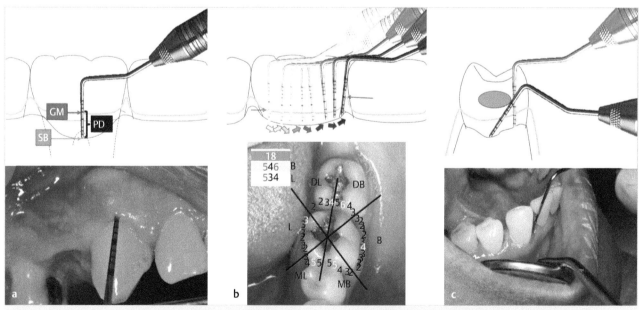

Fig. 2.5 How to probe: (a) Begin at midfacial/lingual, insert gently into sulcus while holding probe parallel to tooth, and determine distance between gingival margin to sulcus floor for probing depth. Round up to next higher millimeter. (b) Walk probe along the sulcus with light force, feeling all areas of the sulcus for any drops and other irregularities in the sulcus. Note probing depths along the way, and identify the highest probing depth in a given sextant as shown. (c) When approaching the interproximal contact, it is important to angle the probe under the contact in order to detect interproximal pocketing, so that pocketing under the contact point is not missed (as shown here). As probing depths are read and recorded, note any areas of significant gingival bleeding that developed in response to probing. Probes will have different millimeter ruler designs as shown here (UNC-15, bottom left; Michigan "O" probe, top row; WHO probe, bottom right), and need to be considered when measuring probing depths.

- ○ *Thin biotype or sensitive, tight gingiva*: Consider a thin, or flat probe (i.e., Goldman-Fox).
- Significance:
  - ○ Sites with deep probing depths have a risk of future attachment loss, which may lead to tooth loss. Typically, deep pocketing relates to localized radiographic bone loss.
  - ○ Sites with probing depths greater than 5 mm are more likely to contain disease-causing bacteria. Complete calculus removal without surgery is also unlikely for these pockets.
  - ○ A complete probing depth chart showing at least 4 to 5-mm pocketing is required for dental insurance reimbursement of periodontal procedures.

Bleeding on Probing

- Method:
  - ○ Note the appearance of blood from the sulcus while probing.
  - ○ Use a consistent definition of gingival bleeding (i.e., profuse gingival bleeding upon touch).
  - ○ For efficiency, record together with pocketing (i.e., bleeding-5–2–3).
  - ○ On paper charts, bleeding is often recorded as a dot above the probing depth number associated with the site where bleeding occurred.
- Significance:
  - ○ Bleeding on probing occurs typically with deep probing depth or visible inflammation.
  - ○ Bleeding on probing signifies active disease, and a 30% chance of attachment loss within the next year if bleeding encircles the tooth. Contrary, the absence of bleeding indicates a 98% chance that there will not be attachment loss in the near future.

Clinical Attachment Level

- *Method*: There are two methods, depending if there is gingival recession present (see ▶ Fig. 2.6, ▶ Video 2.6).
  - ○ *No recession*: Identify cementoenamel junction (CEJ) by running a periodontal probe apically toward the site with the deepest pocket. Find the location where the smooth enamel ends, and the rougher dentin begins. Note the position of the gingiva on the periodontal probe, and determine how much further the probe needs to be inserted to reach the rubbery sulcus floor. This difference is the clinical attachment level (CAL).
  - ○ *Recession*: Identify the CEJ as the junction between white enamel and darker, more yellow-white dentin. Measure the distance from there to the base of the sulcus with a periodontal probe.
- When is it necessary to determine CALs?
  - ○ *Rarely in general practice*: Attachment loss is usually inferred from radiographic bone loss.
  - ○ CALs are usually measured for periodontal research using a stent with grooves that define insertion angle.
  - ○ Attachment levels measurements may be useful for monitoring recession defects.
- Special circumstances:
  - ○ If the CEJ is not detectable, a "relative attachment level" can be measured as distance from the sulcus to another landmark (i.e., restorative margin, cusp tip, or the edge of a stent).
- Significance:
  - ○ CAL equals attachment loss since tooth eruption.
  - ○ Presence of clinical attachment loss is used by periodontal disease classification systems to distinguish between "gingivitis" and "periodontitis."
  - ○ Risk of tooth loss increases sharply after about 8 mm of attachment loss.

Gingival Recession

- *Method*: Gingival recession is only recorded in areas of exposed root surfaces (see ▶ Fig. 2.7, ▶ Video 2.7).
  - ○ Measure distance from exposed CEJ to gingival margin in apical direction.
  - ○ If the CEJ is obliterated by abfraction or restoration, use the restorative or abfraction margin as a landmark to measure recession instead.
- *Special circumstance*: A deep facial/lingual extent of enamel can mimic gingival recession.

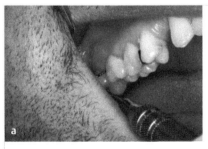
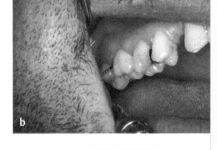
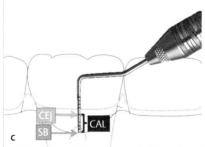
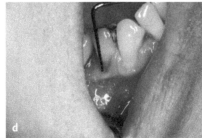

Fig. 2.6 Determining the CAL or attachment loss. (a) Feel with the tip of the periodontal probe for the CEJ, and note the position of the probe. (b) Slide the probe more apical along the root surface until the tip encounters the sulcus base (SB). Note how much further the probe slides into the pocket from the CEJ; this is the CAL or attachment loss since tooth eruption. As with probing depth, the CAL is always rounded up to the next higher millimeter. (c) The CAL is measured from the CEJ to the sulcus base. (d) If the CEJ is exposed through gingival recession, the CAL is easily measured from the CEJ to the base of the pocket, as seen here: probing depth is 2 mm as measured with a UNC-15 probe, recession is 2 mm and the CAL is at 4 mm.

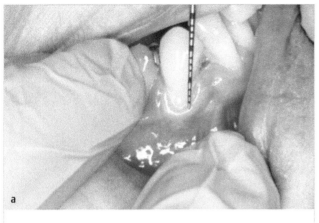

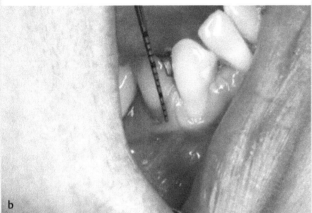

Fig. 2.7 Measuring gingival recession. (**a**) Often, there is gingival recession at the canines, and the CEJ is no longer readily identifiable because of abrasion or a cervical restoration. For recording and monitoring purposes, decide on a readily identifiable landmark such as the apical margin of the restoration, and measure recession as distance from this landmark to the gingival margin. In these cases, the true amount of recession can only be estimated by picturing the original CEJ based on the anatomy of the tooth. (**b**) Gingival recession is readily measured if the CEJ is readily identifiable through the contrast of dark root and bright enamel. Here, recession is the distance between CEJ and gingival margin, rounded up to the next higher millimeter.

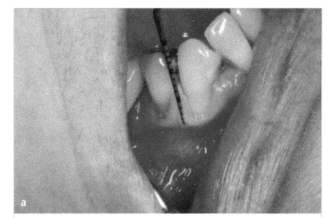

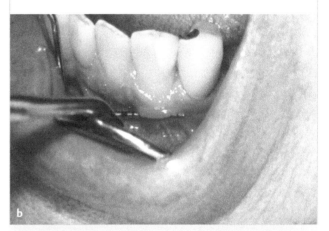

Fig. 2.8 Determining the position of the mucogingival junction and measuring the amount of MGJ in all sites except the lingual surfaces of maxillary teeth. (**a**) Often, the mucogingival junction is clearly visible as a color change from pink to dark pink. The amount of MGJ is simply the distance between the gingival margin and the mucogingival junction, rounded up to the next highest millimeter. (**b**) If the mucogingival junction is not visible, the roll test can identify it. Here, a blunt instrument is placed on the mucosa, and the mucosa is gently pushed toward the teeth. The tissue will bunch up, and the line where the tissue stops folding is the position of the mucogingival junction.

- Significance:
  - On facial and lingual surfaces, the sum of recession and probing depth should equal CAL, since measurement vectors line up parallel to each other.
  - Recession is a consequence of attachment loss, but may not always be caused by periodontitis.
  - Gingival recession predicts a risk of future attachment loss and poses a risk for root caries.
  - Gingival enlargement can be measured similarly. In this case, feel for the CEJ and determine how deep it is below the gingival margin. In periodontal health, the CEJ is located 1 to 3 mm apical to the gingival margin.

Areas of Inadequate Gingiva/Keratinized Gingiva Width/Attached Gingiva

- *Method (▸Fig. 2.8, ▸Video 2.8)*: This is only recorded if an area of inadequate gingiva width is identified.
  - The mucogingival junction is identified either through visual inspection (where the pink gingiva meets the darker colored mucosa) or the roll test (the point where

mucosa stops moving if mobilized with either finger pressure or the side of a periodontal probe). For research purposes, the mucogingival junction can also be identified with Schiller's iodine, which darkly stains mucosa.
  - The amount of keratinized gingiva width (MGJ) is the distance between gingival margin and mucogingival junction. The amount of attached gingiva is the difference between the local MGJ and the local probing depth.
- Significance:
  - While not required, presence of at least 2 mm of attached gingiva leads to better gingival health and esthetics around teeth with subgingival restorations.
  - Presence of at least 2-mm MGJ around implants favors gingival health and good esthetics around implant-supported restorations.

Areas of Furcation Involvement

- Method (▸Fig. 2.9, ▸Video 2.9):
  - A curved Nabers probe is used to gently probe the furcation area of a tooth, and determine how far it can be inserted with gentle pressure and light rotation.

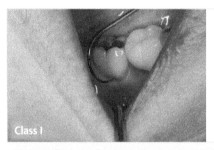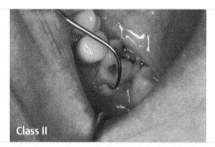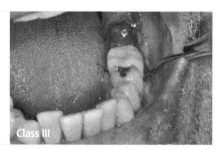

Fig. 2.9 Glickman furcation Classes I, II, and III.

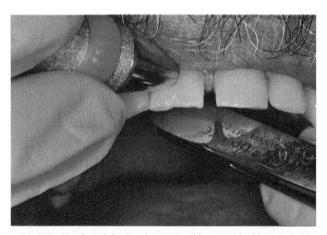

Fig. 2.10 Tooth mobility can be assessed by using the blunt ends of two instruments to check if a tooth visibly moves compared to the surrounding teeth.

○ *Any tooth with multiple roots should have all furcation entrances assessed.* Maxillary molars (buccal, distolingual, and mesiolingual); mandibular molars (buccal and lingual); and maxillary premolars (mesial and distal).
○ Among various classification systems, the Glickman furcation classification is most commonly used (see ▶ Fig. 2.9).
  – *Class I*: The furcation entrance can be felt, but there is no horizontal component.
  – *Class II*: The probe slides into the furcation area with a horizontal component. If the probe is tugged back, it will "hook" under the tooth in contrast to a Class I.
  – *Class III*: The furcation area connects under the tooth to another furcation entrance, forming a tunnel. Most likely, there will be at least two furcation entrances where the probe slides more than halfway under the crown of the tooth.
  – *Class IV*: There is a clearly visible, exposed furcation tunnel.
• Special circumstance:
  ○ On paper charts, the typical notation for furcation involvement is to draw a wedge next to the odontogram tooth symbol at the affected furcation area for Class I, a stroked triangle for Class II, and a filled triangle for Class III.
• Significance:
  ○ Teeth with exposed furcation entrances are difficult to clean and maintain, and therefore have a poorer prognosis than teeth without furcation involvement.
  ○ Deep Class II furcation involvement triples the chance of tooth loss, and Class III furcation involvement leads to the 7-fold increased chance of future tooth loss.[14]

Tooth Mobility

• Method (▶ Fig. 2.10, ▶ Video 2.10):
  ○ One tooth at a time is held on buccal and lingual surface with the tip of a blunt instrument (i.e., mirror handle), and an attempt is made to move the tooth buccolingually. Tooth movement is observed against the neighboring tooth cusps, and felt with the instrument handles. If mobile, an attempt is made to rotate the tooth and depress it into the socket while avoiding lateral movement.
  ○ Miller grade tooth mobility classification scheme is the most widely used.
    – *Grade I*: Any slight observable movement.
    – *Grade II*: Significant horizontal movement up to 1 mm from the resting position.
    – *Grade III*: Tooth movement greater than 1 mm from resting position, or ability to rotate or depress tooth into socket.
• Special circumstances:
  ○ Mandibular incisors display minor tooth mobility in most patients.
  ○ Loose crowns and fixed partial dentures can be loose even if the supporting tooth is not.
  ○ Dental implant-supported restorations that display any mobility have failed.
• Significance:
  ○ Tooth mobility predicts future attachment loss and tooth loss.
  ○ Teeth with mobility are poor candidates for indirect restorations and should never be used as abutments for removable partial dentures.
  ○ Generally, teeth displaying grade III mobility are removed at the onset of treatment.
  ○ Severe tooth mobility is usually caused by the loss of bone support from severe periodontal disease or traumatic injury. Occlusal trauma, short/resorbed roots, periodontal/periapical inflammation, and orthodontic therapy usually cause minor to moderate tooth mobility.

Plaque Level

• Method:
  ○ Plaque disclosing should never be done prior to oral cancer screening and clinical photographs.
  ○ Visual assessment of teeth either by air drying teeth and looking for off-white, rough plaque, or after disclosing plaque with indicator solutions (see ▶ Fig. 2.11a,b, ▶ Video 2.11).
  ○ For periodontal disease, only plaque at the gingival margins and in pockets is relevant.
  ○ Many plaque scoring methods exist such as Greene-Vermillion simplified oral hygiene index, Quigley-Hein

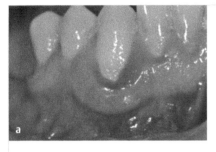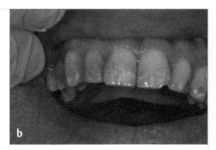
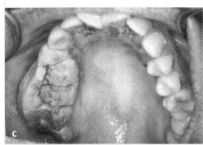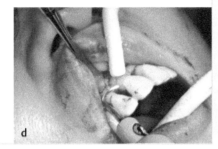

Fig. 2.11 Plaque and calculus. (a) If plaque is heavy, it presents as readily visible granular, white to yellow deposits on root tooth surfaces that does not rinse off with water spray and usually is associated with an adjacent erythematous, swollen gingival margin. (b) Plaque disclosing solutions can readily highlight more subtle plaque accumulation. For periodontal diagnostic purposes, only plaque near the gingival margin is considered an etiologic agent of periodontal diseases. (c) Off-white relatively soft supragingival calculus can be found sometimes in large amounts. (d) Subgingival calculus is often much smaller in volume (as seen here, exposed during periodontal surgery near the tip of a curette), more difficult to detect, and is often black to green in color forming dense, hard clumps on a root surface.

as modified by Turesky, Gilmore & Glickman, and the various modifications of the Navy Plaque Index.
- Significance:
  - Plaque is a clinical sign of bacterial colonization.
  - Plaque levels correlate well with bleeding on probing, but are not predictive for future attachment loss.
  - Consistently low plaque levels correlate with long-term restorative success.

Calculus Level

- Method:
  - Clinically observe off-white to yellow hard supragingival calculus, most likely at tooth surfaces opposing salivary duct openings. Brown-black or dark-green calculus is formed subgingivally (see ▶ Fig. 2.11c,d, ▶ Video 2.12).
  - Feel for roughness, ledges, and clicks on a root surface with the sides of the tip of a fine calculus explorer. This can also be done with a periodontal probe with lower accuracy.
  - Very large pieces of calculus will present as pointed root surface irregularities interproximally on radiographs (see ▶ Fig. 2.12, ▶ Fig. 2.13). Solid masses of facial or lingual calculus will appear as irregular radiopaque material overlaying root surfaces near the CEJ.
- Significance:
  - Root surfaces contaminated with calculus feel very rough, producing clicks when the probe is dragged across the calculus piece. Endotoxin-contaminated root surfaces feel slightly sticky, or have a gritty texture similar to sandpaper. Clean surfaces feel glassy smooth or have a satin-like texture.
  - Periodontal therapy aims to completely remove calculus and contaminated cementum from all root surfaces.
  - Clinical licensing exams usually require a certain number of calculus pieces to be present for an acceptable exam patient, and a passing involves removing all calculus to smooth surface.

2.5 Using Radiographic Imaging and Adjunctive Tests

Radiographic findings should correlate with clinical findings and uncover hidden hard tissue conditions that may have been missed during the clinical exam. Adjunctive tests are useful for the diagnosis of unusual periodontal disease or periodontal disease unresponsive to previous treatment.

2.5.1 Radiographic Assessment

A thorough radiographic evaluation is essential to a comprehensive periodontal exam as it provides information on the supporting bone and periodontal ligament (see ▶ Video 2.13). For patients with periodontal health or mild periodontal disease, bitewing radiographs that clearly show interproximal bone level are sufficient as long as radiographs clearly show interproximal bone levels. For patients who show signs of significant attachment loss or gingival recession, periapical radiographs should clearly show the entire root and surrounding bone of periodontally involved teeth. Radiographs should be viewed in a quiet viewing area with low ambient light and a good quality monitor (or viewbox for conventional radiographs). New radiographs should always be evaluated for signs of oral pathology prior to focusing on teeth. For periodontal assessment, the following factors should be evaluated.

Alveolar Crest Contour

- *Method*: Evaluate the alveolar crest found interproximally between teeth. On panoramic radiographs and bitewing radiographs, crestal bone should be parallel to the CEJ and occlusal table.
- *Significance*: Deviations indicate enhanced periodontal disease that was modified by unique local contributing factors.

Horizontal Bone Loss

- *Method*: Evaluate the distance between the CEJ of teeth and crestal bone (see ▶ Fig. 2.12a).
- *Special circumstance*: Patients with thick biotype may have appearance of mild bone loss in the absence of clinical signs of past or current periodontal disease.
- *Significance*:
  - If distance is less than 2 mm, there likely is no bone or attachment loss.
  - Radiographic bone loss may underestimate attachment loss as attachment loss precedes alveolar bone loss by about 6–8 months.

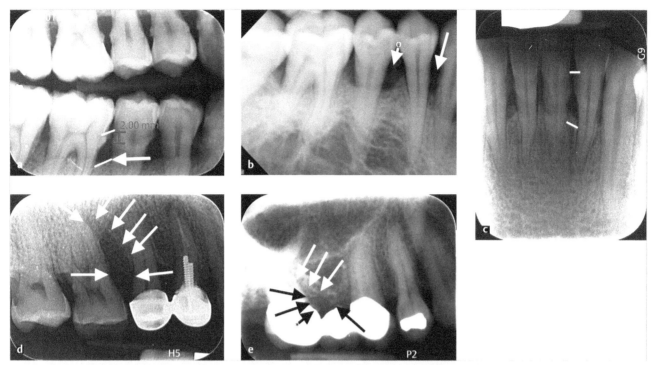

Fig. 2.12 Bone defects caused by periodontal disease as seen on radiographs. (**a**) Horizontal bone loss mesial to tooth no. 30 and around the premolars. To identify horizontal bone loss, visualize the CEJ of each tooth and connect them (*top white line*). Compare this with the crestal bone level (*bottom white line*), which should be parallel to it. If the distance between the CEJ and bone is greater than 2.0 mm (*red bar*), there is bone loss. Also, note the radiographic appearance of heavy calculus (*next to red bar*). (**b**) Accentuated bone loss, or a "0-wall defect" (*single white arrow*), and a circumferential bone defect encircling a premolar (*white arrow* marked with "O"). (**c**) Shallow 1-wall defect. Note that line connecting CEJs and bone level are not parallel. (**d**) Likely a deep 2-wall defect: Note the deep J-shaped interproximal wall of the bone defect(*white arrows*), and *one* faint, flat outline of the remaining crestal bone (*black arrows*). (**e**) Likely a moderate-deep 3-wall defect: Note the ramp-like interproximal wall of the defect (*white arrows*), and the presence of *two* faint outlines of buccal and lingual walls of the defect converging (*black arrows*) at the tip of the interproximal wall. Also note the radiographic calculus (*arrow with star*) at the opening of the bone defect.

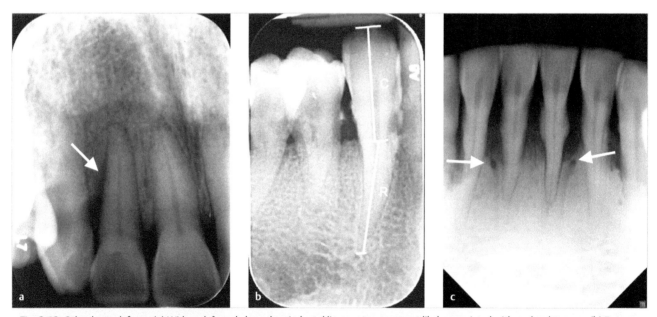

Fig. 2.13 Other bone defects. (**a**) Widened, funnel-shaped periodontal ligament space, most likely associated with occlusal trauma. (**b**) Determining crown-to-root ratio. The amount of root structure "R" within the bone should be more than the amount of tooth structure "C" outside of bone. (**c**) Nutrient canals (*white arrows*) associated with severe inflammation. Note the heavy radiographic calculus around the roots.

Vertical Bone Loss

- *Method*: Adjust brightness and contrast to evaluate edges of wedge-shaped bone interproximal radiolucencies at the alveolar crest. The floor and mesial/distal wall have the highest radiopacity, followed by buccal and lingual walls. The number of walls names the defect type (0, 1, 2, and 3 wall defects). A crater is a 2-wall defect consisting of a buccal and lingual wall, and will clinically appear as two radiographic ridge crests with an associated deep pocket on both adjacent tooth surfaces. Along with walls, note depth and width of each defect (see ▶ Fig. 2.12).
- *Special circumstance*: Occlusal trauma and unusual root anatomy can produce narrow bone defects.
- *Significance*:
  ○ Vertical bone defects indicate local factor(s) exacerbating periodontal disease.
  ○ The higher the number of walls, and the deeper the defect, the more likely regenerative therapy will have beneficial effects.

Bone Quality

- *Method*: Subjectively judge radiopacity compared to tooth enamel, density of trabeculation, and thickness of crestal bone.
- *Significance*: Dark radiolucent bone with few trabecula is a soft bone prone to rapid bone loss. Bone density in mandible correlates well with overall bone density in patient.

Periodontal Ligament/Lamina Dura

- *Method*: Observe the darker radiolucent area between lamina dura. It should be very thin and uniform around all teeth.
- *Significance*:
  ○ Widened or funnel-shaped space usually indicates occlusal trauma in adults (see ▶ Fig. 2.13a).
  ○ Orthodontic treatment usually produces widened periodontal ligament.
  ○ Systemic sclerosis can produce generalized ligament widening, and squamous cell carcinoma can produce isolated widening of periodontal ligament.

Crown-to-Root Ratio

- *Method*: Determine ratio of the tooth length outside of bone, and the tooth length from the apex to the most coronal alveolar crest level (see ▶ Fig. 2.13b).
- *Special circumstance*: Crown-to-"root" ratio does not apply to dental implants.
- *Significance*: Teeth with a crown-to-root ratio worse than 1:1 are poor candidates for bridge and denture abutments.

Root Quality/Anatomy

- *Method*: Subjectively evaluate tooth roots. Check the teeth for any unusual root anatomy, such as dilacerations, twinning, dens invaginatus, taurodontia, microdontia, and any cemental, dentinal, or enamel hyper/hypoplasia, and judge if these have been exposed or exacerbated by periodontal disease.
- *Significance*:
  ○ Teeth with short, single, and conical roots are more likely to display tooth mobility.
  ○ Teeth with thin, ribbon-shaped roots are likely to break during tooth removal.
  ○ Multirooted teeth with pronounced root trunks, long roots, and curved roots require near complete bone loss for the onset of tooth mobility.

Nutrient Canals

- *Method*: Look for small round radiolucent "holes" near the crestal bone, which connect to a faint darker linear feature in the bone (see ▶ Fig. 2.13c).
- *Significance*: Nutrient canals are blood vessels that typically feed into heavily inflamed tissues, but may also be a variant of normal anatomy. If associated with heavily inflamed tissues, scaling and root planing may elicit more than unusual bleeding. During surgery, nutrient canals can cause heavier bleeding when the overlying tissue is removed, and it is useful to anticipate this prior to surgery.

Local Factors Influencing Periodontal Disease

- *Method*: Check each tooth for signs (see ▶ Fig. 2.14, for example).
  ○ *Residual calculus*: Wedge-shaped or thorn-shaped root surface projection
  ○ *Furcation involvement*: Darkening of the interradicular bone in the furcation area for furcations oriented buccally and lingually. A darkened radiographic "furcation arrow" as this is called likely indicates a class II or class III furcation involvement, and usually appears sometime after clinical detection of furcation involvement.
  ○ *Root concavities*: Most commonly are seen interproximally with a doubled lamina dura line in the area of the root concavity showing buccal and lingual edges.
  ○ Enamel pearls are round projections found typically on maxillary second and first molar with a radiodense cap that is similar to enamel.
  ○ Cervical enamel projections may appear as tiny radiodense triangle on mandibular molars with the apex pointing at the furcation, and may be associated with a U-shaped area of associated bone loss on the facial or lingual side of a tooth.
  ○ Crowding/tipping of teeth.
  ○ *Caries*: Primary interproximal caries will produce triangle-shaped radiolucencies pointed toward the pulp chamber and centered between contact point and CEJs. Buccal or lingual Class V lesions often produce ovoid subtle radiolucencies near the neck of the tooth, and occlusal caries sometimes produces subtle radiolucencies at the dentin-enamel junction underneath the occlusal table.
  ○ *Overhangs*: Very radiodense restorative material protruding from a tooth surface.
  ○ *Rough margins*: Sometimes seen on radiographs as irregularly shaped tooth surface.
  ○ *Open margins*: There is a radiographic gap or dark space between restoration margin and tooth.
  ○ Bulky crown contours.
  ○ *Root fractures*: May be seen as dark line that either runs horizontally across a tooth surface or vertically. Horizontal root fractures may be inconsequential for tooth longevity if they are closer to the root apex and if there is no widened area of radiolucency around it. Vertical root fractures usually become infected and produce large areas of radiolucency and clinical bone loss.

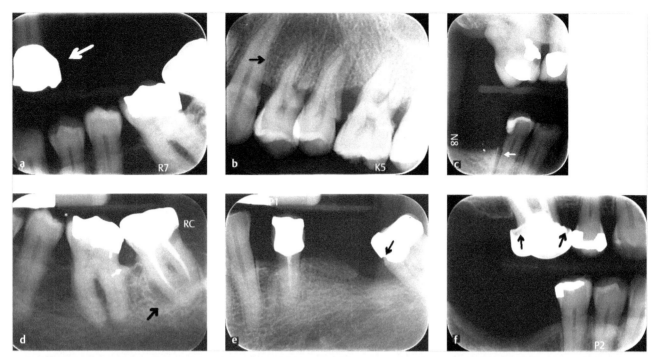

Fig. 2.14 Various local factors that contribute to periodontal disease. (**a**) Bulky restorations such as extracoronal retention grooves for partial denture attachment (*arrow*) are difficult to clean and lead to gingival inflammation. (**b**) A flat, slightly concave distal root surface of the canine (*black arrow*), heavy radiographic calculus (wedge-shaped areas as shown next to *white arrow*), and multiple furcation involvement (premolars and molars) associated with more severe bone loss. (**c**) Cemental tear (*white arrow*) and irregular shaped molar roots. (**d**) Diastema associated with minor defect (*white asterisk*), dentin ridges on the molars (*white arrow*), recurrent caries under a steel crown (RC) and a periapical lesion associated with failed root canals (*black arrow*). (**e**) Open margin (*black arrow*) and (**f**) overhanging margins of a steel crown associated with enhanced bone loss. A periapical radiograph shows severe bone loss associated with this tooth.

○ *Cemental tears*: Occasionally seen radiographically as a thin sliver of root surface that has become separated from the main body of the tooth.
○ *Biologic width invasion*: Suggested by radiographs that show restorative material close to the alveolar crest (<2 mm). Clinically, the same area shows persistent signs of inflammation despite low plaque levels.
○ *Endodontic infections*: Small area of widened periodontal ligament at the apex, round periapical radiolucency centered on the apical foramen of a tooth, or as wide diffuse area of bone loss surrounding the entire tooth root. Any of these radiographic findings should correlate with pulp vitality tests that show pulpal necrosis for the affected tooth. If the tooth is vital, oral pathology should be suspected.
○ *Occlusal discrepancy*: Seen as steps in the occlusal plane, or as different levels of the marginal ridges
○ Plunger cusps are protruding cusps that point past the occlusal plane at an interproximal contact that is usually weak.
○ *Dental implants*: Very radiopaque, usually screw-shaped objects embedded in bone-supporting dental restorations. A fine line between implant body and restoration indicates the implant platform. The following factors are worth noting:
  – *Bone adjacent to implant*: Radiopaque bone should be in immediate contact with the implant body. Radiolucency around the implant body indicates the lack of bony integration and a failed implant.
  – *Bone level adjacent to implant platform*: Minor bone loss (<2 mm) from platform is common and normal around implants. Larger amount of bone loss suggests peri-implantitis.

  – *Implant platform relative to the CEJ of surrounding teeth*: If distance is excessive (>5 mm), it may be associated with deep probing depth.
  – *Position relative to adjacent teeth/implants*: Close placement (<3 mm between implants, <1.5 mm between teeth) may be associated with interproximal bone loss and gingival recession.
  – *Angulation relative to adjacent teeth*: Excessive angulation (>30 degrees) may be associated with enhanced bone loss.
• *Significance*: Local factors often explain locally exacerbated periodontal disease in form of significant bleeding on probing, deep probing depths, attachment loss, recession, or enhanced bone loss.

2.5.2 Microbial, Genetic Testing, and Other Tests for Unusual Periodontal Disease

While a clinical and radiographic evaluation is sufficient for diagnosing and treatment planning common periodontal diseases, there will be situations where additional tests may be needed.

Microbial Testing

For patients with unusually severe periodontal disease at a young age and absent significant genetic or medical conditions, microbial testing may be useful in detecting unusually aggressive microorganisms. Microbial testing may also be useful in patients where previous attempts of competent periodontal therapy failed to control periodontal disease, and it may be useful for patient education as a type of risk assessment tool. For patient educational purposes, microbial testing has a long history, where the goal is to educate and motivate the patient in controlling the microbial flora in their mouth. This was part of the historical Keyes technique, where a dark field microscope was used to demonstrate live oral microbial flora to patients and spur them into compliance using a specific oral hygiene technique in an attempt to eliminate periodontal infection.

The same educational approach applies when using a DNA test that involves sending a sample to a commercial genetic laboratory (MyPerioPath, OralDNA Labs, Eden Prarie, and Minnesota) to identify the presence or absence of a collection known periodontal pathogens. This can also be done using a chair-side immunological (Evalusite, Eastman Kodak Company, Rochester, New York), biochemical (Perioscan, Sirona, Charlotte, North Carolina), or genetic test (Omnigene DMDx, Omnigene, Inc., Cambridge, Massachusetts; IAI Pado Test 4.5, IAI, Zuchwil, Switzerland) (reviewed in[15]). The disadvantage of any of these tests is that they cannot provide you information about antibiotic susceptibility, which can only be done by culturing the bacteria in the patient sample.

Unfortunately, very few laboratories (only one currently in the United States – Oral Microbiology Testing Services Laboratory at Temple University, Philadelphia, Pennsylvania) offer this service due to the high cost and low profitability of these services. With antibiotic sensitivity testing, it is possible to prescribe antibiotics that may be effective in stopping an aggressive periodontal infection, and repeat testing can confirm the effectiveness of therapy.

For most microbial testing, the greatest problem is sample error, where it is possible that significant microbes are missed out by not sampling the correct area. With culture methods, another problem is that periodontal pathogens are generally sensitive to air and heat, and errors in handling and shipping the sample may kill periodontal pathogens, resulting in an erroneous lab result. For this reason, it is important to follow the instructions for each testing kit carefully, and interpret any obtained results critically. Clinically, the value of test results is rather limited except for the selection of antibiotics and recall interval determination as periodontal treatment methods are not tailored yet to specific microbes and disease-causing microbial genes.

Genetic Testing

While there is a strong genetic component to periodontal disease as suggested by the Minnesota twin study, a genetic predilection for periodontal disease is likely caused by the interplay of many genetic factors. It appears that promoter mutations that lead to the enhanced production of inflammatory messenger molecules including the generally proinflammatory cytokines Interleukin (IL)-1 alpha/beta and IL-6 play a large role in determining whether a patient has a predilection for developing earlier and more aggressive forms of periodontal disease. The most researched genetic factor is the IL-1 beta polymorphism that is associated with a higher risk of developing periodontal disease, where carrying the IL-1 alpha or IL-1 beta polymorphisms increases the odds of periodontitis by about 1.5-fold.[16] In smokers, this polymorphism becomes quite relevant as the odds of periodontitis increase up to 5-fold compared to IL-1 genotype negative nonsmokers, or double the odds compared to IL-1 genotype negative smokers. Carrying the IL-6 polymorphism seems to increase the odds of periodontitis about 1.4-fold in Caucasian and Brazilians populations. The only

commercially available test in the United States that tests polymorphisms is the MyPerioID PST test (Oral DNALabs, Eden Prairie, Minnesota) that tests IL-1 and IL-6 polymorphisms and provides a periodontal risk assessment for patients. While useful for risk assessment and patient education, its clinical value is somewhat compromised as the effect of these polymorphisms on periodontal disease varies between ethnic and geographic groups, and not enough data exists yet for most non-Caucasian groups to assess its usefulness. It also has little effect on treatment planning at this time other than shortening recall intervals since there current periodontal therapy does not contain instruments to redress cytokine expression levels.

Other Tests

Complete periodontal diagnosis may also require other tests such as cone beam CT imagery, pulp vitality tests, and occlusal tests. For example, the diagnosis of endodontic conditions usually requires palpating the tooth and percussing the tooth to check for periapical conditions, and various pulp vitality tests using cold, hot, or electric stimuli. Cone beam CT imagery is often indispensable for implant therapy, and can provide clues on intractable tooth pain and subtle bone conditions. While occlusion should be routinely evaluated during periodic and initial exams, more detailed occlusal assessment using jaw record and mounted models in adjustable articulators may be needed to fully address occlusal issues. Behavioral and psychologic assessment may be needed to investigate destructive oral habits that influence periodontal disease activity, while thorough medical evaluation may be needed for patients with questionable medical health.

2.6 Creating a Problem List for Diagnosis and Treatment Planning

2.6.1 Preparing Information for Disease Identification

For risk assessment and insurance reimbursement, fitting a patient's periodontal condition in the currently recognized periodontal disease classification system is important. One approach to this task is to think where a patient's periodontal conditions falls within the following six dimensions (▶ Table 2.5):
- Severity of inflammation.
- Depth of inflammation.
- Extent of inflammation.
- Local factors contributing to periodontal disease.
- Microbial factors contributing to periodontal disease (if known).
- Systemic factors contributing to periodontal disease.

The patient's periodontal condition then can be matched to the best fitting disease or condition category recognized in the most current periodontal disease classification system (▶ Table 2.5).

2.6.2 Developing a Problem List for Risk Assessment

Besides gathering information needed for periodontal diagnosis, the purpose of periodontal assessment is to create a list of problems that periodontal treatment needs to address. Generally, these problems will fall into three categories:
- Problems that pose a risk during treatment, which require treatment modification.

Table 2.5 Information to consider for periodontal diagnosis

Severity of inflammation	None Erythema Gingival bleeding Tissue sloughing/ulceration Tissue necrosis
Depth of inflammation	None Limited to gingiva/connective tissue Involving alveolar bone crest (bone loss/attachment loss) Deep tissue destruction Destruction extends to orofacial tissues
Extent of inflammation	Number of sites/teeth involved If isolated, list teeth _____
Microbial factors	Plaque (near gingival margin: none, isolated, thin band, heavy) Specific microbes identified _____
Systemic factors	List factors:
Local factors	List factors by tooth:

- Problems that enhance periodontal disease, which need to be eliminated for disease control.

The first problem list identifies potential treatment risks that allows safe management of a patient's conditions, which in turn reduces the risk of medical emergencies and professional liabilities. It also serves as a tool to drive consultations with other medical providers (▶Table 2.6).

2.6.3 Developing a Problem List for Treatment Planning

The second problem list is most important for treatment planning as this list contains the factors that influence periodontal disease development. If treatment can address and remove all these factors, periodontal health most likely can be restored. This list of factors can also be used as a blueprint for the prevention of periodontal disease since ensuring the absence of these factors prevents development of periodontal disease. Typically, these factors are either systemic (▶Table 2.7a) or local (▶Table 2.7b) in nature.

The management of systemic factors almost always involves collaboration with physicians and other health care providers, and treatment, if any, will need to take place outside of a dental office. The exception to this is tobacco counseling for tobacco use, which can be done within a dental setting. While possible to perform in a dental setting, nutrition and lifestyle counseling for obesity treatment should be referred to qualified providers such as registered dietitians.

Unlike systemic factors, local factors can be usually addressed with dental treatment, and in general, each local factor corresponds to specific dental procedures that address each problem.

2.7 Essential Takeaways

- A thorough patient evaluation is required for proper diagnosis and treatment planning. A comprehensive exam

Table 2.6 Factors posing a treatment risk or require special patient management considerations

Adrenal insufficiency	GERD
Anemia	Hepatitis
Angina	HIV w/ low CD4+ count
Anticoagulant therapy	Hypertension
Antidepressants (tricyclics, monoamine oxidase [MAO] inhibitors)	Immunosuppressive agents
Antiplatelet agents	Implanted medical devices
Artificial/prosthetic heart valves	Leukemia/lymphoma
Asthma—severe	Myocardial infarct history
Atherosclerosis	NSAID use
Beta blockers	Organ transplant history
Bisphosphonates	Pacemaker
Bleeding disorders (i.e., hemophila, von Willebrand)	Pregnancy
Calcium supplements	Previous infective bacterial endocarditis
Cancer/chemotherapy/radiation therapy	Prostrate enlargement
Cardiac dysrhythmia	Psychiatric conditions w/functional impairment
Congestive heart failure	Sickle cell anemia
COPD/emphysema	Stroke history
Corticosteroid use	Supplements (garlic, gingko, ginger, fish oil, vitamin E)
Damaged heart valves	Thyroid disorders
Dementia/Alzheimer w/ functional impairment	Thyroid hormone replacement
Diabetes mellitus	Tobacco use
Digoxin	Total joint replacement
Epilepsy	Tuberculosis
	Unrealistic patient expectations

consists of review of medical and dental histories, review of systems, extraoral and intraoral exams, periodontal measurements, and a radiographic survey.
- Pain relief is highest priority; acute infection is next in treatment. A medical and dental history review will reveal risk factors or complications to planned treatment (i.e., is prophylactic antibiotics required?).
- Periodontal considerations involve the general appearance of the gingiva and any mucosal anomalies. Indices include probing depths, BOP, CAL, recession, furcation involvements, tooth mobility, plaque, and calculus levels. The occlusion needs to be examined and evaluated.
- Radiographs should correlate with and corroborate to clinical findings. Vertical bitewings are preferable to conventional horizontal bitewings for enhanced viewing.
- Microbial and genetic testing are limited but may be of value in patients with unusual or intractable disease.
- Periodontal disease can be categorized by noting the severity, the depth, and the extent of inflammation. Consider microbial, systemic, and local factors as well.

Table 2.7 (a) Systemic factors that influence periodontal disease development

Specific factor	Factor	Category
Amphetamines	Medication associated with gingival overgrowth (GO Meds)	Systemic factors
Calcium channel blockers		
Cyclosporine, tacrolimus, and sirolimus		
Dilantin/phenytoin		
Phenobarbital		
Valproic acid		
Anti-HIV medications (some) and gray discoloration	Medications associated with gingival discoloration (GD Meds)	
Minocycline and gray gingival discoloration		
Estrogen replacement	Estrogen replacement	
Xerostomic medications and actual xerostomia	Xerostomia-inducing medication	
Medication known to cause lichenoid reaction and actual lichenoid lesions	Lichenoid reaction-inducing medication	
AIDS	Immunosuppression	
Leukemia/lymphoma		
Chemotherapy		
Radiation therapy and oral mucositis	Radiation-induced mucositis	
Cancer (including oral cancer)	Cancer	
Pregnancy and hormonal changes	Hormonal changes	
Sexually transmitted disease and oral ulcers/growths	STDs	
Stroke and decreased manual dexterity	Manual dexterity issues	
Dementia/Alzheimer and decreased manual dexterity		
Rh./osteoarthritis and decreased manual dexterity		
Decreased manual dexterity		
Rheumatoid arthritis	Rheumatoid arthritis	
Diabetes mellitus	Diabetes mellitus	
Obesity	Obesity	
Poor nutrition	Nutrition	
Genetic conditions	Genetic condition	
IL-1 genotype		
Autoimmune diseases	Autoimmune	
Tobacco use	Self-medication	
Recreational drug use		
Alcohol use		

Table 2.7 (b) Local Factors that influence periodontal disease development

Specific factor	Factor	Category
Plaque	Plaque	Microbial factors
Calculus	Calculus	
Specific microbial infection	Microbes	
Caries	Caries	Restorative factor
Endodontic infection	Endodontic infection	
Nonrestorable teeth (i.e., root tips)	Nonrestorable teeth	
Open contact/diastema and food impaction	Defective restoration	
Open margin		
Overhanging restoration		
Rough restorative surface/fractured restoration/coronal fracture		
Bulky/overcontoured restoration		
Subgingival margin and gingival inflammation		
Deep pocketing, gingival inflammation	Deep pocketing, gingival inflammation	Periodontal factor
Furcation involvement and gingival inflammation	Furcation involvement	
Tooth mobility	Tooth mobility	
Recession, other mucogingival defects	Mucogingival defects	
Implant conditions	Implant conditions	
Crowding, orthodontic appliances	Tooth position issues	Anatomic factors
Rotated/tipped teeth		
Severe Angle Class II and Class III		
Excessive overjet/overbite		
Marginal discrepancy/infra/supraerupted teeth		
Enamel ridges, enamel projections	Anatomic abnormalities	
Root surface concavities		
Enamel pearls		
Cervical enamel projections		
Dentin projections, ridges		
Unusual root/tooth anatomy		
Partially impacted 3rd molars (and other teeth)	Impacted teeth	
Cemental tears	Cemental tears	
Occlusal trauma	Occlusal trauma	Occlusion
Bruxism	Parafunctional habits	Parafunction
Clenching		
Nail-biting		
Pipe chewing		
Piercings		
Other parafunctional habits		

2.8 Review Questions

Case description applies to all the following questions:

A 49-year old male presented for a comprehensive dental exam after he obtained medical and dental insurance coverage through his employer, a local trucking company. He does not report any dental concerns, but reports that he has not had dental care for the last 25 years and has not seen a physician for the last 10 years. He is not aware of any health condition or allergies, but says he gets thirsty often in the heat, drinks a lot of milk "to say hydrated and keep bones and teeth healthy." He is planning to get a medical evaluation as well, but his medical appointment is next month, due to the physician's long appointment waitlist. After consenting to the exam, a dental assistant recorded his vital signs as 270 lbs., 5'2", 159/92 mm Hg, and pulse 74/min. He excuses himself after this "to go to the bathroom" since he is nervous about the dental visit. The dental assistant tells you that this is the third bathroom visit of the patient, and is starting to feel annoyed by it.

A month later, the following lab results are available from the patient's physician:
- Fasting glucose: 139 mg/dL (normal < 100).
- HbA1c: 8% (normal < 5).
- Platelet 230,000 (normal 150–300,000) per microliter
- WBC 5000 (normal 4500–10,000) per microliter.
- Hematocrit: 45% (normal 40–45%).
- Creatinine: 1.2 mg/dL (normal 0.6–1.2).
- Prostate specific antigen (PSA): 2 ng/mL (normal < 4).

The clinical presentation (▶Fig. 2.15) and radiographs (▶Fig. 2.16) are shown in these figures.

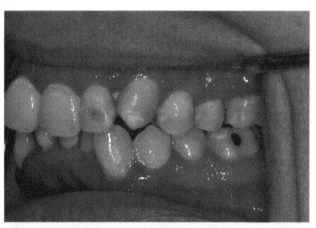

Fig. 2.15 Photograph at initial exam for review case.

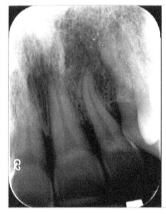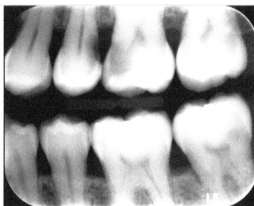

Fig. 2.16 Pertinent radiographs for review case.

Findings in the periodontal chart for the involved quadrant are as follows:

Maxilla facial		9	10	11	12	13	14	15	16
	PD	839	837	827	725	626	648	645	
	BOP	1 1	111	1 1	1		1		
	CAL	6 7	5	5	5		6		
	GR								
	MGJ								
	Furc								
	PLQ	3	3	3	3	3	3	3	
Maxilla lingual	PD	435	535	556	638	725	625	767	
	BOP	111		111	1			1	
	CAL				6	5		5 5	
	GR								
	Furc								
	Mobil		1						
	PLQ	3	3	3	3	3	3	3	

Abbreviations: BOP, bleeding on probing; CAL, clinical attachment level; Furc, furcation involvement; GR, gingival recession; MGJ, mucogingival junction; Mobil, mobility; PD, probing depth; PLQ, plaque (0 = none, 5 = heavy).

Learning objective: Assess the systemic context of a patient's periodontal condition.

1. Based on the patient's dental history and CC, which of the following dental conditions is likely found?
   A. Severe caries
   B. Calculus buildup
   C. Missing teeth
   D. Broken teeth

2. The condition LEAST likely to cause risk to oral and systemic health in this case is
   A. Hypertension
   B. Diabetes mellitus
   C. Obesity
   D. Genitourinary problems

3. Evaluate the following statements.
   Statement 1: Diabetes mellitus and obesity increase the likelihood of the patient having significant periodontal disease.
   Statement 2: The HbA1c level in this case suggests a low periodontal disease risk.
   A. Both statements are true
   B. Both statements are false
   C. The first statement is true, the second is false
   D. The first statement is false, the second is true

Learning objective: Evaluate a patient's clinical periodontal condition for current status and local contributing factors.

4. Evaluate the following statements.
   Statement 1: In this case, teeth nos. 13 and 14 have deep caries.
   Statement 2: Caries may contribute to pocketing seen in this area.
   A. Both statements are true
   B. Both statements are false
   C. The first statement is true, the second is false
   D. The first statement is false, the second is true

5. Regarding the mobile tooth no. 10, which of the following is NOT correct?
   A. The observed tooth mobility was less than 1 mm in one direction
   B. Tooth mobility predicts future attachment loss
   C. Teeth with Miller grade I mobility need to be removed
   D. The observed tooth mobility may be related to poor crown-to-root ratio

6. Evaluate the following statements.
   Statement 1: Periodontal pockets should be measured at the line angles and mid-facial/lingual sulcus.
   Statement 2: When probing, you should apply a light force of about 25 g to avoid excessive patient discomfort.
   A. Both statements are true
   B. Both statements are false
   C. The first statement is true, the second is false
   D. The first statement is false, the second is true

Learning objective: Use radiographic imaging and adjunctive tests to corroborate periodontal findings and uncover contributing factors.

7. In this patient, bone level is best observed on:
   A. Bitewing radiographs
   B. Panoramic radiograph only
   C. Periapical radiographs
   D. Occlusal radiographs

8. Which of the following radiographic signs of periodontal disease is MOST DIRECTLY a sign of a local factor influencing periodontal disease at a particular tooth?
   A. Generalized horizontal bone loss
   B. Isolated vertical bone defect
   C. Crown-to-root ratio
   D. Coarse trabeculation

9. Which of the following commercially available methods is BEST suited to identify an effective antibiotic regimen to treat severe periodontal disease?
   A. Genetic
   B. Microbial culture
   C. Enzymatic test
   D. Antibody-based

Learning objective: Prepare a problem list that leads to an etiology-based treatment plan.

10. At the next dental visit, you measure the patient's glucose just prior to the exam, and obtain a value of 122 mg/dL. The patient's diabetes most likely poses a
    A. Hypoglycemia risk during the visit
    B. Infection risk after the exam
    C. Infection risk after invasive periodontal treatment
    D. Risk of periodontal disease recurrence after treatment

11. Which of the following is NOT a factor contributing to periodontal disease in this quadrant?
    A. Bone loss at no. 10
    B. Recurrent caries no. 14 mesial surface
    C. Clinically visible plaque
    D. Tipping of no. 11

12. Which of the following information is LEAST helpful in identifying this patient's periodontal disease?
    A. Presence of type 2 diabetes mellitus in an older male
    B. Moderate to severe generalized attachment and bone loss
    C. Presence of bleeding on probing, but no ulceration of gingival tissue
    D. Lack of radiographic calculus on all radiographs

2.9 Answers

1. **B.** The patient has not had dental care for decades, but appears to have a diet high in calcium. Typically, this would allow for significant accretions of calculus. The CC does not mention anything about pain or broken teeth, which would be the likely consequence of severe caries. Also, most patients complain about loose teeth since it affects speaking and chewing ability as well as appearance. Since this patient has no dental concerns, this seems unlikely.

2. **D.** While not impossible, genitourinary problems seem least likely compared to diabetes, hypertension, and obesity. We know from the case description that the

patient has Stage I hypertension (systolic pressure 160–140 mm Hg), and that the patient likely has a body mass index greater than 30, which could indicate obesity. Given the likelihood of obesity, and symptoms of diabetes mellitus (thirst and frequent urination), the patient may have undiagnosed type 2 diabetes mellitus.

3. **C.** Diabetes mellitus and obesity significantly increase the risk of more severe and widespread periodontal disease as shown in numerous studies, and there is a well-defined mechanism explaining how diabetes mellitus influences periodontal disease. The HbA1c level measures the percent of glycosylated hemoglobin, which is created when consistently high concentrations of blood glucose undergo a Schiff base reaction with hemoglobin. The higher the level of blood glucose, the higher the level of HbA1c becomes as more glucose is available for the reaction. Typically, the target for diabetics is to bring HbA1c level at or under 7%, and it is somewhat elevated in this case suggesting a mildly increased risk for periodontal disease.

4. **A.** The bitewing radiograph shows deep caries on both teeth as interproximal shadowing originating from the interproximal surface. There also are 5 to 6-mm pockets in the area as bacteria from the carious lesions contribute to periodontal inflammation, and the cavitated surfaces provide a rough area that allows plaque maturation. This favors colonization by late colonizers such as *P. gingivalis,* which can set up a microbial ecosystem that is more likely to cause periodontal destruction, as seen with the accentuated radiographic bone loss seen in the area.

5. **C.** Slightly mobile teeth (Miller grade I) can be retained, especially if occlusal trauma is removed and further bone/attachment loss can be prevented with periodontal therapy. Research shows a small, but significant association of tooth mobility with future attachment loss, as tooth mobility may be associated with current attachment loss. Tooth mobility is caused by either loss of periodontal support or damage to periodontal ligament fibers, and the mobility seen here is likely a product of the thin, short root, and significant bone/attachment loss observed here.

6. **D.** Spot-checking pockets at the line angles and midfacial/lingual surfaces likely will miss periodontal pocketing and disease that begins interproximally. Probing with too much force may be accurate but painful for patients, and it is not necessary to inflict that level of discomfort. The key to probing is not to force the probe into the pocket, but to gently work the probe around pieces of calculus and other constrictions.

7. **A.** Bone level measurements are most accurate on bitewing radiographs as X-ray geometry minimizes distortion. In periapical radiographs, X-rays are not perpendicular to the alveolar crest, creating shadows for the buccal and lingual edge of flat interproximal bone seen in posterior regions, which makes it difficult to assess bone levels. Panoramic radiographs can sometimes produce a good image of the interproximal crestal bone, but are liable to distortion from the imaging process. Crestal bone does not show on occlusal radiographs.

8. **B.** An isolated vertical bone defect is typically caused by a local factor associated with the tooth such as furcation entrances, local tooth anatomy, or occlusal factor.

Generalized bone loss is the consequence of factors that generally affect the entire mouth such as poor oral hygiene and medical conditions. Crown-to-root ratio may be affected by local factors, but it is not known from the question if there is horizontal or vertical bone loss affecting crown-to-root ratio. Coarse trabeculation may be either typical for a patient's normal bone anatomy, or the result of mechanical stress on a given tooth, which is not known here.

9. **B.** The best way to find out antimicrobial resistance is to culture microbes in a laboratory in media containing the various amounts of antimicrobial agents. Although DNA tests in theory could identify antimicrobial resistance genes, this is not done for commercially available microbial tests for the oral cavity. Enzymatic tests could identify some agents of antibiotic resistance such as beta-lactamase, but again these are not done by commercial laboratories. Instead, enzymatic tests usually identify metabolic capacity such as Nα-Benzoyl-DL-Arginine-p-Nitroanilide (BAPNA) and hydrogen peroxide breakdown, and serve along with antibody tests to identify certain groups of bacteria.

10. **D.** The patient has mild type 2 diabetes mellitus with borderline glucose levels. Hypoglycemia seems unlikely as the current and past glucose levels suggest mildly elevated glucose levels, and there is no indication of past hypoglycemia episodes. Given the history, it seems unlikely that the patient's immune system is compromised to the point of infection risk, but it is possible that the diabetes may contribute to the patient's periodontal disease.

11. **A.** Bone loss is a consequence of periodontitis, but not a direct cause. Bone loss may lead to increased recession, which may make it more difficult for a patient to clean and maintain teeth. In contrast, the other factors contribute directly to periodontal disease. The generalized plaque (PLQ-3) seen in the chart, and clinically suggests extensive bacterial colonization of teeth, which may be the root cause of periodontal disease seen in this case. Tipping and caries create niches where plaque is allowed to mature and support periodontal disease causing bacteria.

12. **D.** Absence or presence of calculus is least likely of diagnostic value as classification systems for periodontal disease usually use degree and extent of inflammation and tissue damage as distinguishing factors between diseases. In contrast, the most significant finding for periodontal disease diagnosis is the presence of generalized radiographic bone loss (about 3–4 mm) and CAL at about 5 mm in an older patient with a preexisting systemic condition (type 2 diabetes mellitus) associated with a higher risk of severe periodontal disease. Presence of bleeding on probing suggests active disease, and lack of ulceration rules out various rare forms of periodontal diseases.

2.10 Evidence-based Activities

- Search the internet for photographs of the oral cavity and identify local factors that contribute to periodontal disease.
- Pick a systemic condition and find out if it is associated with periodontal disease using the PubMed or EMBASE databases. Debate in class if the observed association is a risk marker or risk factor.

- Pick a contributing factor and propose a mechanism that leads all the way to clinically observable periodontal disease using scientific studies and reviews found in the PubMed or EMBASE databases.
- Go to the University of Texas Health Science Center School of Dentistry at San Antonio's library of critically appraised topics (CAT) at https://cats.uthscsa.edu/ and search for a review on the link between pregnancy outcomes and periodontal disease treatment. Read any CAT you can find, and debate if the conclusion is still correct based on current literature.
- Create a CAT on the effect of occlusion on periodontal disease (or any other topic for which a CAT is not available) following the outline provided by Sauve S, et al. in "The critically appraised topic: a practical approach to learning critical appraisal" (Ann R Coll Physicians Surg Can. 1995; 28:396–398).

References

[1] Ciancio SG. Medications: a risk factor for periodontal disease diagnosis and treatment. J Periodontol 2005;76(11, Suppl):2061–2065

[2] Becker DE, Reed KL. Local anesthetics: review of pharmacological considerations. Anesth Prog 2012;59(2):90–101, quiz 102–103

[3] Shi Q, Xu J, Zhang T, Zhang B, Liu H. Post-operative bleeding risk in dental surgery for patients on oral anticoagulant therapy: a meta-analysis of observational studies. Front Pharmacol 2017;8:58

[4] Napeñas JJ, Oost FC, DeGroot A, et al. Review of postoperative bleeding risk in dental patients on antiplatelet therapy. Oral Surg Oral Med Oral Pathol Oral Radiol 2013;115(4):491–499

[5] Krimmel M, Ripperger J, Hairass M, Hoefert S, Kluba S, Reinert S. Does dental and oral health influence the development and course of bisphosphonate-related osteonecrosis of the jaws (BRONJ)? Oral Maxillofac Surg 2014;18(2):213–218

[6] Infective Endocarditis. 2016; http://www.heart.org/HEARTORG/Conditions/CongenitalHeartDefects/TheImpactofCongenitalHeartDefects/Infective-Endocarditis_UCM_307108_Article.jsp#.WGrkhtIrJQl. Accessed 1/2/2017, 2017

[7] Sollecito TP, Abt E, Lockhart PB, et al. The use of prophylactic antibiotics prior to dental procedures in patients with prosthetic joints: evidence-based clinical practice guideline for dental practitioners—a report of the American Dental Association Council on Scientific Affairs. J Am Dent Assoc 2015;146(1):11–16.e8

[8] Little JW, Falace DA, Miller CS, Rhodus NL. Dental management of the medically compromised patient. 8 ed. St. Louis, Missouri: Elsevier Mosby; 2013

[9] Regezi J, Sciubba J, Jordan R. Oral pathology: clinical pathologic correlations. 7th ed. St. Louis, Missouri: Saunders; 2017

[10] Sheiham A, Nicolau B. Evaluation of social and psychological factors in periodontal disease. Periodontol 2000. 2005;39:118–131

[11] Albandar JM. Epidemiology and risk factors of periodontal diseases. Dent Clin North Am 2005;49(3):517–532, v–vi

[12] Pihlstrom BL. Periodontal risk assessment, diagnosis and treatment planning. Periodontol 2000. 2001;25:37–58

[13] Harrel SK, Nunn ME. The association of occlusal contacts with the presence of increased periodontal probing depth. J Clin Periodontol 2009;36(12):1035–1042

[14] Salvi GE, Mischler DC, Schmidlin K, et al. Risk factors associated with the longevity of multi-rooted teeth. Long-term outcomes after active and supportive periodontal therapy. J Clin Periodontol 2014;41(7):701–707

[15] Mani A, Anarthe R, Marawar PP, Mustilwar RG, Bhosale A. Diagnostic kits: an aid to periodontal diagnosis. J Dent Res Rev. 2016;3(3):107–113

[16] Karimbux NY, Saraiya VM, Elangovan S, et al. Interleukin-1 gene polymorphisms and chronic periodontitis in adult whites: a systematic review and meta-analysis. J Periodontol 2012;83(11):1407–1419

3 Identifying Periodontal Diseases

Abstract

The next step after periodontal data gathering is periodontal diagnosis, which means identification of a patient's ongoing periodontal disease(s) and attempting to understand what factors led to a patient's current periodontal condition. Identifying the patient's ongoing disease(s) is necessary for documentation, treatment planning, billing, and insurance reimbursement. Having an understanding of a patient's periodontal disease is critical to treatment planning, as missing a contributing factor to periodontal disease may cause treatment failure. This chapter will describe a thought process for approaching diagnosis, identifying common and uncommon periodontal diseases, ruling out periodontal disease as a cause of pain or lesions, and developing an etiology-based treatment plan.

Keywords: diagnosis, etiology, treatment plan

3.1 Learning Objectives

- Identify common periodontal diseases.
- Develop an etiology-based treatment plan.
- Identify uncommon periodontal diseases.

3.2 Case

A 62-year old Caucasian female presented to the clinic for a "check-up." She used to see a dentist regularly up to 2 years ago, when crowns were made, but moved to this area recently and wanted to see if everything was still all right. She did not report any immediate concerns, but did report that her gums bled when she flosses and that some teeth are slightly sensitive when she bites down. She uses a medium toothbrush twice a day and does not floss since it makes her gums bleed.

She felt "healthy" and checked off "gastroesophageal reflux disease (GERD)" on the medical history form. When questioned, she reported taking 40-mg Omeprazole once daily for it which rendered her free of symptoms. She also takes 10-mg Simvastatin once a day and 500-mg naproxen occasionally for occasional headaches or muscle pain from her arthritis in her knee and hand joints. She reports having her gall bladder removed 4 years ago because of a "cyst," and that she used to smoke tobacco for 40 years (about 3 packs/week) before quitting it

5 years ago. She also used to drink alcoholic beverages daily, but quit about 10 years ago. She is 5'0" tall and weighs 160 lbs. Her blood pressure is 138/87 mm Hg, pulse is 77/min, and respiration 15 breaths/min.

Extraorally, there were no findings other than fair facial skin that exhibits signs of aging. Temporomandibular joints function normally with no pain and normal open range. Salivary glands are shaped normally, but flow seems to be reduced. Oral mucosal surfaces appear normal other than patches of marginal and papillary erythema such as between teeth nos. 24 and 25. Teeth nos. 5, 9, 11, 12, 21, 23, and 29 have wear facets, and there was an interference between tooth no. 5 distal ridge and tooth no. 29 mesial ridge, that produced a corrective slide into centric occlusion. At the same time, tooth no. 29 appeared to move slightly at occlusal contact, but the fremitus could not be confirmed with light palpation. Teeth are in Angle Class I relationship with about 3-mm overjet and overbite.

Periodontal exam findings revealed numerous deep pockets, generalized bleeding on probing (BOP), attachment loss, and multiple teeth with facial recession. At each tooth, plaque was found in a thin rim of plaque at the gingival margin, and subgingival calculus was found on most interproximal and lingual surfaces. Multiple teeth had caries and there was minor tooth mobility on teeth nos. 6, 24, 29, and 32. The clinical appearance (▶ Fig. 3.1) and radiographs (▶ Fig. 3.2) are shown in these figures.

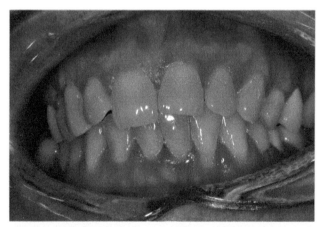

Fig. 3.1 Case facial view.

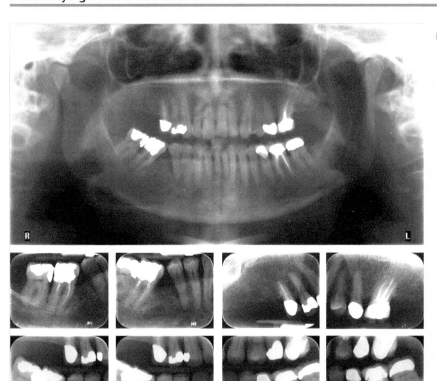

Fig. 3.2 Case radiographs.

Findings in the periodontal chart are as follows:

Maxilla facial		1	2	3	4	5	6	7	8	9	10	11	12	13	14	15	16
	PD				672	434	524	324	323	323	423	423	524	435	636		
	BOP				1	1	1					1	1	1	1		
	CAL				7	2	3	4	3	3	4	4	4	4	6		
	GR					232	231					1	1	121			
	MGJ				333	333	323	323	444	444	323	323	3333	222	222		
	Furc																
	PLQ				4	3	3	3	1	1	1	1	1	1	2		
Maxilla lingual	PD				434	436	645	534	443	324	425	524	434	546	546		
	BOP				1	1	1	1			1	1	1	1	1		
	CAL					6	6	5	4	4	5	5		5	6		
	GR						1				1	1		21	22		
	Furc																
	Mobil						1										
	PLQ				1	1	2	2	1	1	1	2	2	1	1		
Mandible lingual		32	31	30	29	28	27	26	25	24	23	22	21	20	19	18
	PD	646	748		645	424	434	434	434	424	425	424	424	435	537	647
	BOP	1	1		1	1	1	1	1	1	1	1	1	1	1	1
	CAL	4	6		6	4	4	3	3	4	5	4	4	5	7	6
	GR	222	222		1			121	121	121	121	1	2	222		121
	MGJ	444	444		444	444	444	444	434	434	434	444	444	444	444	444
	Furc	2	2												1	1
	PLQ	4	3		2	3	3	3	3	3	3	3	3	3	2	3

Mandible facial															
PD	636	1037		954	425	424	424	524	423	425	424	423	424	436	637
BOP	1 1	1		1	1	1	1	1			1	1	1	1	1
CAL	6	6		9	5	4	4	5	4	5	4	4	4	6	7
GR	2	421		21	1			1	11	131	11	31			
MGJ	999	999		888	777	655	555	555	555	555	557	777	888	999	999
Furc		2												1	1
Mobil				1				1							
PLQ	2	3		1	1	2	2	2	2	2	2	2	2	2	1

Abbreviations: BOP, bleeding on probing (1), suppuration (2); CAL, clinical attachment level; Furc; furcation involvement (Glickman class); GR, gingival recession; MGJ, position of mucogingival junction from margin; Mobil, tooth mobility (Miller grade); PD, probing depths; PLQ, plaque level (0 = none, 5 = heavy).

Table 3.1 Information to consider for periodontal diagnosis in this case

Severity of inflammation	Erythema Gingival bleeding (>10% of sites)
Depth of inflammation	Involving alveolar bone crest (**bone loss/attachment loss** less than 1/3 most teeth, but more than 2/3 of root length for no. 29)
Extent of inflammation	All molars, premolars
Microbial factors	Plaque (did not conduct microbial tests)
Systemic factors	Decreased dexterity, obesity; past use of tobacco and alcohol
Local factors	List factors by tooth: Generalized plaque, calculus, pocketing, and inflammation; No. 4 – biologic width issue No. 5 – caries, abfraction, and recession No. 6 – caries and abfraction recession No. 13 – open margin No. 14 – open margin No. 18 – caries No. 21 – recession and abfraction No. 23 – recession No. 29 – abfraction, heavy occlusal contact; open contact and severe bone loss No. 31 – rough surface, poor contact, questionable margin or recurrent caries, questionable root canal filling, tipping, furcation involvement, and likely not restorable No. 32 – rough surface, poor contact, overhang, caries, tipping, furcation involvement, and likely not restorable

What can be learned from this case?

As discussed in Chapter 2, a patient seeking a "check-up" may have significant dental problems that accumulated since the last period of dental care, as shown in this case.

The most significant information for periodontal diagnosis has been summarized (see ▸ Table 3.1).

Periodontal diseases fall along a spectrum of disease exhibiting a spectrum of inflammation from none (healthy) to most severe leading to tissue die-off, purely local diseases affecting a tooth to systemic illness, superficial disease affecting gingiva to deep bone involvement, and modified by a myriad of microbial, systemic and local factors. Based on the clinical findings, this patient's periodontal disease falls clearly in the middle spectrum of periodontal diseases, neither healthy nor extremely severe. Based on the current International Workshop definitions, this patient's periodontal disease fits the diagnosis of periodontitis, stage III, and grade B.

While naming the disease is important for documentation and treatment justification, the real diagnostic work for most patients is to determine the factors that lead to the disease so that an effective treatment plan can be created. In this case, the factors contributing to the patient's periodontal disease are:

- *Decreased dexterity*: The patient reports arthritis in her hands, which would interfere with efficient oral hygiene.
- *Obesity*: The patient's body mass index (BMI) suggests obesity. This must be verified by physical observation. Obesity is associated with more severe periodontitis.
- The patient's past tobacco and alcohol use may have made periodontal disease more severe in the past, but is no longer an active contributor.
- Plaque has been recorded on most teeth. Plaque is the clinical sign of microbial colonization of tooth surfaces, and needs to be treated in order to control gingival inflammation.

- Calculus is visible on lingual surfaces of mandibular incisors and radiographically on posterior teeth, and presents a plaque-retentive surface that the patient cannot clean.
- Caries presents a source of bacterial irritants and a rough, non-cleansable surface on many teeth:
  - *No. 5*: Recurrent, under mesio-occlusal-distal (MOD) amalgam, associated with isolated enhanced **bone loss.**
  - *No. 6*: Recurrent under distal amalgam, associated with isolated enhanced bone loss.
  - *No. 18*: Recurrent under distal crown margin, associated with bone loss and pocketing.
- *Nonrestorable teeth nos. 31 and 32*: Heavily restored; have defective restorations exceeding the past furcation level. This, along with poor crown-to-root ratio, makes restoration unlikely.
- Food impaction is possible as there are many open contacts and diastemas, but the patient did not report "food getting stuck." Given the uncertainty of food impaction, it is unknown how much it may have played a role in development of the periodontal disease seen at tooth no. 29.
- Open margins at teeth nos. 13 and 14: Open margins retain plaque, cause gingival inflammation, and are associated with an increased bone loss in this case, as seen at tooth.
- *Biologic width impingement is possible at no. 4*: Crown is close to apical crest, and there is some local bone loss.
- Multiple deep pockets, mostly in the posterior region and generalized BOP.
- Slight tooth mobility at tooth no. 6 is most likely related to occlusion as bone support is normal. Slight tooth mobility at teeth nos. 29 and 32 is due to severe loss of bone support.
- *Gingival recession at teeth nos. 5, 6, 12, 21 and 23*: Associated with abfractions, and also inflamed because of marginal plaque build-up.
- Tipping of no. 31 likely causes plaque retention in this area and may have contributed to furcation exposure.
- Mesial root concavities at teeth nos. 5 and 12 present plaque-retentive areas associated with pocketing.
- Wear facets, matching abfraction, and fremitus at tooth no. 29 suggest occlusal trauma.

The corresponding treatments for these contributing factors are as follows:
- *Decreased dexterity*: Oral hygiene instruction: use electronic toothbrush instead of a manual brush, preferably one with a wide handle. Consider using an electronic flosser (i.e., Hummingbird), and antiseptic mouthwash to reduce plaque levels.
- *Obesity*: Encourage patient to lose weight.
- *Nonrestorable teeth*: Remove teeth nos. 31 and 32.
- *Plaque*: Oral hygiene instruction (see above).
- *Calculus*: Scaling and root planing in all quadrants, 4+ teeth.
- *Caries*: Crowns for teeth nos. 5, 6, and 18 for better interproximal contact and appearance.
- *Open margins*: Replace crowns at teeth nos. 13 and 14.
- *Biologic width impingement at tooth no. 4*: Osseous surgery will solve the problem (see below).
- *Deep pocketing/inflammation*: If scaling and root planing is not effective, osseous surgery may be needed in all quadrants. A regenerative procedure may benefit tooth no. 29.

- *Mobile teeth*: Wait and see if mobility improves. Tooth no. 29 may need to be removed.
- *Gingival recession at teeth nos. 5, 6, 12, 21, and 23*: Connective tissue grafting.
- *Tipping of teeth*: Removal of teeth nos. 31 and 32 solves this problem.
- *Root concavities at no. 5*: Odontoplasty prior to restoration may make the tooth more cleansable.
- *Occlusal trauma*: Occlusal analysis and adjustment, limited where needed.

Missing teeth need to be replaced and the patient needs to be maintained:
- *Missing teeth*: Either removable partial dentures or implant-supported restorations, depending on the patient's wishes and ability to commit to an expensive and long therapy.
- Periodontal maintenance every 3–4 months.

Some patient factors that may affect treatment are as follows:
- *Naproxen use*: Although this medication may increase bleeding tendency, it is unlikely to be a risk in this case given the infrequent use.
- *Hypertension*: Long-term risk for stroke, heart disease, and dementia. Counsel patient to strive for lower blood pressure. Monitor prior to invasive treatment, and postpone treatment in case of severe, symptomatic hypertension.
- *Atherosclerosis*: Patient has long-term risk of in-office medical emergency.
- *GERD*: The patient may feel uncomfortable reclining in a supine position.

3.3 Identify Common Periodontal Diseases

After thorough assessment, the next step in periodontal treatment is periodontal diagnosis, the identification of the disease(s) present and identification of the factors that lead up to the disease(s). Periodontal diagnosis aids:
- Justification of treatment for insurance reimbursement.
- Treatment planning as procedures are often tied to specific diseases and conditions.
- Prediction of future disease activity (prognosis), which determines long-term dental treatment.

3.3.1 The Six Dimensions of Periodontal Diseases

In order to prepare for periodontal diagnosis, consider data from the periodontal exam and organize the findings a long the following six dimensions that describe periodontal diseases:
- Severity of inflammation.
- Depth of inflammation.
- Extent of inflammation.
- Microbiologic factors.
- Systemic factors.
- Local factors.

In order to match a patient's individual periodontal disease(s), consider summarizing the clinical data first along the following dimensions:

Severity of Inflammation

Periodontal inflammation fills a spectrum from pristine, healthy, pink, firm, and tight gingival margins over various levels of redness to rapid tissue die-off. Clinically, rate the worst level of inflammation seen at the gingival margin during the periodontal exam (▶Table 3.2).

Depth of Inflammation

The second dimension of periodontal disease is how deeply the tissue is damaged. Mild periodontal diseases affect only superficial tissues and are generally curable with no loss of tissue, whereas severe periodontal diseases cause lasting tissue damage including tooth loss. Based on clinical measurements, rate the depth of inflammation and tissue damage for the worst site along this spectrum (▶Table 3.3).

Consider if this is representative of the entire mouth, or if it reflects a unique local factor, such as a tooth fracture or failed root canal treatment. Also note if the depth of tissue damage is evenly distributed across all teeth, or is affecting few teeth or tooth types. For eventual disease grading, consider past loss in terms of the size of attachment loss over the last 5 years, or percent bone loss/year.

Extent of Inflammation

The third dimension of periodontal disease is the extent of inflammation, and subsequent tissue damage. While the generalized tissue damage is suggestive of mouth-wide local factors such as poor oral hygiene or systemic conditions (i.e., tobacco use), the localized tissue damage usually indicates a unique local factor that exacerbates periodontal disease. Analyze the pattern of deep pockets, attachment loss, or bone loss, and note if this affects only molars (excluding 3rds) and incisors. If it does not, calculate the percentage of teeth with attachment/bone loss to describe disease as localized or generalized (▶Table 3.4).

While the first three dimensions of periodontal disease mostly help in identifying the periodontal disease, the last three inform treatment planning and allow for grading the complexity of periodontal disease.

Microbiome

The fourth dimension of periodontal diseases is the make-up of the microbial community that makes up the disease. In most cases, no microbial testing is done and one has to subjectively judge the virulence of the microbial flora as shown below (▶Table 3.5 top row).

Microbial testing should be performed whenever there is attachment/bone loss that is much more severe than anticipated for a patient's age and if there are no known local factors that could explain the observed disease activity. This usually includes:

- Children, adolescents, and adults under age 30 with significant attachment/bone loss.
- Adult patients who continue to experience attachment/bone loss despite competent periodontal treatment.

If microbial test results are available, the microbiome's influence on disease activity can be rated as follows (▶Table 3.5 bottom row).

▶ **Table 3.2** The first dimension of periodontal disease: severity of inflammation

Rate the worst level of inflammation seen in the gingival margins along this spectrum

No inflammation at all	Marked redness (erythema)	Shedding of papilla tip
		Ulceration
Mild redness (erythema)	Readily apparent BOP	Gray film of necrotic tissue
	Cyanosis	
Minimal BOP	Slight shedding	Loss of gingiva to bone
		Bone die-off
Health	Inflamed	Necrotic
	(Gingivitis/periodontitis)	(Necrotizing periodontitis)

Abbreviations: BOP, bleeding on probing with light pressure (0.25 N); Cyanosis, dark red/purple/slightly blue appearance of marginal tissue; Shedding, increased white cell debris appears of gingival papilla tip.

Table 3.3 The second dimension of periodontal disease: depth of inflammation and tissue damage

Rate the worst area of tissue damage seen clinically and radiographically

No/minimal pocketing	Deep pocketing (5+ mm)			
No attachment loss (CAL = 0)	Possible/Early attachment loss (CAL = 1–2 mm)	Definite attachment loss (CAL = 3–4 mm)	Severe attachment loss (CAL = 5+ mm)	Severe attachment loss (CAL = 5+ mm)
No bone loss	<15% bone loss	<33% bone loss	>33% bone loss	
No tooth loss			<5 teeth lost*	5+ teeth lost*
Health Gingivitis	Stage I Periodontitis	Stage II Periodontitis	Stage III Periodontitis	Stage IV Periodontitis

Abbreviations: CAL, interdental clinical attachment level; attachment loss not due to other factor (i.e., tooth loss).

* Tooth loss due to periodontal disease; should include teeth that are about to be lost.

Table 3.4 The third dimension of periodontal disease: extent of inflammation

Rate the extent of the disease by how many teeth have attachment/bone loss:

Only molars or incisors involved	Involves most/all tooth types

If there is no molar/incisor pattern, calculate % of involved teeth:

<30% of teeth involved	30+ % of teeth involved (9+ teeth in a complete dentition without 3rd molars)
Localized	Generalized

Table 3.6 The fourth dimension of periodontal disease: systemic influence

Nonsmoker	< 10 cigarettes/day	10+ cigarettes/day
Normal HbA1c levels	HbA1c < 7.0% (with history of diabetes)	HbA1c ≥7.0% (with history of diabetes)
Grade A: slow rate of progression	Grade B: moderate rate of progression	Grade C: rapid rate of progression

Rate the level of systemic involvement along the following spectrum:

Not necessarily used for grading periodontal disease, but other systemic factors that may enhance or protect against periodontal disease. These include:

Good overall health	Obesity
Healthy lifestyle, nutrition	Osteoporosis
Good self-care	Rheumatoid arthritis
	Emotional stress, depression
	Malnutrition
	Recreational drug use
	Immunosuppressive meds.
	HIV infection
	Leukemia
	Sickle cell disease
	Hormonal change (Pregnancy)
	Genetic polymorphisms (i.e., IL-1)

Systemic Factors

The fifth dimension of periodontal disease are the systemic background and possible contributing factors (see ▶ Table 3.6 for factors, and how they relate to periodontitis grading). As with microbial factors, for most patients, no specific test results will be available, and the systemic contribution to a patient's periodontal disease needs to be estimated from the medical history.

Key factors to be recollected are:
- *Smoking history*: Cigarettes/day.
- *Diabetes mellitus history*: HbA1c level.

If a patient's severity of attachment/bone loss cannot be explained by the presence of local factors or unusual microbes

Table 3.5 The fourth dimension of periodontal disease: microbial virulence

Heavy plaque/calculus, but low level of disease activity	Plaque/calculus level seems appropriate for disease activity	Marked tissue destruction in absence of significant plaque/calculus; tissue destruction continues despite plaque/calculus removal

Rate the level of virulence along the following spectrum:

Oral streptococci	Fusobacteria species	A. actinomycetemcomitans
Actinomyces species	Prevotella species	Large number spirochetes
Low bacteria count	Small % P. gingivalis (1–2%)	P. gingivalis + T. forsythia
		Enteric or staphylococci bacteria
		Large number yeasts (candida)
		Large number entamoeba
		Large number viruses
Grade A: slow rate of progression	Grade B: moderate rate of progression	Grade C: rapid rate of progression

Abbreviations: A. actinomycetemcomitans, Aggregatibacter actinomycetemcomitans; *P. gingivalis,* Porphyromonas gingivalis; *T. forsythia,* Tannerella forsythia.

and there is no known systemic factor that could explain the observed level of periodontal disease, the patient should be sent for a comprehensive physical exam.

Local Factors

The local factors that explain locally enhanced pockets, attachment loss, or bone loss comprise the sixth dimension of periodontal disease. Generally, factors that cause locally enhanced periodontal disease either favor plaque retention or induce chronic tissue trauma.

Case complexity and treatment difficulty increase with the number of complicating local factors (▶ Table 3.7).

3.3.2 Everyday Periodontal Diagnosis

Even though many periodontal diseases exist, in day-to-day practice, identifying a patient's periodontal disease means choosing from the following four choices:
- Health.
- Gingivitis.
- Periodontitis.
- Other diseases.

If a patient presenting for an initial exam has not received periodontal treatment within the last year, the decision tree for diagnosis could be this (▶ Fig. 3.3).

Essentially, if there is no sign of significant BOP, the patient most likely has a form of periodontal health. If there is more than minimal BOP, the patient most likely either has periodontitis or gingivitis, depending on signs of attachment /bone loss attributable to periodontal disease in the presence of typical signs, symptoms, and medical history of common periodontal

Table 3.7 The sixth dimension: local factors contributing to periodontal disease

Bacterial	Restorative	Periodontal	Anatomical	Trauma
Calculus**	Caries	Deep pocketing	Crowding	Occlusal trauma
	Endodontic infection	Inflammation	Ortho. appliances	Bruxism
	Nonrestorable teeth	Furcation	Rotated teeth	Clenching
	Food impaction	Tooth mobility	Tipped teeth	Nail-biting
	Open margin	Recession	Severe angle II	Pipe chewing
	Overhang	Mucogingival Defect	Severe angle III	Piercings
	Subgingival margins	Implant conditions	Excess overjet	Other parafunctional habits
	Rough surface		Excess overbite	Other injury
	Fracture		Margin discrepancy	
	Bulky/overcontoured		infra/supra-erupted	
	Biologic width issue		Enamel ridges	
	Hyposalivation		enamel projections	
			Root concavities	
			Enamel pearls	
			Cervical projections	
			Dentin ridges	
			Unusual anatomy	
			Partially impacted	
			Cemental tears	
			*Missing teeth	

* Missing teeth may or may not contribute to periodontal disease. Removal of teeth may eliminate local periodontal disease, but can also lead to malposition of adjacent teeth and occlusal trauma that favors tissue destruction.
** Supragingival calculus that is not in contact with gingiva may not produce gingival irritation as it is too distant to have an effect.

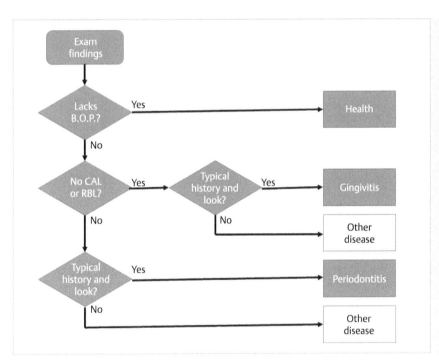

Fig. 3.3 Typical decision tree for diagnosis of common periodontal disease. BOP = significant bleeding on probing (>10% of sites). CAL = interdental clinical attachment level greater than zero, and explainable by the patient's periodontal disease. RBL = radiographic bone loss, typically a distance greater than 2 mm between the cemento-enamel (CEJ) junction and alveolar bone crest.

diseases. If the signs and symptoms are unusual for common periodontal disease (i.e., pain, tissue ulceration, not responsive to oral hygiene), or a medical condition is present that is associated with severe periodontal disease, the patient most likely has some periodontal disease other than periodontitis or gingivitis.

If a patient was seen recently for periodontal treatment, the patient may have achieved "periodontal disease remission" if recent treatment markedly improved BOP and pocketing. Alternatively, if signs and symptoms of periodontal disease have not changed much since the beginning of treatment, the patient still may have ongoing periodontal disease as diagnosed for untreated patients.

Health

Patients rarely present with periodontally healthy tissues during an initial exam, and this is the goal of periodontal treatment. There are four possible "healthy" outcomes in periodontal therapy (▶ Table 3.8).[1]
- *Pristine periodontal health*: There is no sign of inflammation anywhere, and there is no evidence of past tissue damage in the form of increased pocketing, attachment loss, or bone loss. This is exceedingly rare.
- *Clinical periodontal health*: There is at most minimal inflammation (minor erythema or minimal BOP) and no evidence of deeper tissue damage such as pocketing, attachment loss, or bone loss.

- *Periodontal disease stability (healthy, but reduced periodontium)*: There is, at most, minimal inflammation, but evidence of past disease activity in the form of attachment/bone loss.
- *Periodontal disease remission (controlled periodontal disease)*: Treatment significantly reduced inflammation, depth, and extent of periodontal disease, but contributing local, microbial, or systemic factors have not fully been controlled.

Clinical Relevance

Patients with clinical or pristine periodontal health have a low risk of periodontal disease, and treatment mostly consists of periodic evaluation every 6–12 months to ensure the absence of disease, and possible removal of any irritating factors.

Patients with periodontal disease stability and remission have a higher risk of disease recurrence and need frequent evaluation every 3–4 months (or sooner in the most high-risk cases) to check for disease progression and control factors that may re-initiate active disease.

Gingivitis

Gingival inflammation (gingivitis) is most often caused by dental plaque,[2] and is the most common periodontal disease in otherwise healthy children, adolescents, and young adults. For the diagnosis of gingivitis,[3] there must be significant BOP present, but no sign of attachment loss or radiographic bone loss that is attributable to the periodontal disease. Ulceration or severe pain is not a feature of gingivitis. Plaque-induced gingivitis resolves with control of plaque, and local and systemic factors. Gingivitis can be modified by several medical conditions, and other gingival conditions such as pigmentation or enlargement can be present in addition to gingivitis as shown in ▶ Table 3.9. Gingivitis can be called localized if less than 30% of sites have BOP, and this may suggest a local contributing factor.

Attachment/bone loss can be present if caused by trauma (i.e., aggressive tooth brushing, tooth abfraction, and smokeless tobacco), orthodontic treatment, or malposition of teeth. In these conditions, bone and attachment loss is usually seen on the facial side of teeth in areas of gingival recession. Loss of teeth can also cause bone loss, gingival recession, and attachment loss on adjacent remaining teeth.

Clinical Relevance

Signs and symptoms of gingivitis can be removed completely with the removal of local and systemic irritating factors. Typically, for simple plaque-induced gingivitis, this involves regular oral hygiene instruction and periodontal prophylaxis every 3 to 6 months depending on the level of plaque/calculus build-up seen at each recall visit. If initial plaque control and

Table 3.8 Forms of periodontal health

Severity of inflammation	Depth of inflammation	Diagnosis	Needs treatment other than preventive?
No inflammation at all	No pocketing No attachment loss No bone loss	Pristine periodontal health	No
No/minor erythema Minimal BOP	No pocketing No attachment loss No bone loss	Clinical periodontal health	No
No/minor erythema Minimal BOP (reduced)	No pocketing Has attachment loss	Periodontal disease stability	No
Erythema (reduced) BOP (reduced)	Pocketing (reduced) Has attachment loss	Periodontal disease remission	Maybe

Table 3.9 Gingivitis

Severity of inflammation	Depth of inflammation	Systemic factors Local factors	Diagnosis
Erythema Bleeding on probing	Minimal pocketing No attachment loss No bone loss	None	Gingivitis, plaque induced + …
Erythema Bleeding on probing (both more severe than expected based on plaque level)		Local factors: • Hyposalivation • Subgingival restorative margin defect	+ Enhanced by oral factors
		Systemic conditions: • Hormonal change (Pregnancy) • Oral contraceptives • Diabetes mellitus • Leukemia • Smoking • Malnutrition	+ Enhanced by systemic factors
Erythema Bleeding on probing	Enlarged pockets Enlarged papilla (may have attachment loss, bone loss from co-existing periodontitis)	Systemic conditions: • Medication associated with gingival enlargement*	+ Drug-influenced gingival enlargement

* Typical medications are: calcium channel blockers, cyclosporine, phenytoin, valproic acid derivatives, and methamphetamines.

prophylaxis do not resolve gingivitis within the first 2 weeks of treatment, and if there are no local or systemic factors that can explain the condition, then diagnosis of other periodontal diseases, such as allergic reaction, autoimmune disease, systemic infection, or neoplastic disease, should be considered.

Periodontitis

Periodontitis slightly affects less than half of adults, and is very common in older adults. The key for diagnosis of periodontitis is the presence of interdental attachment loss attributable to periodontal disease on at least two nonadjacent teeth. Attachment loss associated with the following conditions specifically does not count toward the diagnosis of periodontitis:

- Gingival recession linked to trauma (i.e., aggressive brushing).
- Root caries.
- Distal surface of 2nd molars adjacent to a malpositioned or extracted 3rd molar.
- Endodontic infections draining through a periodontal pocket.
- Vertical root fractures.

Ulceration or visible necrosis of gingiva and underlying tissues are not features of periodontitis, but are typical of another disease group, the "necrotizing periodontal diseases." Patients with periodontitis will not have a medical history of the following rare conditions (▶Table 3.10), which may produce severe attachment loss as part of the manifestations of the medical condition.[4]

Periodontitis is also staged according to disease severity, as follows (▶Table 3.11) using severity, depth, and extent of inflammation:[5]

Staging may be increased depending on treatment complexity. The following may justify increasing stages I and II cases to stage III:

- 6+ mm probing depths.
- Class II or III furcation involvement.
- 3+ mm deep vertical bone defect(s).

Likewise, stage III may be increased to stage IV if rehabilitation of the failed dentition is complicated by:

- **Bite collapse** or drifted/flared teeth.
- Grade II or III tooth mobility.
- Masticatory dysfunction (i.e., **bruxing** and clenching).

Table 3.10 Medical conditions/syndromes that may produce severe attachment loss

Genetic disorders	Genetic disorders (cont'd)	Neoplasms
Down	Angioedema	Gingival squamous cell carcinoma
Leukocyte adhesion deficiency	Glycogen storage disease	Odontogenic tumors
Papillon-Lefèvre	Gaucher disease	Periodontal tissue neoplasms
Haim-Munk	Hypophosphatasia	Metastic tumors
Chediak-Higashi	Hajdu-Cheney	Granulomatosis with polyangiitis
Congenital neutropenia (Kostmann)	Aplastic anemia	Langerhans histiocytosis
Cyclical neutropenia	Acquired conditions	Giant cell granulomas
Chronic granulomatous disease	AIDS	Hyperparathyroidism
Hyperimmunoglobulin E diseases	Acquired neutropenia	Systemic sclerosis
Cohen syndrome	Epidermolysis bullosa acquisita	Vanishing bone disease
Dystrophic epidermolysis bullosa		
Kindler		
Plasminogen deficiency		
Ehlers-Danlos (type IV, VIII)		

Table 3.11 Periodontitis stages

Severity of inflammation	Depth of inflammation	Extent of inflammation	Diagnosis
Erythema	CAL = 1–2 mm	<30% teeth OR Molar/incisor pattern	Periodontitis, stage I, localized
Bleeding on probing	<15% bone loss		
	No tooth loss yet	>30% teeth	Periodontitis, stage I, generalized
	CAL= 3–4 mm	<30% teeth OR Molar/incisor pattern	Periodontitis, stage II, localized
	15–33% bone loss		
	No tooth loss yet	>30% teeth	Periodontitis, stage II, generalized
	5+ mm CAL	<30% teeth OR Molar/incisor pattern	Periodontitis, stage III, localized
	>33% bone loss		
	<5 teeth lost	>30% teeth	Periodontitis, stage III, generalized
	5+ mm CAL	<30% teeth OR Molar/incisor pattern	Periodontitis, stage IV, localized
	>33% bone loss		
	>5 teeth lost	>30% teeth	Periodontitis, stage IV, generalized

Table 3.12 Periodontitis grading

Grade	A	B = default grade	C
Disease progression	Slow	Moderate	Rapid
Over past 5 years (preferred measure)	No loss	≤2 mm	>2 mm
% radiographic bone loss/age (indirect measure)	<0.25%/year	0.25–1.0%/year	>1.0%/year Molar, incisor pattern in child/adolescent
Microbiome	Heavy plaque/calculus, but low level of inflammation	Typical plaque/calculus level	• Destruction exceeds what is expected of plaque level • Presence of *A. actinomycetemcomitans* • Atypical microflora • No response to plaque control
Systemic	Nonsmoker Normoglycemic	Smoker <10 cigs/day HbA1c <7.0%	Smoker > 10 cigs/day HbA1c ≥ 7.0%
Other factors that may be considered for grading he disease			
Systemic	Overall health Healthy lifestyle	Presence of controlled medical conditions	Obesity Osteoporosis Rheumatoid arthritis Stress Specific genotypes Serum/saliva markers
Local	Smooth, convex tooth/restoration surfaces	Normal tooth/restoration anatomy	Severe caries Occlusal trauma Malformed roots

Note: The grade is determined by the presence of factors in the rightmost column of this table.

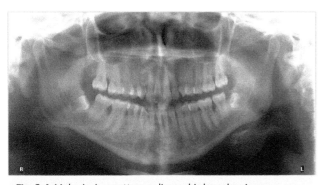

Fig. 3.4 Molar-incisor pattern radiographic bone loss in an otherwise healthy 17-year old high school athlete of Hispanic background. Microbial testing did not show evidence of colonization with *A. actinomycetemcomitans,* but a high proportion of staphylococcal and enteric bacteria which is unusual for typical periodontal disease.

- Less than 20 remaining teeth (or 10 opposing pairs); lack of suitable abutment teeth.
- Severe ridge defect in edentulous area.

The patient's periodontitis also needs to be graded, which judges the speed of disease progression. Preferably, disease progression should be determined by evaluating attachment/bone loss over the last 5 years. However, since this is impractical in most new patients, disease progression can be estimated by calculating yearly bone loss (% of bone loss divided by patient age) or judging the risk from the microbiome, systemic, and local factors. The default periodontitis grade is "B," and increased or decreased as suggested in the following table (▶ Table 3.12).

Clinical Relevance

Determining the stage and grade of a patient's periodontitis feeds into determining the prognosis, and ultimately the aggressiveness of needed treatment. For example, grade C may suggest a need for systemic antibiotics during scaling and root planing for improved outcome. Grade C may also suggest a quicker turn to periodontal surgery compared to grades A and B, and a more aggressive maintenance regimen with more frequent recall visits and increased use of antiseptic irrigation.

Staging a patient's periodontal disease may also influence treatment philosophy. For example, stages I and II will most likely benefit from periodontal therapy including pocket-reduction surgery. In contrast, patients with stage IV periodontitis will most likely require some form of denture therapy. Implant therapy in patients with a history of stage III or IV periodontitis may be difficult due to lack of bone.

Aggressive Periodontitis

Earlier classification systems recognized disease entities called "Aggressive Periodontitis," "Early onset periodontitis," or "Localized juvenile periodontitis." These were forms of periodontitis that produced rapid attachment, bone, and tooth loss early in otherwise healthy children and adolescents. The most common variant produces a molar/incisor loss pattern that was also associated with *A. actinomycetemcomitans* bacteria, and more frequent in patients of African or Mediterranean ancestry (see ▶ Fig. 3.4). However, researchers and clinicians currently cannot agree on specific disease criteria for these conditions,[6] and these conditions are currently diagnosed as "Periodontitis, grade C."

Other Disease

While health, gingivitis, and periodontitis apply as periodontal diagnosis to almost every patient seen in an average practice, it is necessary to be alert for other types of periodontal disease. In addition to gingivitis and periodontitis, a patient may have a local periodontal disease superimposed on a general background of periodontal disease for a specific site, tooth, or implant:

- Abscesses of the periodontium:
  - Either present as localized swelling or fistula draining a milky, purulent liquid.
  - Source of abscess is removed from the tooth's root canal system, and the tooth is either vital or shows no sign of root canal failure.
  - Diagnosed by location of the abscess:
    - Within the gingiva, but without signs of bone loss: Gingival abscess.
    - Within alveolar bone, with signs of bone loss: Periodontal abscess, often within furcation area of molars.
- Periodontal-endodontic lesions:
  - May present as localized swelling or fistula draining a milky, purulent liquid.
  - May have a large J-shaped area of bone loss on side of tooth.
  - Tooth is necrotic or has failed root canal.
  - Often has deep pocket to apex.
- Peri-implant disease:
  - Gingival inflammation at a dental implant. If the bone level at the implant is stable, this is called **peri-implant mucositis**.
  - May show progressive bone loss and implant exposure. This is called **peri-implantitis**.
- Traumatic injuries producing ulcers or cuts in the gingiva.

There are also very rare periodontal diseases that present with unique signs and symptoms:
- Necrotizing periodontal disease:
  - These display severe, excruciatingly painful inflammation that produces progressive tissue necrosis starting from the interdental papilla margin.
- Medical conditions that manifest as unusually severe periodontal disease (see ▸ Table 3.10).
- Oral pathology that happens to produce gingival ulcers or unusually intense erythema.
  - Microbial infections (i.e., herpes, varicella, coxsackievirus; tuberculosis; and histoplasmosis).
  - Autoimmune disease (i.e., pemphigus vulgaris, pemphigoid, erosive lichen planus, …).
  - Allergic reactions.
  - Oral neoplasms (i.e., squamous cell carcinoma).

3.3.3 Classification Systems of Periodontal Diseases

Different generations of dentists used different classification systems for periodontal diseases. It is therefore useful to know the equivalent names of periodontal diseases and conditions when communicating with other dentists or reading periodontal research articles. Periodontal disease names became standardized in the late 1970s with classification schemes endorsed by the American Academy of Periodontology, and were named after the year they were developed.

- Periodontitis (2018 classification) includes the following:
  - The common periodontal disease causing gradual attachment/bone loss in older adults alternatively known as follows:
    - Chronic periodontitis (1999 classification).
    - Adult periodontitis (1986, 1989 classifications).
    - Chronic marginal periodontitis (1977 classification).
  - And the rapidly progressive variant (Periodontitis, grade C) causing attachment/bone loss in children, adolescents, and young adults is termed as follows:
    - Aggressive periodontitis (1999 classification).
    - Juvenile periodontitis (1977, 1986 classifications).
    - Early onset periodontitis (1989 classification).
- Necrotizing periodontal diseases were called alternatively as follows:
  - Necrotizing ulcerative gingivitis, periodontitis (1999 classification).
  - Acute necrotizing ulcerative periodontitis (1989 classification).
  - Necrotizing ulcerative gingiva-stomatitis (1986 classification).
- Refractory periodontitis (1986, 1989 classifications) is a condition where periodontal disease continues to cause tissue destruction despite competent therapy. This is no longer recognized as a separate disease.

3.4 Develop an Etiology-based Treatment Plan

For the majority of patients presenting with gingivitis and periodontitis, the most important aspect of diagnosis is the identification of contributing factors and planning treatment that attempts to address all of these factors.

3.4.1 Recognizing Contributing Factors

The most important aspect of a periodontal exam is to identify all contributing factors that lead to a patient's periodontal disease. This has to be done by a thorough periodontal exam that reviews medical history, examines both extraoral and intraoral tissues for signs of systemic and oral disease, records the current periodontal state and examines all local factors that may contribute to periodontal disease (Chapter 2). This should have led to a careful evaluation of the three dimensions of periodontal disease that explain the development of the current disease from a microbiological, systemic, and local view.

In order to identify the factors that lead to a patient's current periodontal disease, identify patterns of inflammation, pocketing and bone/attachment loss first, and then judge how these are related in the following order:
- Systemic factors.
- General factors in the oral cavity (general plaque and calculus level).
- Local factors unique to each site.

3.4.2 Identifying and Judging the Influence of Systemic Factors

Systemic factors influence the general rate of disease progression for all sites in the mouth. Evaluate systemic factors as follows:
- Consider the following factors that could contribute to periodontal disease (▶Table 3.13) and match these with the patient's health history.
- Consider the average disease progression of periodontal disease and judge if the patient's average bone/attachment loss is more severe than expected for the patient's age (see ▶Fig. 3.5).
- If more severe than expected for a patient's age, the patient's systemic factors may have contributed to the patient's periodontal disease in a significant manner, and should be addressed as part of treatment planning.

Table 3.13 Systemic factors contributing to gingivitis/periodontitis

Common	Uncommon	Requires testing
Tobacco use	Rheumatoid arthritis	IL-1 genotype
Diabetes mellitus (Hb A1c >7%)	Immunosuppressive meds	Elevated serum CRP
Obesity	Chronic kidney disease	
Stress or anxiety	HIV/AIDS	
Osteoporosis (T-score <–2.5)	Crohn's disease	
Smoked Marijuana Use	Leukemia	
If oral hygiene affected by: • Stroke • Dementia • Arthritis • Gout If excessive BOP observed: • Pregnancy • Puberty • Oral contraceptives	Neutropenia Malnutrition Down syndrome Other rare genetic conditions associated with periodontal disease	

3.4.3 Identifying and Judging the Influence of Generalized Local Factors

Evaluate oral factors that affect the entire mouth:
- Evaluate plaque and calculus:
  ○ Unless there is no BOP, pocketing, or attachment loss, plaque and calculus will explain some degree of present periodontal disease.
- Check for xerostomia (and xerostomia-inducing medications):
  ○ Xerostomia enhances plaque formation and caries.
- Check for presence of parafunctional habits (i.e., bruxism, clenching):
  ○ If there is associated tissue damage (worn teeth/severe attrition; tooth or restoration fractures; enlarged masticatory muscles; maxillary exostoses or generalized thickening of lamina dura and alveolar bone), it may also play a role explaining the patient's periodontal disease.

3.4.4 Identifying and Judging the Influence of Local Factors

Often, there will be local variations in periodontal disease severity that cannot be explained by systemic factors and local factors that affect the entire mouth. Local contributing factors that are specific to certain teeth can be identified by looking for local variations in periodontal disease severity:

Using Bone Loss as a Clue for Local Factors

For most patients with local disease severity variations, this will suffice to uncover relevant local factors.
- Evaluate radiographic bone level:
  ○ If the bone level is uniform (and parallels the cemento-to-enamel junction [CEJ]), plaque, calculus, and possible systemic factors may explain the patient's periodontal disease. Clinically, this will be apparent as uniform pocket depths and attachment levels (within 1–2 mm).

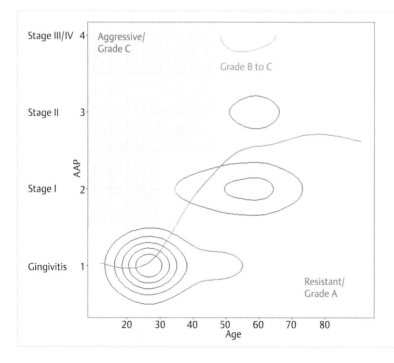

Fig. 3.5 A tool for grading periodontal disease progression. This is a density plot of periodontal diagnoses versus age of 2135 patients seen at the Western University Dental Center from 2010 to 2013 (as created in R). The *blue line* represents the average periodontal disease severity for a given age. For grading periodontal disease, look up age of a given patient, and note the expect disease severity as indicated by the *"white"* shading. If a given patient's disease severity is higher than average *(red-orange shading)*, the disease is progressing at a more aggressive pace (grade C). If it is lower than average, the patient is likely resistant against periodontal disease (grade A). Systemic conditions that contribute to periodontal disease may produce a somewhat higher than expected disease severity ("grade B to C")

Table 3.14 Local factors that may explain enhanced bone/attachment loss

Restorative factors	Evidence of occlusal trauma	Anatomical factors	Implant-related factors
Caries	Fremitus	Furcation involvement	Adjacent implant platform too
Endodontic infection	Heavy wear facets	Crowding	deep relative to CEJ (>5 mm)
Nonrestorable teeth	Plunger cusp	Rotation	Adjacent implant platform too
Food impaction	Heavy contact	Tipping	close to tooth (<2 mm)
Open margin	Fracture	Enamel/Dentin ridge	Extruded cement
Overhang	Widened PDL	Cervical projection	Peri-implantitis
Subgingival margins	Funnel-shaped PDL	Enamel pearl	
Rough surface	Circumferential bone loss	Infra/super-erupted	
Fracture		Adjacent impacted tooth	
Bulky/overcontoured			
Biologic width issue			

- o If there are vertical bone defects, tooth-specific local factors are likely responsible for the enhanced bone loss.
- Evaluate each tooth for the following local factors (▶Table 3.14).
- Determine if the local factor is immediately adjacent to the bone defect, attachment loss, or pocket associated with the tooth.
  - o If the affected tooth is restored, check the restoration radiographically and clinically for restorative contributing factors (▶Table 3.14). Generally, the bone will attempt to remain at a distance of 3 mm from the most apical portion of a subgingival restorative margin or carious lesion, creating an area of bone loss at deep cervical restorations or caries.
  - o Typically, local bone defects are seen at posterior teeth. If a bone defect is seen in the absence of restorative factor, it is useful to check the occlusion for signs of occlusal trauma (▶Table 3.14), as occlusal trauma is a common contributing factor to periodontal disease.

If there are no occlusal interferences or restorative factors that could explain a local bone defect, unfavorable root anatomy may be another factor to consider. Bone defects at molars are typically associated with furcation entrances, while bone defects at maxillary premolars may be attributable to deep mesial and distal root concavities.

- Unfavorable implant-tooth relationships (▶Table 3.14) may also cause localized bone loss.
- 1st molar/incisor pattern bone loss in young individuals suggests aggressive disease.
  ▶Fig. 3.6 illustrates how the presence of localized bone loss provides a clue for identifying local contributing factors.

Using Pocketing as a Clue for Local Factors

Alternatively, since local increases in probing depths usually correspond to local underlying bone defects, variations in pocket depths can be used as a clue for identifying contributing factors:
- When evaluating sites with deep pocketing (5 mm or greater), consider what caused the pocketing:
  - o Is the pocketing due to swelling of the gingiva? Compared to previous exams (if available), the attachment level will be unchanged. There will also be no change in bone level, and there may not be bone loss. The gingiva will appear more swollen and may cover more of the tooth.
    - Inflammatory swelling usually correlates to plaque/calculus levels.
    - Medication-induced enlargement produces firm and rubbery gingival papilla tips, and is associated with typical medications (see ▶Table 3.9).

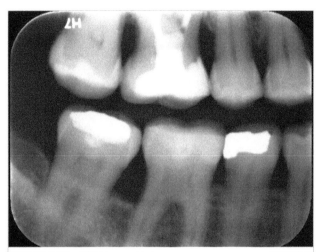

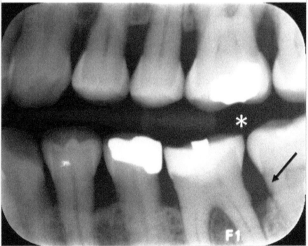

Fig. 3.6 Local factors cause local destruction. In this case, pocketing was limited to 3 to 4 mm pocketing around all teeth except for the interproximal area between teeth nos. 18 and 19, where 9-mm pocketing was found, and the distal side of no. 30, where there was a 5-mm pocket. This is also reflected in the radiographs as there is a significant 2-wall defect at the distal side of no. 19 (*black arrow*), but only a shallow area of accentuated bone loss distal to no. 30. The stark difference in disease presentation of teeth with the same anatomy is explained by local factors unique to no. 19: the open contact (marked with a *star*), and likely strong occlusal forces as evidenced by the excessive wear of the occlusal surface of no. 19. These unique factors likely lead to food impaction and enhanced accumulation of plaque as evidenced by the small piece of radiographic calculus, and worse periodontal disease than anywhere else in the mouth.

- Is the pocketing due to attachment/bone loss?
- Consider the distribution of pocketing:
  - If generally deepened with no significant variation throughout the mouth (i.e., 4–6 mm pocketing for all teeth), it is most likely related to plaque and calculus.
    - Moderate deep generalized pocketing (5–6 mm) with low plaque/calculus level may be associated with diabetes mellitus or pregnancy.
    - Unusually severe pocketing at a young age may be due to significant underlying systemic disease (see ▶Table 3.13, uncommon factors).
  - If there is significant variation in pocketing, local factors as shown in ▶Table 3.14 are most likely responsible for these. If there is a 1st molar/incisor pattern to the disease, it may indicate aggressive forms of periodontitis (i.e., grade C).

Using Inflammation as a Clue for Local Factors

Inflammatory changes in the gingiva (i.e., erythema, BOP) can provide a quick way to identify some local contributing factors not found through bone loss/pocketing analysis:

- Is the inflammation generalized (i.e., BOP on most/all teeth)?
  - If adjacent to significant plaque or calculus, most likely due to plaque and calculus.
  - In absence of significant plaque or calculus, most likely due to systemic factors:
    - Hormonal changes (i.e., pregnancy, puberty, menopause).
    - Diabetes mellitus.
    - Allergic reaction, if the inflammation is diffuse throughout the oral cavity and recent in onset with known trigger.
    - *Autoimmune condition*: Inflammation may also produce unusual signs of disease (i.e., ulceration, white patches) that are independent of plaque and not typical of periodontal disease. Most likely, the diagnosis will require a biopsy.
- Is the inflammation localized to some teeth?
  - If associated with pocketing, it often indicates subgingival calculus or other local contributing factors (▶Table 3.14).
  - If associated with a subgingival restoration or implant-supported restoration, marginal erythema commonly indicates a defective margin such as an open margin or under/overcontoured profile.
  - If associated with an unrestored tooth and minimal pocketing, it may indicate a local root defect such as a pitted root surface or pronounced groove.
  - Diffuse erythema on the facial gingiva mesial to maxillary canines in the absence of other local factors (▶Table 3.14) may indicate mouth breathing. Usually, the facial profile of the patient will show an up-curled upper lip.

Using Gingival Recession as a Clue for Local Factors

Gingival recession provides a way to identify local factors that may not be detected otherwise:

- Gingival recession involving interproximal spaces is most likely due to periodontitis, and contributing factors identified as described for bone loss and pocketing.

- Localized facial/lingual recession may be due to:
  - *Ectopic tooth position*: Tooth protrudes outside of arch.
  - *Past orthodontic therapy*: Most orthodontic therapies produce a small amount of facial gingival recession, and the amount may be significant if a tooth was significantly tipped or moved facially during therapy.
  - *Aggressive brushing*: Patient uses a hard brush or scrubs teeth aggressively. This affects most likely the canines, and there may be a shallow, broad area of facial tooth wear.
  - *Smokeless tobacco*: Area of recession is adjacent to area where tobacco is usually placed by patient.
  - *Occlusal trauma*: Gingival margin has receded to apical margin of abfraction defect on a tooth with a heavy excursive contact.
  - *Clasp trauma*: Recession is caused by chronic contact with ill-fitting partial denture clasp.
  - *Past injury*: Site was injured either during dental treatment or another form of accident causing permanent recession that patient can remember.

Using Tooth Mobility as a Clue for Local Factors

Tooth mobility may be a sign of occlusal trauma:

- Evaluate tooth mobility and compare it with available radiographs.
  - Tooth mobility is most likely due to loss of support if the following is seen radiographically:
    - Poor crown-to-root ratio.
    - Short conical or slender roots.
    - Severe bone loss around the mobile tooth.
  - Tooth mobility is most likely due to primary occlusal trauma if the following is seen:
    - Widened periodontal ligament space.
    - Funnel-shaped periodontal ligament.
    - No or minor interproximal bone loss.
  - Minor tooth mobility (Miller grade I) on isolated teeth can be caused by endodontic or periodontal abscesses producing a distinct area of bone loss at the apex or the side of a tooth root.

Clinically, tooth mobility caused by primary occlusal trauma will be relatively mild (Miller grade I) and there will be other signs of occlusal trauma such as heavy centric or interference contacts on affected teeth.

3.4.5 Creating a Comprehensive Periodontal Treatment Plan

Following the process of recognizing contributing factors to periodontal disease, create a list of factors that need to be addressed. The general rules for addressing these factors are as follows:

- There is usually a corresponding treatment for each contributing factor.
- Systemic and generalized factors are addressed first.
- More complex and definite treatment is performed later.
- Once treatment is complete, there always needs to be long-term follow-up and maintenance.

The details of treatment planning are explained next.

Pretreatment Considerations

Prior to dental treatment, systemic contributing factors and any medical factors that complicate the treatment should be considered. Usually, this requires collaboration with a patient's primary physician for the following conditions (▶Table 3.15) with a consultation to assess the impact on dental care and determine the need for antibiotic prophylaxis or other treatment modifications as described in textbooks for dental management of medically complex patients.

For periodontal treatment, it may be worthwhile to consult with a physician on modifying medical treatment for the following conditions (▶Table 3.16).

Initial Treatment

Initial treatment aims to control periodontal disease by removing as many contributing factors as possible. This begins with controlling common modifiable systemic factors and local factors (▶Table 3.17[7]):

- Remove any clearly hopeless teeth (see Chapter 4—extraction decisions).
- If acute endodontic infections are present and the affected tooth is restorable, begin the root canal therapy, and provisionalize completed root canal therapy with core-build up material.
- If any plaque is present, provide oral hygiene instructions.
- If a patient uses tobacco and this is not done elsewhere, provide tobacco-cessation counseling.
- If there is an evidence of caries activity, provide nutritional counseling.
- If plaque or calculus is present, plan according to disease:
  - Prophylaxis for patients with gingivitis. If calculus is heavy, a "scaling" procedure may be used.
  - Scaling and root planing for patients with periodontitis. This is usually planned for each quadrant with deep pockets and by the number of teeth in each quadrant with deep pockets (4+ mm).
  - If this is an aggressive form of periodontitis (grade C), prescribe systemic antibiotics (i.e., 250-mg Amoxicillin and 250-mg Metronidazole every 8 hours for 1 week).
  - In case of generalized BOP, consider additional oral irrigation with iodine or antiseptic mouthrinse.
- If a patient has parafunctional habits, consider behavior-modifying techniques.
- If caries is present, remove caries and restore with direct restorations.
  - Composite/amalgam/glass ionomer definite restoration wherever feasible.
  - Core build-up for the provisional restoration of larger caries.
- Remove and replace defective direct restorations. Consider the need for crown-lengthening procedures (Chapter 6) for defective restorations with subgingival margins.
- If occlusal trauma is present, analyze the occlusion and decide if limited or comprehensive adjustment is needed.
- Re-evaluate the periodontal condition.

Surgical Treatment

Surgical periodontal treatment attempts to reduce pocketing if nonsurgical treatment failed to eliminate pocketing. This is done because pocketing poses a risk for disease progression as plaque cannot be predictably eliminated from deep pockets. Periodontal surgery can also be used to correct root anatomy defects and aid the restoration of teeth by providing better access. Surgical periodontal treatment may be attempted also to make furcation entrances more cleansable, reduce gingival recession, increase the amount of keratinized gingiva, augment bone, and place implants as a part of implant therapy.

With surgical treatment, several treatment choices that are all valid may exist, and it is difficult to predict what type of periodontal surgery may be needed at the initial exam visit. Generally, the type of periodontal problem (a.k.a., local factor associated with disease) determines the surgical treatment (see ▶Table 3.18):

- *Deep pocket depths*: If probing depths are greater than 5 mm at the initial exam, it likely seems that pocket-reduction surgery is needed after initial therapy. The type of pocket-reduction surgery usually depends on the type of bone defects associated with the deep pockets (see Chapter 6):
  - If there are no bone defects, gingival flap surgery may suffice.
  - If there are shallow bone defects (i.e., 1–2 mm deep), osseous surgery may be effective.
  - *Deep bone defects (3+ mm)*: Add regenerative surgery using bone grafts, membranes, or biologic agents to the osseous surgery already planned for the quadrant.
- *Furcation involvement*: Usually, it is only a concern if associated with deep pockets, and treated for pocket reduction. Furcation areas can also be definitely treated with treated with biologic shaping, hemisection, and root amputation (see Chapter 7).

Table 3.15 Conditions that usually require consultation with a patient's physician

Adrenal insufficiency	COPD/emphysema	Implanted medical devices
AIDS/HIV	Corticosteroid therapy	Leukemia/lymphoma
Alcohol abuse	Damaged heart valves	Myocardial infarct history
Anemia	Cardiac dysrhythmia	Obesity, morbid
Angina	Congestive heart failure	Organ transplant history
Anticoagulant therapy	COPD/emphysema	Pacemaker
Antiplatelet agents	Corticosteroid therapy	Poor nutrition
Artificial/prosthetic heart valves	Damaged heart valves	Psychiatric conditions
Asthma—severe	Dementia/Alzheimer	Recreational drug use
Atherosclerosis	Diabetes mellitus	Rh./Osteoarthritis
Autoimmune diseases	Epilepsy	Sexually transmitted disease
Bacterial endocarditis history	Genetic conditions	Sickle cell anemia
Bleeding disorders	GERD	Stroke
Cancer	Hepatitis	Thyroid disorders
Chemo/radiation therapy	Hypertension	Total joint replacement
Cardiac dysrhythmia	Immunosuppressive agents	Tuberculosis
Congestive heart failure		

Table 3.16 Systemic factors associated with periodontal disease that may be modified by a patient's physician

Specific factor	Suggested change
Amphetamines	If possible, switch medication if the current patient medication causes gingival overgrowth
Calcium channel blockers	
Cyclosporine, Tacrolimus, Sirolimus	
Dilantin/Phenytoin	
Phenobarbital	
Valproic acid	
Anti-HIV medications (some) and gray discoloration	If possible, consider switching medication. Discoloration usually is permanent.
Minocycline and gray gingival discoloration	
Estrogen replacement	If possible, change medication or contraceptive method
Xerostomic medications and actual xerostomia	If possible, change medication; consider pilocarpine
Medication known to cause lichenoid reaction and actual lichenoid lesions	If possible, change medication
AIDS	Successful medical treatment also helps resolve periodontal disease. Supportive periodontal therapy (gentle antiseptic mouth wash)
Leukemia/lymphoma	
Chemotherapy	
Radiation therapy and oral mucositis	
Cancer (including oral cancer)	Extract questionable teeth; Maintenance after therapy
Pregnancy and hormonal changes	End of pregnancy usually resolves problem. Supportive periodontal therapy (cleanings,
Sexually transmitted disease and oral ulcers/growths	Medical treatment resolves problem. Supportive periodontal therapy
Stroke and decreased manual dexterity	Modify oral hygiene method
Dementia/Alzheimer and decreased manual dexterity	
Rh./Osteoarthritis and decreased manual dexterity	
Decreased manual dexterity	
Diabetes mellitus	Encourage best possible glycemic control
Obesity	Consider medical weight management
Poor nutrition	Consider referral to registered dietitian
Genetic conditions	No change. Supportive periodontal therapy; more aggressive periodontal therapy with IL-1 genotype
IL-1 genotype	
Autoimmune diseases	Successful medical treatment may help resolve problem. Supportive periodontal therapy
Tobacco use	Consider referral for counseling/addiction therapy
Recreational drug use	
Alcohol use	

- *Soft tissue defects*: Most commonly, gingival recession is treated with connective tissue grafting, but can also be treated with various other techniques. Lack of keratinized gingiva is often treated with a free gingival graft (see Chapter 8).
- Tooth mobility is often treated as an occlusal problem, and may involve splinting along with occlusal analysis and adjustment (see Chapter 9).

If surgical periodontal therapy lasts longer than 3 months, the patient should also receive maintenance treatment (▶Table 3.19). This helps to control periodontal disease in areas that have not received surgical treatment yet, and helps to maintain improvement gained from periodontal surgery. One way to accomplish this is to schedule surgeries, postop visits, and maintenance visits in a pattern for each quadrant:

- Surgery in quadrant.
- Postop visit (1 week after surgery).
- Evaluation and maintenance (6 weeks after surgery).
- Wait another 6 weeks, and start next quadrant.

Table 3.17 Initial therapy treatment planning

Factor	Treatment	CDT code
Hopeless teeth of no value	Extraction (no complication expected), by tooth	D7140
	Surgical extraction (has complicating factors), by tooth	D7210
Partially impacted teeth	Removal of impacted tooth—soft tissue, by tooth	D7220
	Removal of impacted tooth—partially bony, by tooth	D7230
Acute root canal infection	Root canal treatment, by tooth	D3310. D3320, D3330
	Retreatment of failed root canal treatment, by tooth	D3346
	Core build-up, by tooth	D2950
Caries/nutrition issue	Nutrition counseling	D1310
Tobacco use	Tobacco cessation counseling	D1320
Plaque Aggressive brushing	Oral hygiene instruction	D1330
Calculus	If gingivitis:	
	and low-moderate calculus: prophylaxis	D1110
	and high amount of calculus: scaling	D4346
	If periodontitis:	
	1–3 teeth with 4+ mm pockets, per quadrant	D4342
	4+ teeth with 4+ mm pockets, per quadrant	D4341
	Oral irrigation, per quadrant	D4921
Caries	Direct restorations, per surfaces and teeth	(various)
Open margin	Provisional crown, per tooth (if not part of definite crown)	D2799
Overhang		
Rough surface		
Open contact		
Fracture		
Bulky contour		
Occlusal trauma	Occlusal analysis	D9950
	Occlusal adjustment, limited	D9951
	Occlusal adjustment, complete	D9952
	Re-evaluation	D0120

Maintenance

Once periodontal disease has been successfully treated, treatment must focus on preventing more disease with the appropriate maintenance procedure at the appropriate time interval based on risk (see Chapter 4). Once periodontal disease is controlled, definite treatment of remaining disease-contributing factors that require more complex therapy can be completed. The general sequence of more complex treatment after surgical periodontal therapy is as follows (▶ Table 3.19):

• Orthodontic therapy if needed (or feasible).
• Indirect restorations.
• Implant therapy (or/and removable partial dentures if needed).
• Occlusal guard (if needed).
• Long-term preventive strategies to prevent recurrent caries (i.e., fluoride application).

Long-term prevention of periodontal disease consists of continuing monitoring and removal of new contributing factors to periodontal disease. At a minimum, this consists of continued removal of plaque and calculus deposits. The appropriate procedure depends on the initial diagnosis (▶ Table 3.19):

• *Gingivitis*: Prophylaxis.
• *Periodontitis*: Periodontal maintenance.

The frequency of these procedures needs to be determined for the risk of disease progression (see Chapter 4). Generally, the frequency of evaluation and maintenance follows the original diagnosis at first, can be shortened or lengthened once the patient's periodontal disease behavior is better known:

• *Health*: Evaluation and prophylaxis every 6 to 12 months depending on calculus build-up.
• *Gingivitis*: Evaluation and prophylaxis every 4 to 6 months depending on the level of inflammation.
• *Periodontitis*: Evaluation and periodontal maintenance every 3 months.

Table 3.18 Basic surgical periodontal treatment overview

Factor	Factor detail	Treatment	CDT code
Residual deep pocketing, Inflammation after nonsurgical treatment	No bone loss	Gingivectomy, 1–3 teeth	D4212
	excess gingiva gingival overgrowth	Gingivectomy, 4+ teeth	D4211
	No bone defect, single site distal-most tooth	Distal wedge/proximal wedge	D4274
	No bone defect or anterior maxilla	Gingival flap, 1–3 teeth, per quadrant	D4241
		Gingival flap, 4+ teeth, per quadrant	D4240
	Shallow bone defect and not anterior maxilla	Osseous surgery, 1–3 teeth, per quadrant	D4261
		Osseous surgery, 4+ teeth, per quadrant	D4260
	Deep bone defect*	+ Bone graft, and/or	D4263
		+ GTR (resorbable), and/or	D4266
		+ biologic materials	D4265
Enamel projections		+ Odontoplasty**, or	D9971
Root concavities		hemisection (mandibular teeth), or	D3920
Enamel pearls		root amputation (maxillary molars)	D3450
Cervical projections		may also require new crown, core-build up, RCT for furcation treatment, depending on case	(various)
Dentin ridges			
Unusual anatomy			
Furcation involvement			
Cemental tears			
Gingival recession	Single, isolated facial/lingual*	Lateral pedicle flap, per tooth, or	D4270
		Connective tissue graft, per tooth	D4273
	Several facial/lingual*	Connective tissue graft, or	D4273
		Allodermal matrix graft	
	Many facial/lingual	Allodermal matrix graft	D4275
Mucogingival defect	Not anterior maxilla	Free gingival graft, first tooth	D4277
	Anterior maxilla (unlikely)	Connective tissue graft or allodermal matrix graft	D4273 or D4275
		Periodontal re-evaluation	D0120
		Postoperative visit	D0171

* The surgery used for these defects depends on defect anatomy, patient characteristics and surgeon preference.
**Odontoplasty may be performed simply as part of osseous surgery in some cases.
Abbreviation: GTR: guided tissue regeneration. For convenience, most often resorbable membranes are used.

3.5 Identify Uncommon Periodontal Diseases

Some patients will have additional periodontal diseases that overlay existing gingivitis or periodontitis, or have other diseases that happen to manifest themselves in the periodontal tissues. For diagnosing these conditions, it may be useful to identify the key characteristic that distinguishes the condition or disease from ordinary gingivitis or periodontitis:
- BOP, pocketing, or bone loss around implants.
- Localized severe bone loss to apex/near apex on a single tooth.
- Localized tissue soft swelling or fistula tract.
- Firm, rubbery enlargement of interdental papillae unresponsive to initial plaque control.
- Patchy severe erythema unresponsive to initial plaque control.
- Ulceration.
- Tissue necrosis.
- Severe pain.

Based on this key characteristic, differential diagnoses can be made and ruled out one-by-one.

Table 3.19 Periodontal maintenance phase

Factor	Factor detail	Treatment	CDT code
Prevent further disease by removing plaque, calculus	Gingivitis/health	Prophylaxis	D1110
	Periodontitis	Periodontal Maintenance	D4910
Caries risk		Fluoride varnish application	D1206
		Application of interim caries arresting medication (silver diamine)	D1354
		Xylitol supplements	
		Antiseptic rinse	
		Nutrition counseling	
Crowding		(Finish) Orthodontic therapy	(various)
Ortho. appliances			
Rotated teeth			
Tipped teeth			
Severe Angle II			
Severe Angle III			
Excess Overjet			
Excess Overbite			
Margin discrepancy			
infra/supra-erupted			
Provisionalized teeth		Inlays, onlays, per tooth	(various)
Open margin		Crowns, per tooth	
Overhang		Pre-fabricated posts	
Rough surface			
Open contact			
Bulky contour			
Missing teeth		Implant therapy, and/or	
		Fixed partial dentures, and/or	
		Removable partial dentures	
Bruxism		Occlusal guard	D9940
Clenching			
		Periodontal re-evaluation	

* The surgery used for these defects depends on defect anatomy, patient characteristics and surgeon preference.
**Odontoplasty may be performed simply as part of osseous surgery in some cases.
Abbreviation: GTR: guided tissue regeneration. For convenience, most often resorbable membranes are used.

3.5.1 Bleeding on Probing, Pocketing, or Bone Loss around Implants

Implants should be surrounded by healthy tissue that tightly adapted to the implant with minimal probing depths and no BOP. However, implants may develop disease analogous to periodontal disease, and the following is needed for diagnosis:
- Clinical findings (BOP, pocket depths).
- Bone relative to implant platform (at platform, within 2 mm of it, greater than 2 mm).
  - If available, radiographs of the same implant can be taken since implant placement.
- Time of implant placement (within months, last 1–2 years, more than 5 years ago).

The differential list of possible implant diagnoses includes the following conditions:
- Peri-implant mucositis.[8]
- Peri-implantitis.[9]
- Other conditions:
  - Pocketing caused by deep placement relative to surrounding teeth or implants.
  - Improper implant position.
  - Bone loss caused by placement or restoration techniques.
  - Failure of implant components.
  - Bone loss centered around the apex of the implant.

Peri-implant Mucositis

This is condition may develop as a result of poor oral hygiene around implants or defective implant restorations that retain plaque. Its key characteristics are as follows (▶Fig. 3.7):
- Clinical signs:
  - Significant erythema, BOP; suppuration may be present.
  - May show increased pocketing.
  - Visible plaque accumulation or presence of plaque-retentive factors.
- Radiographic signs:
  - No or minimal bone loss around the implant platform (less than 2 mm).
  - If past radiographs are available, no additional bone loss since restoration.
- Implant and restoration have been in place for at least several weeks.

Usually, nonsurgical periodontal therapy also is effective for treating peri-implant mucositis.

Peri-implantitis

This condition develops in about 30 to 50% of implants about a decade after placement. This condition usually is associated with a history or periodontitis, infrequent maintenance, smoking or diabetes.

Key characteristics are as follows (▶Fig. 3.7):
- *Clinical signs*: Same as peri-implant mucositis including high plaque level.
- *Radiographic signs:*
  - Significant bone loss around the implant platform (2 mm or more).
  - Progressive bone loss over time.
- Implant was placed and restored more than 2 years ago.

Treatment usually requires surgical therapy, but it is unclear yet which method is most effective.

Other Conditions

Other, relatively uncommon conditions may cause inflammation, pocketing, and unusual bone loss around implants. These conditions can be identified as follows.

Pocketing Caused by Deep Placement Relative to Surrounding Teeth or Implants

Clinically, there will be increased probing depths, and may be signs of inflammation depending on the probing depth. Radiographically, bone level is near the platform, but the platform is located much more apical compared to the bone level of surrounding teeth or implants.

Improper Implant Position

Clinical and radiographic signs will depend on the implant position:
- *Too far buccal*: Implant restoration will likely appear longer than surrounding teeth or have gingival recession, or the implant may show as a dark gingival shadow.
- *Too far distal/mesial*: This is apparent radiographically, and not a concern as long as it allows proper restoration and does not create a hygiene problem.
- *Tipped*: This will be apparent radiographically and not a concern as long as the implant is restorable and does not create an esthetic or mechanical issue. Tipped placement of the implant may be mandated by the existing bone, but should not exceed 30 degrees.

Bone Loss Caused by Placement or Restoration Techniques

Clinically, this becomes apparent within weeks or months after the last implant procedure, and usually causes rapid bone loss or implant mobility as the implant fails to osseointegrate. Common causes are as follows:
- Overheating alveolar bone with improper drilling technique (caused by dull burs, too much pressure, and not enough irrigation).
- Lack of primary stability during placement.
- Heavy occlusal load during healing on immediately restored implants.
- Extruded cement after cementation of implant restoration.

Failure of Implant Components

Clinically, failure of implant components usually results in mobility of the implant restoration, and may produce

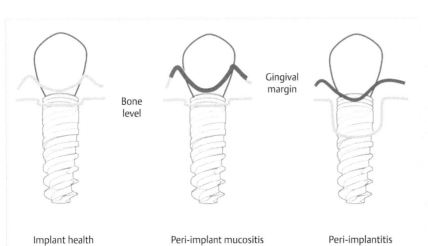

Bone level

Gingival margin

Implant health

Peri-implant mucositis

Peri-implantitis

Fig. 3.7 The two main peri-implant diseases are peri-implant mucositis, which produces swollen, erythematous inflamed tissue around implants with no bone loss, and peri-implantitis, which results in bone loss around implants.

inflammation, pocketing, or bone loss. Radiographically, fracture of an implant component will be apparent, and usually this will be retaining screw inside the abutment.

Bone Loss Centered Around the Apex of the Implant

This will appear as radiolucent change around the apex of an implant reminiscent of a root canal infection in teeth. Typically, this occurs at sites with a history of recurrent root canal infections.

3.5.2 Localized Severe Bone Loss to Apex/Near Apex on a Single Tooth

Isolated severe bone loss to the apex most commonly suggests endodontic disease, and requires endodontic tests such as pulp vitality tests and percussion testing for diagnosis. The differential list of conditions causing isolated severe bone loss to the apex are:
- Perio-endodontic lesions (most common).[10]
- Root fractures.
- Periodontal abscess (rare).
- Local malignant neoplasms (exceedingly rare).

Perio-endodontic Lesions

Perio-endodontic lesions are not as common as purely endodontic infections, and may develop either from preexisting deep pockets, endodontic infections, or combinations of both (▶ Fig. 3.8). Key characteristics are as follows:
- Clinical:
  - Isolated very deep probing depths (i.e., 10+ mm) and attachment loss that reaches toward the apex. Absence of calculus within the pocket suggests primary endodontic origin.
  - Pulp vitality tests demonstrate questionable pulp vitality or there is a reason to doubt the success of previous root canal therapy (i.e., deep recurrent caries).
- Radiographic:
  - Large, often J-shaped area of bone loss reaching and wrapping around the apex. The shape and degree of radiolucency can range from very subtle if the lesion

is developing or surrounded by dense cortical bone, to easily identifiable long-standing lesions (see ▶ Fig. 3.9, for radiographic variations).
  - If previously treated, defective root canal treatment (i.e., short; has voids, low-density filling; signs of transportation, ledging; contains broken instrument).

Treatment is either by tooth removal or attempting root canal treatment, followed by the pocket-reduction surgery or root amputation/hemisection.

Root Fractures

Vertical root fractures typically produce complete and wide bone loss around the fractured tooth, and the fracture may be obvious on radiographs. Fine fractures may be detected with transillumination or by endodontic microscopy using dyes. If the fracture is recent, it may be associated with a narrow, deep pocket. Fractured teeth are not restorable and need to be removed.

Periodontal Abscess

Periodontal abscesses are much less common than endodontic abscesses. Key features are as follows:
- Clinical:
  - Deep probing depths and presence of purulent discharge when initially probing the area.
  - Deep pocket usually contains calculus at the base of the pocket.
  - Vital pulp or no reason to doubt success of previous root canal treatment.
- Radiographic:
  - Bone loss is centered away from apex, usually the side of the root or at a furcation.
  - If previously treated, no apparent deficiency in root canal treatment and restoration.
  - Abnormal root anatomy such as an enamel pearl or furcation grooves may be seen.

Immediate treatment is by scaling and root planing and possible antibiotics if there are systemic signs of infection (i.e., fever, lymph node swelling). Teeth with recurrent periodontal abscesses may need to be removed.

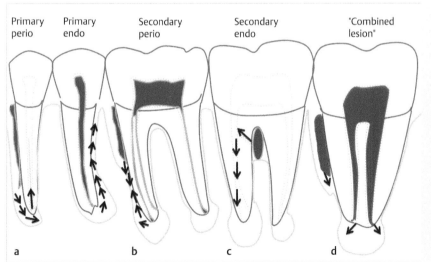

Primary perio | Primary endo | Secondary perio | Secondary endo | "Combined lesion"

a   b   c   d

Fig. 3.8 Different types of perioendodontic lesions based on origin (Simon Glick Frank classification): lesions of primary periodontal origin are caused by severe periodontitis reaching the apex. Lesions of primary endodontic origin are caused by pulpal infection. Lesions of secondary periodontal origin are caused by an endontic infection that then fuses with bone loss caused by periodontitis. Lesions of secondary endodontic origin are caused by periodontal diseases that compromise blood supply. "Combined lesions" happen when there are two independent endodontic and periodontic lesions found on the same tooth. (a-d) Perioendodontic lesions can have varied radiographic appearances.

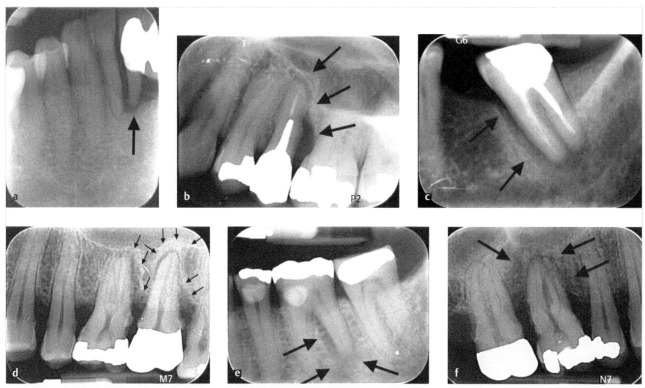

Fig. 3.9 It is important to recognize perioendodontic lesions on radiographs as their appearance ranges from obvious to very subtle as shown in this range of examples. (Most obvious **a** to least obvious **f**, lesions indicated by *arrows*). All teeth with lesions had very deep pocketing reaching to the apex, and questionable pulp vitality. (**a**, **c**, and **e**) are most likely endodontic in origin given the round periapical area of bone loss and low amount of generalized bone loss at other teeth. (**b**) Lesion suggests root fracture or perforation at post level. (**d**) Likely of periodontal origin as suggested by calculus, generalized bone loss, and narrow area of periapical bone loss. (**f**) Lesion is likely the combined result of periodontal disease (calculus, furcation involvement, unusual root anatomy) and endodontic infection (distal caries with pulpal involvement).

Local Malignancy

While exceedingly rare, this is a possibility if the other differential diagnoses have been ruled out and if the local bone loss is not explainable as a consequence of unique local anatomy or occlusal trauma. Likely key features are as follows:

- Clinical:
  - Does not improve with endodontic and periodontal therapy.
  - *Shows other unusual signs and symptoms that slowly become worse*: Pain, gingival ulceration, swelling, discoloration, and displacement of tooth.
- Radiographic:
  - *Shows signs of malignancy*: Tooth resorption, loss of crestal bone and lamina dura, and invades and destroys adjacent structures.

Any lesion that does not respond to periodontal and endodontic therapy, or does not heal properly after extraction, needs to be biopsied for diagnosis.

3.5.3 Localized Soft Tissue Swelling or Fistula Tract

The typical differential for solitary soft tissue swelling from common to rare includes the following:
- Endodontic abscesses.
- Gingival abscesses.[10]

- Pericoronitis.
- Periodontal abscesses.[10]
- Various neoplasms.

Endodontic Abscesses

This is by far the most common cause of localized tissue swellings and fistula tracts. Key features are as follows:
- Clinical:
  - Soft tissue swelling in mucosa usually on buccal side, near the root apices.
  - Soft tissue swelling is adjacent to nonvital teeth.
  - Typically adjacent to a tooth with severe caries or other form of pulp exposure.
  - Often contains fistula tract that can be probed with a gutta-percha point.
- Radiographic:
  - Typically presents as radiolucent area centered at apex of tooth (▶ Fig. 3.10).
  - Gutta-percha point inserted into fistula points toward apex.

Treatment is by root canal treatment of adjacent nonvital teeth, which should resolve the fistula.

Gingival Abscesses

If foreign material, such as hard food fragments or toothbrush bristles, becomes lodged in oral mucosa, it may form a superficial abscess. This and periodontal abscesses are one of the few

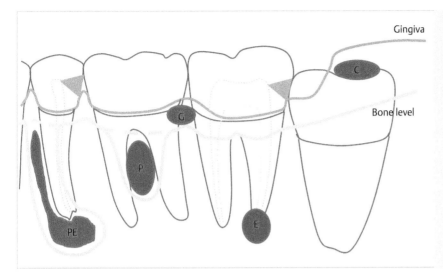

Fig. 3.10 Abscess types. C—periocoronal abscess found under operculum partially covering a partially erupted tooth. E- endodontic abscess on a tooth with caries extending to the pulp. G—gingival abscess that is often caused by impacted foreign objects such as seeds, and stay outside of the alveolar bone. P—periodontal abscess that causes bone loss below the surrounding bone level. PE—combined periodontal-endodontic lesion.

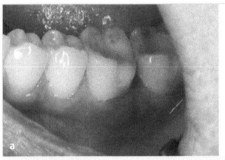

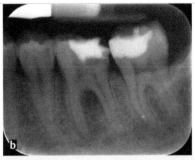

					PLQ
					Mobil
					Furc Inv
					MGJ
					AGR
B B	B B B	B B B	B B B		Bleed/S
					CAL
2 1 2	3 2 3	3 2 3	4 2 4	5 5 4	PD
22	21	20	19	18	17
					PLQ
					Calc. surf
					Furc Inv
					MGJ
					AGR
B		B B B B			Bleed/S
					CAL
2 1 2	2 1 3	3 1 3	4 6 4	4 3 4	PD

Fig. 3.11 Periodontal abscess clinical view, probing data and radiograph. (**a**) A 21-year old healthy female presented with a painful swelling on tooth no. 19, which displays a small fistula and drains purulent discharge. (**b**) A radiograph shows bone loss in the furcation area, which along with moderately deep pocketing (**c**) into the furcation area and same area of the fistula suggesting a periodontal abscess. Incidentally, this tooth also had a large restoration impinging on the pulp chamber. As consequence, a periapical lesion is forming, and it may fuse with the existing periodontal bone loss to form a combined periodontal endodontic lesion. The tooth was extracted since the patient was not interested in saving the tooth.

periodontal diseases that can cause significant pain. Key features are as follows:

- Clinical:
  - Typically, isolated soft tissue swelling near the gingival margin or on cheek mucosa near the occlusal plane (▶Fig. 3.10).
  - Typically, the patient recalls recent onset of swelling and significant pain.
  - Usually, the swelling contains a foreign body.
  - Adjacent teeth are vital.
  - Older abscesses may show superficial purulent material or a fistula.
- *Radiographic*: No sign of bone loss.

Treatment involves scaling and root planing adjacent teeth, and removing the foreign object.

Pericoronitis

Pericoronitis may be seen as a variant of a gingival abscess that is located under the tissue flap overlying a partially erupted tooth. Key features are as follows:

- Clinical:
  - Swollen, inflamed tissue flap overlying a partial erupted tooth (▶Fig. 3.10).
  - Tissue flap may have tooth marks from opposing tooth.

  - Severely painful, especially if the patient closes.
- Radiographic:
  - Partially erupted tooth in area of painful tissue flap.

Periodontal Abscess

Calculus in deep periodontal pockets may become enclosed by overlying gingiva and form an abscess (see ▶Fig. 3.11 for case). Key features are as follows:

- Clinical:
  - Deep probing depth with suppuration when tissue is probed initially.
  - Causes pain.
  - Typically, there is underlying periodontitis with a history of deep pockets or furcation involvement.
  - Tooth is vital or has been treated previously with high-quality root canal treatment.
- Radiographical:
  - Localized deep bone loss; often within a furcation entrance.
  - No periapical bone loss.

Neoplasm

Solitary tissue swellings that slowly enlarge may also be created by neoplasms. If a single localized swelling cannot be explained as result of either endodontic or periodontal infection, it should be biopsied and analyzed by an oral pathologist for malignancy.

3.5.4 Firm, Rubbery Enlargement of Interdental Papillae

Interdental papilla may enlarge for the following reasons from common to rare:
- Inflammation caused by plaque and calculus.
- Drug-induced gingival enlargement.
- Hereditary gingival enlargement (very rare).
- Malignant infiltrate (very rare).

As soft tissue condition, there is usually no radiographic sign of this condition. In any case, any gingival enlargement that is not resolving through periodontal therapy should be biopsied for diagnosis.

Inflammation Caused by Plaque and Calculus

This is common, but resolves usually with nonsurgical periodontal treatment. Key features are as follows:
- Clinical:
  ○ Typical signs of periodontitis or gingivitis.
  ○ Bulbous smooth, erythematous papilla tips.
  ○ Visible plaque near gingival margin or plaque-retentive factor (i.e., open margin).
  ○ Nonsurgical periodontal therapy largely resolves the condition.
- *Radiographic*: May see radiographic calculus or open margin.

Drug-induced Gingival Enlargement

Key features are as follows:
- Clinical:
  ○ Typically produces firm, rubbery papilla. Papilla may have pebbly texture.
  ○ Patient takes medication associated with gingival enlargement:
    – Cyclosporin, phenytoin/dilantin, calcium channel blockers, and amphetamine.
  ○ Nonsurgical periodontal therapy resolves inflammation, but not the enlargement and pocketing at the site.
  ○ Plaque control slows down the growth of papillae, or may prevent further growth.
- *Radiographic*: May have thickened gingival shadow.

Hereditary Gingival Enlargement

Rare genetic conditions, such as hereditary gingival fibromatosis, may cause slow down enlargement of the papillae and gingival margin independent of plaque level. Key features are as follows:
- Clinical:
  ○ Slow generalized growth of gingival margin.
  ○ Results in "gummy smile," and gingiva may completely cover teeth.
  ○ May have family history of enlarging gums.
  ○ Biopsy reveals excess connective tissue matrix, but normal cells and little inflammation.
- Radiographic:
  ○ Thick gingival shadow.

Malignant Infiltrate

It is unlikely that generalized gingival enlargement is caused by a local neoplasm, which usually forms a solid tissue mass. The exception to this are forms of leukemia, where malignant cells may infiltrate the gingiva around teeth, causing slow enlargement. In a dental setting, this should be extremely rare because, most likely, leukemia will be detected by a patient's physician prior to onset of oral signs and symptoms. Key features likely are as follows:
- Clinical:
  ○ Gingival enlargement.
  ○ May have spontaneous gingival bleeding.
  ○ Patient will have signs and symptoms of leukemia (weight loss, proclivity to infections, bruising, and fatigue).
  ○ Incisional biopsy will reveal malignant leukocyte infiltrate.
- *Radiographic*: May have progressive crestal bone loss and root resorption

3.5.5 Patchy Severe Erythema

Common periodontal diseases respond to plaque control with decreased inflammation. If gingival erythema does not resolve after low plaque levels have been achieved, it is most likely due to other disease processes. Generally, this is uncommon, and is caused by the following rare conditions:
- Allergic reactions.
- Autoimmune conditions.
- Localized infections and granulomas not caused by plaque.
- Localized malignancy or premalignant lesions.

In order to diagnose these conditions, a thorough history and biopsy of the affected area is needed. Usually, there is no radiographic evidence as these conditions affect soft tissue, not hard tissue. Generally, the steps to diagnose the conditions are to first have the patient avoid spicy foods and use a bland oral hygiene regimen, and then biopsy affected areas if the erythema does not resolve within 2 weeks.

Allergic Reactions

Allergic reactions in the oral cavity are uncommon, but may be triggered by foods, oral hygiene materials, or dental materials. Key features are as follows:
- Usually produces generalized to patchy erythema throughout mouth.
- May be accompanied by a generalized burning sensation.
- Usually, the patient remembers recent onset of the condition, and a possible trigger (i.e., last dental visit; ate a certain food or used a new toothpaste).
- Condition resolves on its own with bland food and gentle oral hygiene without toothpaste and mouth rinse within 1 to 2 weeks.

Autoimmune Reactions

Many different autoimmune conditions may manifest themselves early in the gingiva as this area is subject to frequent mechanical trauma from eating and chemical attack by bacteria. These conditions include lichenoid reactions toward oral medications and restorative materials as well as rare to very rare autoimmune conditions such as pemphigus vulgaris, mucous membrane pemphigoid, lichen planus, and lupus erythematosus. Generally, management of these conditions requires a complete physical exam by the patient's physician and further medical management. Local lesions can be treated with the application of topical steroids.

Key features are as follows (see ▶ Fig. 3.12):
- Patchy erythema starting at the gingival margin and extending possibly to the vestibular mucos.
- May also show white scarring, or thin white tissue slough.
- Rubbing gingiva or mucosa may result in blister formation or loss of superficial tissue layer (Nikolsky sign).
- Often, patients complain of a burning sensation.
- Gradual onset, and slow worsening of the condition.
- Incisional biopsy reveals abnormal findings suggestive of specific diseases:
  - Intraepithelial blister formation: Pemphigus vulgaris.
  - Separation of connective tissue and gingival epithelium: Pemphigoid.
  - Band of lymphocyte infiltrates in lamina propria and sawtooth rete pegs: Lichen planus and lichenoid reactions.
  - Perivascular lymphocyte infiltrates: Lupus erythematosus.

Localized Infections and Granulomas not Caused by Plaque

Although rare, single localized patches can be caused by granulomas and infections not typically associated with oral disease. This may include the following:
- Focal infections caused by bartonella species, mycobacterium species (tuberculosis), neisseria species (gonorrhea), treponema species (syphilis), histoplasma species (histoplasmosis), or other microorganisms. This is usually seen in severely immunocompromised patients (i.e., AIDS).
- Granulomatous reactions to oral bacteria, such as pyogenic granuloma, peripheral giant cell fibroma, and peripheral ossifying fibroma.

In this case, a lesion that does not respond to plaque and calculus removal and oral hygiene instruction after 2 weeks should be biopsied. Histology may provide enough information for a diagnosis, or suggests a further microbial culture of the lesion. There are no other unifying characteristics.

Localized Malignancy or Premalignant Lesions

Although it is very unlikely that oral malignancy will result in multiple erythematous patches, it is possible in some conditions such as erosive lichen planus. Incisional biopsy of these patches may reveal squamous cell carcinoma or severe epithelial dysplasia.

3.5.6 Ulceration

Ulceration is highly unusual for periodontal disease, and most likely caused by other disease processes. Unless there is an obvious explanation for the ulceration from the patient's history or disease presentation, persistent ulcerative lesions should be biopsied in order to investigate the presence of malignancy or autoimmune disease. The following conditions may produce gingival ulcers from common to rare:
- Trauma.
- Autoimmune diseases.
- Viral diseases.
- Malignant neoplasms.

Trauma

Trauma is a common cause of single ulcers and lacerations in the mouth, and usually it is readily identified as the patient will remember the incident (▶ Fig. 3.13). Key characteristics are as follows:
- Usually, a single isolated ulcer.
- Usually remembers when and what caused the ulcer. The offending agent could be heat (i.e., hot food; a hot handpiece head), chemical (i.e., bleach from a root canal procedure), or mechanical (i.e., broken denture clasp; floss cut).
- Ulcer will close on its own at a rate of 0.5 to 1 mm/day unless re-injured.

Autoimmune Diseases

Autoimmune diseases may produce shallow irregular ulcers if they damage the basement membrane or overlying epithelium. A biopsy is required for diagnosis (see Section 3.5.5).

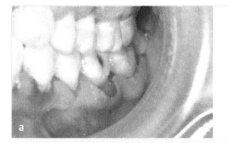 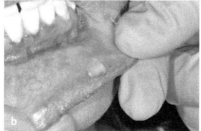 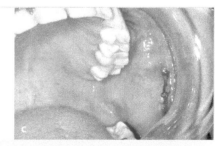

Fig. 3.12 Pemphigus vulgaris case: a 31-year old Hispanic female presented complaining of sore gums, and clinical evaluation revealed widespread shallow ulcerations (**a**) and blisters (**b**) in the oral cavity. Simply rubbing the cheek mucosa with the back side of a mouth mirror caused stripping of the mucosa, leaving a bleeding ulcer, which is considered a positive Nikolsky sign (**c**).

Viral Diseases

Viral infections, such as herpes, varicella, and coxsackie, produce clusters of shallow round ulcers that may be extremely painful, and resolve within 2 weeks. The patient's history, and distribution of ulcers may provide clues for the origin:

- *Varicella*: Ulcers may outline dermatome; usually seen in older adults ("shingles").
- *Herpes*: May be seen as primary herpetic gingivostomatitis in young children with ulcers covering entire gingiva; rare in adults, and usually suggests immunocompromised state (i.e., AIDS).
- *Coxsackie*: Lesions also on extremities (hand foot and mouth disease).

Malignant Neoplasms

Neoplasms generally produce a single ulcer within an area of enlarged tissue, unless there is severe metastatic disease. Generally, there will be a history of a slowly enlarging tissue mass that eventually ulcerates in the center. Often, these ulcers will be painless and go unnoticed for years.

3.5.7 Tissue Necrosis

Tissue necrosis or tissue die-off is highly unusual in the oral cavity, especially if it is not provoked by recent trauma (i.e., surgery trauma). Tissue necrosis will present with the following characteristics in the mouth:

- Severe pain.
- Intense mouth odor.
- Area(s) where tissue has disappeared. The tissue adjacent to this area will have a gray, friable rim, followed by intense erythema, and normal appearing tissue.

The only condition apart from trauma that causes progressive tissue necrosis, starting from the papilla tip and progressing down the alveolar bone, is necrotizing periodontal diseases.[10] Generally, these conditions are called based on the degree of tissue destruction:

- *Necrotizing gingivitis*: Loss of interdental papilla epithelium (see ▶ Fig. 3.14, for mild case).
- *Necrotizing periodontitis*: Exposure of interdental bone.
- *Necrotizing stomatitis*: Loss of tissue extends into vestibule.
- *Orofacial gangrene/noma*: Loss of tissue extends onto facial tissues.

Generally, these necrotizing periodontal diseases are triggered by severe stress, malnutrition, or immunocompromised state (i.e., AIDS, chemotherapy).

For urgent dental treatment, necrotic lesions should be gently debrided with local anesthesia until bleeding occurs, and a broad-spectrum antibiotic, such as 875-mg Augmentin twice a day for 1 to 2 weeks should be prescribed. The underlying systemic condition predisposing the patient to necrotizing periodontal disease should be addressed and reversed with improved nutrition, rest, and control of any immunosuppressive conditions.

3.6 Essential Takeaways

- Periodontal disease presents in various manifestations and complexities. Gingivitis and periodontitis are the most common and prevalent in the population.
- Influences such as severity of inflammation, depth of inflammation, and extent of inflammation as well as

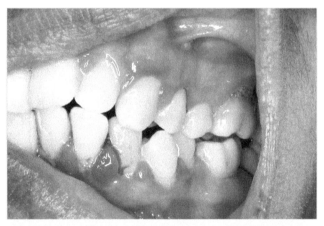

Fig. 3.14 Necrotizing periodontitis. Severe gingival inflammation bordering on necrotizing periodontal disease in a 44-year old otherwise healthy female complaining of pain and mouth odor. Very heavy subgingival calculus causes intensely inflamed tissue that produces milky exudate and light sloughing at the papilla tips that suggests the beginning of necrotizing periodontal disease.

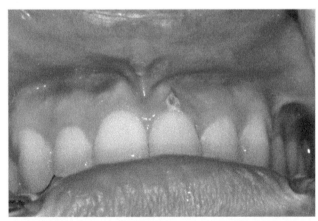

Fig. 3.13 Ulceration as a result of bleach and mechanical trauma during root canal treatment.

microbial, systemic, and local factors will establish a diagnosis of health, gingivitis, or the various stages and grades of periodontitis.

- Periodontal disease is categorized according to the American Academy of Periodontology classification system. Stages I to IV of this disease are related to the depth of inflammation previously described as mild, moderate, or severe. Grading from A to C is related to the virulence or rate of disease progression as slow, moderate, or rapid. The default is grade B.
- Peri-implant mucositis and peri-implantitis are implant analogs to gingivitis and periodontitis in natural teeth. Terminology has changed as the classification system changed.
- Appropriate treatment (nonsurgical vs. surgical) can be instituted by accurate diagnosis from the groupings. Surgical treatment is instituted after nonsurgical therapy has failed to eliminate pocketing.
- Disease classification is subject to change. Knowledge and definitions evolve due to the multi-factorial and dynamic nature of periodontal disease.

3.7 Review Questions

For the following questions, consider this case.

A 27-year old refugee presents to you with a concern about pain in several teeth and loose front teeth. He denies having any medical conditions, using medications or supplements, and does not have any allergies. He saw a dentist 4 years ago for the removal of loose and painful teeth, and received "some other work" back then from a free dental clinic. He smokes one pack of cigarettes per day, and brushes his teeth as shown by the previous dentist. He does not floss unless he feels food gets stuck between his teeth. Given his young age, microbial sampling was performed with the following results:

A. actinomycetemcomitans not detectable

Campylobacter: not detectable

F. nucleatum: 0.5%

P. gingivalis: 1.5%

P. intermedia: 0.3%

T. forsythia: 1.2%

Spirochetes: 0.4%

Enteric rods: not detectable

Staphylococci: not detectable

Beta streptococci: not detectable

Yeasts: 0.1%

Here is the patient's condition (see ▸Fig. 3.15 for clinical appearance and ▸Fig. 3.16 for radiographs).

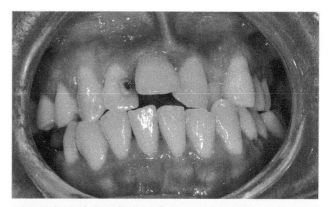

Fig. 3.15 Facial view of review case.

Findings in the periodontal chart are as follows:

Maxilla facial	1	2	3	4	5	6	7	8	9	10	11	12	13	14	15	16
PD	524	524	524	524	425	425	423	426	524	423	324	523	323	646	436	534
BOP	111	111	111	111	111	111						111	111	111	111	111
CAL	1	1	1	1	1	1		1	1					1	1	1
GR																
MGJ	334	435	536	647	757	757	767	646	646	678	647	646	434	646	646	634
Furc																
PLQ	3	3	3	3	3	3	3	3	3	3	3	3	3	3	3	3
Maxilla lingual																
PD	335	536	536	635	525	523	324	669	623	322	322	323	323	325	537	744
BOP	111	111	111	111	111	111	111				11	111	111	111	111	111
CAL																
GR																
Furc																
Mobil				1					1							
PLQ	3	3	3	3	3	3	3	3	3	3	3	3	3	3	3	3

Mandible lingual	32	31	30	29	28	27	26	25	24	23	22	21	20	19	18	17
PD	324				424	423	323	323	423	324	223	434	435	435	537	723
BOP	11				111							111	111			
CAL															2	3
GR																
MGJ	999	999	999	999	999	999	999	997	799	999	999	999	999	999	999	999
Furc																
PLQ	3	3	3	3	3	3	3	3	3	3	3	3	3	3	3	3
Mandible facial																
PD	324				424	423	323	323	423	324	424	425	423	324	427	663
BOP	111				111							111	111	111	111	111
CAL																
GR																
MGJ	646	988	969	766	969	969	767	767	989	867	979	969	978	746	635	643
Furc																
Mobil	1						1	1	1			1	1	1	1	
PLQ	3			3	3	3	3	3	3	3	3	3	3	3	3	

Abbreviations: BOP, bleeding on probing (1), suppuration (2); CAL, clinical attachment level; Furc, furcation involvement (Glickman class); GR, gingival recession; MGJ, position of mucogingival junction from margin; Mobil, tooth mobility (Miller grade); PD, probing depths; PLQ, plaque level (0 = none, 5 = heavy).

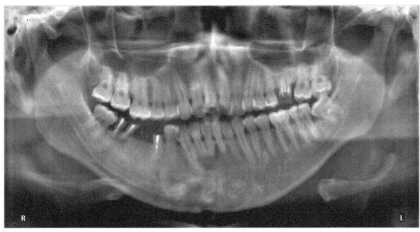

Fig. 3.16 Relevant radiographs for review case.

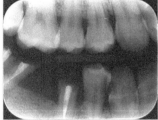
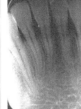
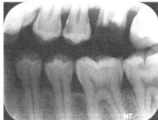

Learning objective: Identify common periodontal disease.

1. This patient has generalized inflammation. This patient does not have attachment loss.
   A. Both statements are true
   B. Both statements are false
   C. The first statement is true, the second is false
   D. The first statement is false, the second is true

2. No local contributing factors, other than plaque, are evident on the photograph. The microbial test shows the presence of red complex bacteria.
   A. Both statements are true
   B. Both statements are false
   C. The first statement is true, the second is false
   D. The first statement is false, the second is true

3. The patient's periodontal disease is best described as:
   A. Healthy
   B. Dental biofilm-induced gingivitis
   C. Periodontitis
   D. Other disease

4. If this patient was considered to have periodontitis, what stage would it be?
   A. Stage I
   B. Stage II
   C. Stage III
   D. Stage IV

5. If the patient was considered to have periodontitis, what grade would it be?
   A. Grade C
   B. Grade B
   C. Grade A

Learning objective: Develop an etiology-based treatment plan.

6. What preventive treatments should this patient receive? (Select all that apply.)
   A. Oral hygiene instruction
   B. Nutritional counseling
   C. Tobacco cessation counseling
   D. Fluoride varnish

7. What is the appropriate procedure to initially remove plaque and calculus in this patient?
   A. Periodontal maintenance
   B. Prophylaxis
   C. Scaling
   D. Scaling and root planing

8. What other treatments are needed for initial periodontal therapy in this patient? (Select all that apply.)
   A. Extraction of teeth nos. 14, 29, and 31
   B. Orthodontic treatment
   C. Direct restoration of teeth nos. 12 and 13 caries
   D. Fabricate an occlusal guard

9. Pocketing persists after initial therapy at teeth nos. 4 and 5. What pocket-reduction surgery would be most appropriate?
   A. Gingival flap surgery
   B. Osseous surgery
   C. Osseous surgery and bone grafting
   D. Gingival flap surgery and guided tissue regeneration

10. During maintenance phase, which of the following procedures should be performed in this case?
    A. Prophylaxis
    B. Periodontal maintenance
    C. Orthodontic therapy
    D. Implant therapy

Learning objective: Identify uncommon periodontal diseases.

11. Fifteen years after implant placement to replace missing no. 30, 3-mm bone loss is found relative to the implant platform along with 8-mm pockets, but there is no BOP. This condition is called:
    A. Healthy peri-implant tissue
    B. Peri-implant mucositis
    C. Peri-implantitis
    D. Other peri-implant condition

12. If the patient presented with a fever, severe pain, tissue sloughing, and slight loss of interdental papilla tissue surrounded by gray tissue margins, this would be a sign of:
    A. Periodontitis, stage IV, grade C
    B. Necrotizing periodontal disease
    C. Periodontal abscesses
    D. Autoimmune disease

3.8 Answers

1. **C.** Gingival bleeding is observed in a little more than half the sites, indicating generalized periodontal inflammation as it affects more than 10% of sites. Most teeth have recorded attachment loss, which correlates with minor bone loss.

2. **D.** Several local factors are present as seen on the photograph: interproximal caries at tooth no. 7, malpositioned teeth nos. 8 to 11. The microbial counts show highest numbers for *P. gingivalis*, spirochetes, and *T. forsythia*, which are the red complex bacteria.

3. **C.** The periodontal condition is not healthy as there is generalized BOP. Bone and attachment loss rule out gingivitis. Other than the relatively young age, there are no indications of unusual disease, such as ulceration, tissue necrosis, or localized tissue swellings.

4. **C.** Even though this patient could be stage I or II based on minimal attachment loss (1–2 mm most teeth with the exception of no. 18 with 3-mm CAL), this patient has 6-mm deep pockets and is likely to lose more teeth because of caries, which indicates higher treatment complexity, hence the higher disease severity. While the patient will lose some teeth, no severe factors are apparent that would preclude replacing the missing teeth.

5. **A** or **B.** This patient has a higher disease activity than expected for the age, and heavy tobacco use favors more rapid attachment loss. Grade B may be considered as the indirect evidence for bone loss appears less than 1% per year. The patient is clearly not resistant to disease as she shows significant disease at a relatively young age.

6. **A, B, C, D.** All the choices would be appropriate. Smoking is a contributing factor to periodontal disease and should be addressed with tobacco cessation counseling. The patient has significant caries on multiple teeth, and the resultant high caries risk should be approached with nutritional counseling, oral hygiene instruction, and fluoride varnish.

7. **D.** The patient has periodontitis and needs initial therapy, so scaling and root planing are needed. Prophylaxis is reserved for patients who either a periodontal healthy or have mild gingivitis. Severe gingivitis caused by heavy calculus buildup is treated with scaling as there are no exposed root surfaces.

8. **A** and **C.** The root tip nos. 14, 29, and 31 are not restorable and should be removed prior to scaling and root planing to facilitate treatment. Caries removal of teeth nos. 12 and 13 is part of initial therapy and should be done after scaling and root planing. Orthodontic therapy should not be done if there is an active disease. There is no evidence of parafunctional habits in the case description to warrant fabrication of an occlusal guard.

9. **A.** There are no discernable bony defects in the area. Since there are no bony defects that can be removed, osseous surgery is not appropriate. Since there are no deep defects, bone grafting and guided tissue regeneration are not predictable and are most likely not appropriate for this case.

10. **B, C,** and **D.** Prophylaxis is not appropriate as the patient has periodontitis. Periodontal maintenance is used to control long-term periodontitis, and orthodontic therapy should be performed to improve the occlusal function. Implant therapy at last can replace missing teeth.

11. **C.** Bone loss is not seen with peri-implant health or peri-implant mucositis. Since there is no other description given, a diagnosis of peri-implantitis must be assumed given the pocketing and bone loss.

12. **B.** Pain, fever, and tissue necrosis (loss of tissue, gray margins) indicate necrotizing periodontal disease. Necrosis is not a feature of severe periodontitis, and an abscess would produce purulent discharge. Although tissue sloughing can be seen with some autoimmune conditions, the tissue stays alive in these conditions, producing erythema and possible bleeding surfaces.

3.9 Evidence-based Activities

- Debate if periodontal diagnosis should rely on clinical attachment level, bone loss, or pocket depth/BOP.
- Debate what healthy periodontium means and how much inflammation do you have to see in order to determine the presence of periodontal disease.
- Go to the University of Texas Health Science Center School of Dentistry at San Antonio's library of critically appraised topics (CAT) at https://cats.uthscsa.edu/, and search for a review periodontal disease diagnosis. Read any CAT you can find, and debate if the conclusion is still correct based on current literature.

- Create a CAT on the uses of salivary biomarkers to detect periodontal disease (or any other topic for which a CAT is not available) following the outline provided by Sauve S. et al. in "The critically appraised topic: a practical approach to learning critical appraisal" (Ann R Coll Physicians Surg Can. 1995; 28:396–398).

References

[1] Lang NP, Bartold PM. Periodontal health. J Periodontol 2018;89(Suppl 1):S9–S16

[2] Murakami S, Mealey BL, Mariotti A, Chapple ILC. Dental plaque-induced gingival conditions. J Periodontol 2018;89(Suppl 1):S17–S27

[3] Trombelli L, Farina R, Silva CO, Tatakis DN. Plaque-induced gingivitis: Case definition and diagnostic considerations. J Periodontol 2018;89(Suppl 1):S46–S73

[4] Albandar JM, Susin C, Hughes FJ. Manifestations of systemic diseases and conditions that affect the periodontal attachment apparatus: Case definitions and diagnostic considerations. J Periodontol 2018;89(Suppl 1):S183–S203

[5] Tonetti MS, Greenwell H, Kornman KS. Staging and grading of periodontitis: Framework and proposal of a new classification and case definition. J Periodontol 2018;89(Suppl 1):S159–S172

[6] Fine DH, Patil AG, Loos BG. Classification and diagnosis of aggressive periodontitis. J Periodontol 2018;89(Suppl 1):S103–S119

[7] CDT 2018: Dental Procedure Codes. Chicago, Illinois: American Dental Association; 2018

[8] Heitz-Mayfield LJA, Salvi GE. Peri-implant mucositis. J Periodontol 2018; 89(Suppl 1):S257–S266

[9] Schwarz F, Derks J, Monje A, Wang HL. Peri-implantitis. J Periodontol 2018; 89(Suppl 1):S267–S290

[10] Herrera D, Retamal-Valdes B, Alonso B, Feres M. Acute periodontal lesions (periodontal abscesses and necrotizing periodontal diseases) and endo-periodontal lesions. J Periodontol 2018;89(Suppl 1):S85–S102

4 Predicting Tooth Longevity

Abstract

Data gathered during periodontal assessment also helps to answer questions about prognosis that are highly relevant to patients and practitioners: what is the likelihood of tooth loss without treatment? How likely will treatment prevent tooth loss? Will treatment work? Is it worth the effort to treat? Which teeth will most likely be lost? Is the patient better off without certain teeth? Which teeth should be removed? How difficult will it be to remove teeth?

This chapter will describe thought processes that can help answer these questions and provide guidance for treatment planning and extractions.

Keywords: prognosis, extraction decisions, informed consent

4.1 Learning Objectives

- Judge how likely a patient will lose teeth.
- Judge how likely periodontal treatment will succeed.
- Determine which teeth should be removed.
- Weigh benefits and risks of tooth removal, tooth replacement, and tooth retention.

4.2 Case

A 47-year old female African American patient presents to you to get "periodontal work and anything else needed done." She states that she could not take care of her teeth for a while, and would like to keep them as long as possible now that she has dental insurance. She also would like to "improve her smile." She used to be seen by a corporate dental chain office until about 15 years ago when she lost her job. She reports that her gums bleed when she flosses and that floss catches between her teeth. She also tells you that she clenches her teeth, especially when driving. She brushes her teeth twice a day with a soft brush and fluoridated toothpaste, flosses twice daily, and rinses with an antiseptic mouthwash.

She checks off "high blood pressure" on the medical history form and lists "Amlodipine" as the only medication she is taking. She does not report any allergies, but records "gall bladder removal" under the surgery item on the form. When questioned, she reports that she had her gall bladder removed 2 years ago after experiencing severe pain, and her blood pressure presented a problem for the surgery. Since then, she is taking amlodipine once a day, but does not experience any side effects. She used to smoke cigarettes about a pack every day for 20 years, before she quit 2 years ago after the surgery. She denies taking any recreational drugs, but says she treats herself and drinks a few glasses of wine once a week with friends.

Vital signs: 5' 11", 230 lb, blood pressure 138/93 mm Hg, pulse 79 beats per minute.

The intraoral exam reveals significant periodontal disease as evidenced through bleeding on probing, pocketing, attachment loss, recession, and tooth mobility. The majority of posterior maxillary teeth are missing, and mandibular molars have begun to migrate into this space. Fremitus was noted on maxillary incisors nos. 8 and 9. See ▶ Fig. 4.1, for clinical appearance and ▶ Fig. 4.2, for radiographs.

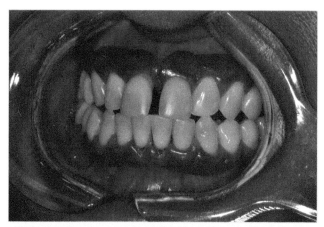

Fig. 4.1 Facial view.

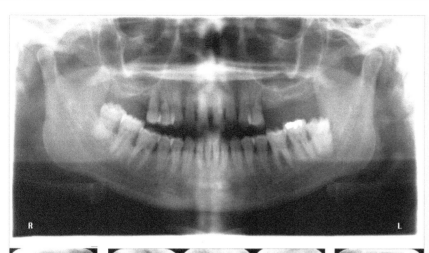

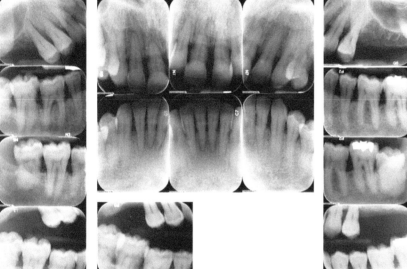

Fig. 4.2 Radiographic series.

What can be learned from this case?

This case presents more severe periodontal disease than the cases presented earlier in this book, and the patient already is missing some teeth. If the patient wants to "improve her smile," then part of addressing this chief complaint will be the need to replace missing teeth and prevent more teeth from getting lost, which of course involves "periodontal work." So, what will be the "periodontal work?"

For this, we need to look at this case methodically, identifying the periodontal disease and its contributing factors, and developing a treatment plan as presented in Chapters 2 and 3. Starting with the periodontal diagnosis, we evaluate the six dimensions of this patient's periodontal disease (▶ Table 4.1).

The clinical findings are typical for periodontitis, such as bleeding on probing, pocketing, attachment loss, bone loss, tooth mobility, and gingival recession. The amount of attachment or bone loss is more severe than the average attachment loss seen at this age, and a possible explanation for this is her past history of heavy tobacco use. Given the current disease trajectory of this patient with above-average attachment loss, the risk of future attachment loss seems higher than average.

The systemic and local contributing factors in this case are shown in ▶ Table 4.2.

Using the tables from Chapter 3, the etiologies listed here translate into the following treatment (▶ Table 4.3).

The initial part of the treatment plan is specific and clear, but becomes tentative toward the end. This is common with treatment planning complex cases as the later definite restorative treatment plan depends on the outcome of initial disease control, which may me be worse or better than anticipated.

For prognosis, the following questions need to be asked:
- What is the likelihood of tooth loss?
- Will treatment reduce the chance of tooth loss?
- Should teeth be removed?

Findings in the periodontal chart are as follows:

Maxilla facial		1	2	3	4	5	6	7	8	9	10	11	12	13	14	15	16
	PD				543	536	535	536	635	444	424	635	536				
	BOP				1	1	1	1	1	1	1	1	1				
	CAL					3	4				2		8				
	GR								112				22				
	MGJ				454	555	666	999	999	999	999	989	667				
	Furc																
	PLQ				2	2	2	2	1	1	2	2	2				
Maxilla lingual	PD				535	536	645	535	657	756	535	535	545				
	BOP				1	1	1	1	1	1	1	1	1				
	CAL				8	8			10	8		6					
	GR																
	Furc																
	Mobil				1	1			2	2							
	PLQ				1	1	1	1	2	2	1	1					

Mandible Lingual		32	31	30	29	28	27	26	25	24	23	22	21	20	19	18	17
	PD	655	645	658	646	745	646	645	524	535	435	435	545	535	435	537	557
	BOP	111	111	111	111	11	111	11	1	1	1	1	11	111	111	111	111
	CAL	5	8	7	5	6	6	6	7	7	5	5	5	5	5	8	4
	GR								222	212			1			111	
	MGJ	999	999	999	999	999	999	999	999	999	999	999	999	999	999	999	999
	Furc		1													1	
	PLQ	2	2	2	2	2	2	2	2	2	2	2	2	2	2	2	2
Mandible facial	PD	568	945	656	645	635	434	635	535	524	526	645	536	535	637	549	447
	BOP	111	111	111	111	111	111	111	111	111	111	111	111	111	111	111	111
	CAL	7														8	9
	GR																
	MGJ	666	999	766	878	768	989	989	989	979	879	979	999	899	989	998	866
	Furc																
	Mobil		1					1	2	2	1						
	PLQ	3	3	2	2	2	1	1	2	2	1	1	2	2	2	3	3

Abbreviations: BOP, bleeding on probing (1); CAL, clinical attachment level; Furc, furcation involvement (Glickman class); GR, gingival recession; MGJ, position of mucogingival junction from margin; Mobil, tooth mobility (Miller grade); PD, probing depths; PLQ, plaque level (0 = none, 5 = heavy).

4.2.1 What is the Likelihood of Tooth Loss?

Given the disease trajectory, tooth loss is unlikely in the short term (5 years) in this case. In the long term, the maxillary premolars (teeth nos. 4, 5, and 12) and central incisors (teeth nos. 8 and 9) have the highest risk as they have the most severe attachment loss, largest amount of bone loss, preexisting tooth mobility, and worst crown-to-root ratio of all teeth along with simple, coni-cal-shaped, relatively short tooth roots. The mandibular canines will be the least likely teeth to be lost given their good level of bone support, long root length, low amount of attachment loss, and absence of most periodontal disease-associated factors.

4.2.2 Will Treatment Reduce the Chance of Tooth Loss?

Systemic factors in this patient are likely not an impediment to periodontal treatment. The patient has hypertension, but not to a degree that poses a high risk for a myocardial infarct or stroke during dental treatment. The patient's local contrib-uting factors can be partially controlled. Plaque and calculus can most likely be treated with oral hygiene instruction and scaling and root planing, and pocket-reduction surgery can be effective. However, furcation treatment may be more dif-ficult, and the patient has multiple occlusal conditions (Class III relationship, severe bone loss complicating orthodontic

Table 4.1 Information to consider for periodontal diagnosis

Severity of inflammation	Erythema Gingival bleeding—has BOP for at least one site every tooth
Depth of inflammation	Involving alveolar bone crest (bone loss/attachment loss)
Extent of inflammation	Generalized—all teeth are involved to a similar degree regarding bleeding on probing and bone loss
Microbial factors	Plaque—plaque scores 1–2 per tooth; visible at margin; likely has typical microflora associated with periodontitis
Systemic factors	Former tobacco user (20 pack years, quit 2 years ago) Hypertension—mild Calcium channel blocker use—but don't see gingival enlargement
Local factors	Listed by tooth: No. 4: tooth mobility; possible interference contact no. 30, root concavity No. 5: tooth mobility; radiographic calculus (D), root concavity No. 7: radiographic calculus No. 8: tooth mobility, radiographic calculus, short conical root No. 9: tooth mobility, radiographic calculus short conical root No. 11: small caries into dentin (M), radiographic calculus No. 12: radiographic calculus, root concavity; may have interference contact with no. 19 No. 17: partially erupted, radiographic calculus No. 18: supraerupted, radiographic calculus, furcation involvement No. 19: radiographic calculus No. 20: radiographic calculus No. 21: radiographic calculus No. 23: radiographic calculus, tooth mobility No. 24: radiographic calculus, short root, tooth mobility, anterior position, possible interference contact No. 25: radiographic calculus, short root, tooth mobility, anterior position, possible interference contact No. 26: radiographic calculus, tooth mobility No. 28: radiographic calculus No. 29: radiographic calculus No. 30: radiographic calculus, furcation involvement No. 31: radiographic calculus, supraeruption No. 32: radiographic calculus, possible caries (O+M), rotated tooth

Table 4.2 Contributing factors

Systemic	Microbial	Local restorative	Local periodontal	Local anatomical	Local trauma
None currently; Previous tobacco use	**Plaque** **Calculus**	Caries	**Deep pocketing,** **Inflammation** **Furcation** **Tooth mobility** **Recession**	Rotated teeth Tipped teeth Margin discrepancy infra/supra-erupted Root concavities Cemental tears	Occlusal trauma

Note that this list does not include past tobacco use as this is no longer something that need to be addressed, and that it does not list hypertension or calcium channel blockers as these are not problems that need to be addressed for periodontal treatment in this case (Hypertension does not cause periodontal disease. This patient does not show signs of drug-induced gingival overgrowth). It also does not mention short conical roots as these do not contribute to periodontal disease development, but allow attachment loss to produce loose teeth much quicker than for teeth with longer roots.

therapy) that may not be correctable. Therefore, periodontal treatment may produce some improvement in inflammation and pocketing, but the restoration of periodontal health is questionable.

4.2.3 Should Teeth Be Removed?

Removal of the supraerupted mandibular 2nd and 3rd molars would likely simplify periodontal treatment, as it will remove four teeth with significant pocketing, and allow better access to the distal surface of the first molar. Even though the incisors have short roots and a significant amount of bone loss, it may be best to maintain these teeth with conservative periodontal therapy. Removal of these teeth will result in a difficult implant therapy scenario involving significant vertical and horizontal tissue loss.

4.3 Judging How Likely a Patient Will Lose Teeth

For most patients, keeping their teeth is the primary motivation for dental care. The ability to accurately predict and then ensure tooth survival is key to maintaining the continued trust of patients.

4.3.1 Prognosis—What Does it Mean?

There are three basic types of questions that need to be asked:
- How likely is tooth loss?
  - Without treatment, how quickly would the patient's periodontal condition deteriorate?
  - Without treatment, how fast will the patient loose teeth?
  - What is the likelihood of tooth loss for each tooth?

Table 4.3 Etiology-based treatment plan

Factor	Treatment	Timing
Plaque	Oral hygiene instruction	0
Calculus	Scaling and root planing	3
Occlusal trauma	Occlusal analysis Occlusal adjustment (limited or complete—depending on extent of tooth surface modifications needed)	6
Tooth mobility	Extra/intracoronal splinting where appropriate (see Chapter 9)	7
	Periodontal re-evaluation	8
Deep pocketing furcation involvement	Pocket reduction surgery (see Chapters 6, 7), if nonsurgical therapy did not eliminate these	10
Root concavities	+Odontoplasty	10
Recession	Corrective soft tissue surgery (Chapter 8)	11
	Periodontal re-evaluation	
Rotated teeth Tipped teeth infra/supraerupted	Orthodontic therapy (if feasible)	20
	Indirect restorations (if needed)	21
	Implant therapy to replace missing teeth (if needed/desired)	22
	Periodontal maintenance	30

- How likely will periodontal treatment succeed?
  - How aggressive should the treatment be?
  - How likely will the proposed treatment succeed in eliminating periodontal disease?
  - How likely will the proposed treatment work in saving a given tooth?
  - Which teeth are most suitable for restoration in the long term?
- Which teeth need to be removed?
  - Are there teeth that should be sacrificed for improved survival of key teeth?
  - Are there teeth that should be sacrificed to create a better dental implant site?
  - For teeth that should be removed, how likely is it that the site becomes suitable for dental implants?
  - For teeth that should be removed, could immediate implant therapy be an option?
  - For teeth that should be removed, what is the risk of surgical complications at a given site?
  - For sites where teeth need to be removed, how likely are long-term complications without tooth replacement?

The answer to these questions require extrapolation of the current periodontal condition into the future based on the patient's evidence of past periodontal disease activity, and the prognosis can change depending on the success of dental treatment. Usually, periodontal prognosis is worse at the beginning of treatment and improves with treatment. For instance, a patient may present with severe periodontal disease, poor oral hygiene, and several slightly mobile teeth initially. At the onset of treatment, the risk of tooth loss seems high and the chance of treatment success low given the initial appearance. However, if this patient develops good oral hygiene and tissues respond favorably to treatment, pocketing, tooth mobility, and inflammation, it results in a better chance of tooth survival.

4.3.2 Tooth Loss in Untreated and Treated Periodontitis

It is useful to understand typical tooth loss rates caused by periodontal diseases. Generally, patients with untreated periodontal disease loose teeth at a rate of 0.4 to 0.6 teeth/year, whereas periodontal treatment greatly reduces the chance of tooth loss to 0.02 to 0.2 teeth/year depending on the frequency and quality of periodontal maintenance.

However, these average tooth loss rates are misleading in that tooth loss rates are not constant across the years. Instead, tooth loss rates accelerate after 45 years of age,[1,2] as attachment loss from periodontitis accumulates. As attachment loss accumulates, rates of tooth loss are slow, but then accelerate with increased attachment loss in severe periodontitis (▶ Fig. 4.3).

Since tooth loss rates are averages, it also obscures the important fact that only about 20% of patients experience continued periodontal destruction while most patients experience little disease activity. Patients with continued disease activity have been described as "downhill" or "extreme downhill" compared to "well-maintained" patients, since they have tooth loss rates exceeding 0.2 teeth/year even despite frequent recall or surgical procedures performed by a periodontal specialist. This means that there is a small subset of patients who need stringent periodontal maintenance with frequent exams, counseling, and quality preventive care in an attempt to slow down tooth loss rates.

Lastly, average tooth loss numbers also obscure the fact that periodontal disease is not a gradual process, but happens in episodic spurts of disease activity at every site. As periodontal assessment only provides a snapshot of current conditions, it may underestimate disease activity at a given visit. Therefore, prognosis becomes more accurate if a patient's periodontal condition is periodically assessed over several years.

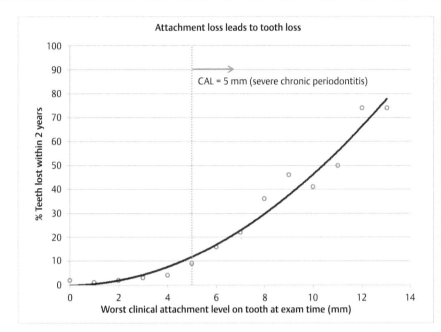

Fig. 4.3 CAL-tooth loss attachment loss brings an accelerated risk of tooth loss (modeled on data from Gilbert GH et al. 2002). Tooth loss increases in a parabolic fashion (R^2 = 0.96), with the risk of tooth loss within the next 2 years exceeding 10% in patients with severe periodontitis. The risk approaches 100% after 13 mm of attachment loss as attachment loss encroaches on the root apex and all bony support is lost on teeth with short roots.

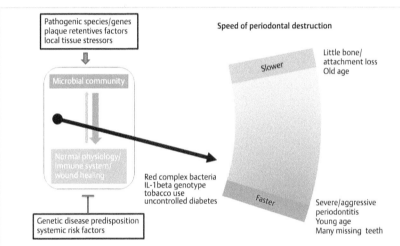

Fig. 4.4 Factors that favor the development of periodontal disease such as pathogenic bacteria and a diminished immunity/wound healing hobbled by systemic disease or genetic factors lead to faster periodontal tissue destruction.

4.3.3 Judging the Speed of Periodontal Deterioration and Setting an Appropriate Recall Interval

Recognizing patients who are at risk of disease progression is the key to decide how aggressive periodontal treatment needs to be, and how often patients should be seen for periodic exams. For example, a "well-maintained" patient experiences either no disease or mild disease that causes little attachment or bone loss over decades of time. These patients either lack periodontal pathogens or are resistant to periodontal disease as a consequence of good genetics, self-care habits, and good overall health. Most likely, these patients respond well to nonsurgical treatment in general practice and require little preventive treatment that is spaced out over 6 to 12 month intervals. In contrast, "downhill" and "extreme downhill" patients have a high risk for disease progression, and will likely need fast-paced treatment that includes surgical treatment and frequent periodontal maintenance.

To predict the speed of disease progression or risk of future attachment loss, consider each dimension of periodontal disease (▶ Fig. 4.4):

- *Depth of inflammation*: Attachment/bone loss: Speed increases with increasing amount.
- *Severity of inflammation*: Bleeding or suppuration: Speed increases with increased severity.
- *Extent of inflammation*: General disease loss suggests an increased risk for all teeth, whereas local disease suggests a tooth-related contributing factor and less overall risk of future disease.
- *Presence of systemic risk factors including genetic risk factors*: Which diminish bone deposition, wound healing, or immune response, leads to faster attachment/bone loss.
- *Presence of pathogenic bacteria/high "red complex" bacteria counts*: High counts equal higher disease activity and risk of attachment/bone loss.
- *Presence of local contributing factors*: Aids in the development of disease. This can be seen in locally enhanced areas of bone loss associated with furcation involvement or overhanging restorations.

Some additional factors can provide additional data for assessing future disease progression:
- *Missing teeth excluding third molars*: The more teeth are missing, the higher the risk for additional tooth loss, partially because of the higher risk of occlusal trauma and fracture.
- *Age*: Given the same attachment/bone loss, older patients have less risk of future attachment/bone loss as older age suggests slower disease progression.
- *Dental history*: Sporadic dental care may suggest a noncompliant patient who is unlikely to follow through with preventive care and has a higher risk of attachment/bone/tooth loss.

Considering these factors, a patient can be judged as low, medium, and high risk for future disease, which then correlates to the required aggressiveness of treatment and recall interval (▶Table 4.4).

Alternatively, several risk calculators are available that suggest the appropriate recall interval:
- *Periodontal risk assessment model:* Uses age, number of teeth, missing teeth, bleeding on probing, sites with more than 5-mm probing depth, tobacco use, bone loss, and systemic/genetic factors (i.e., diabetes) to judge the risk of periodontal disease progression as low, medium, or high.[3] This is a simple, free, web-based calculator that immediately returns the risk category and suggested recall interval. See http://www.perio-tools.com/PRA/en/index.asp.

- Periodontal Risk Calculator uses age, tobacco history, diabetes history, probing depth, bleeding on probing, presence of restorations below the gingival margin, root calculus, radiographic bone height, furcation involvement, vertical bone defects, and history of periodontal surgery to calculate a score from 1 (low risk) to 5 (high risk). This is available at http://www.previser.com that produces detailed reports that can be used to educate patients about periodontal risk and the effect of treatment. As of writing, this tool is completely web-based and requires setting up a free user account before use.

4.3.4 Judging How Fast a Patient Will Lose Teeth

Tooth loss can happen as a consequence of caries, physical trauma (i.e., occlusal trauma that fractures teeth), dental treatment strategy (i.e., 3rd molar removal, removal of premolars for orthodontic therapy), or periodontitis.

Consequently, tooth loss pattern falls into three time periods: imminent, short-term, and long term.
- Imminent tooth loss likely as part of initial dental treatment:
  - Teeth that are fractured, severely carious (i.e., root tips), not restorable (i.e., severe caries, caries in furcation entrance), not treatable with root canal therapy, not usable for restorative treatment (i.e., severely tipped, supraerupted teeth), or diseased teeth that are of no relevance to the patient (i.e., carious 3rd molars).

Table 4.4 Subjective risk of periodontal disease progression

Characteristic	Low risk	Medium risk	High risk
Attachment/bone loss	None to mild grade A periodontitis	Mild to moderate grade B periodontitis	Severe grade C periodontitis
Bleeding/suppuration	None	Isolated bleeding	Generalized
Extent	None	Few teeth	Generalized
Systemic background	Healthy	Mild systemic disease Light smoker	Poor systemic health Heavy smoker Diabetes (HbA1c > 9%) Positive IL-1beta genotype
Microbiological finding	Low plaque level No red complex	Intermediate plaque Some red complex	High plaque level >2% red complex
Local factors	None	Few	Many Heavily restored teeth Complex restorations
Missing teeth Reason for tooth loss	None other than 3rds Malposition/ortho.	1–5 teeth Caries	>6 teeth (no 3rds) Periodontal disease
Age	Mild attachment loss at age 65+	Average attachment loss for given age	Moderate or severe attachment loss before 40 years
Dental history	Regular preventive care	Some gaps of dental care	No or sporadic care
Treatment strategy	Conservative Mostly nonsurgical Can "wait and see"	Intermediate May need limited surgical treatment	Aggressive Move quickly to surgical treatment
Extractions needed	Unlikely	Possible	Likely
Periodontal referral needed	Unlikely	Maybe for surgical procedures if desired	Patient likely will benefit from consultation with specialist
Recall	6–12 months	4–6 months	3 months or less

Note: For a given patient, risk of periodontal disease progression can be estimated by checking the patient's characteristics against this table, and judge which category is the best fit for a patient.

- Teeth with near complete bone loss or severe tooth mobility (i.e., grade III).
- Teeth that need to be intentionally removed in preparation for orthodontic or restorative treatment.
- Nonhealthy teeth in preparation for chemo/radiation therapy.
- Short-term tooth loss likely within the next year or two:
  - Teeth with caries, if no restorative treatment is done and no caries management performed.
  - Presence of severe periodontal disease is attributable to severe genetic or acquired systemic conditions (i.e., AIDS, hypophosphatasia).
  - Presence of some forms of aggressive periodontal disease and dental abscesses.
- Long-term tooth loss expected in years to decades from now:
  - Teeth with chronic forms of periodontal disease. The timing of tooth loss can be extrapolated from the past history of attachment/bone loss to the point when attachment loss reaches the root apex. Attachment loss accelerates if there is:
    - Severe attachment loss > 5 mm.
    - Severe tooth mobility (Miller grade III especially).
    - Loss of adjacent teeth.
    - Furcation involvement.
    - Deep pocketing > 5 mm.
    - Bleeding on probing.
    - Short root length.
    - Occlusal trauma.

This is reflected in ▶ Table 4.5, which presents a quick method to estimate tooth longevity.

4.3.5 Judging the Prognosis for each Tooth

Judging the speed of tooth loss also provides an estimate of the likelihood of tooth loss and restorative potential. One important aspect of treatment planning is to evaluate each tooth and decide if it should be removed at the onset of therapy. Removing teeth of questionable value can simplify treatment and quickly reduce disease burden. Teeth can be categorized based on the likelihood of tooth survival and usefulness for therapy according to the McGuire prognostic system (▶ Table 4.6).

Deciding on these categories may be difficult as many factors need to be considered. Generally, prognosis is easiest and most accurate for good/excellent teeth and applied easiest on single-rooted teeth. For individual tooth prognosis, the following should be considered:
- Caries/restorability:
  - Restorability depends on the skill and confidence of the operator, and is best determined by removing caries, old restorations, and unsupported tooth structure, and

Table 4.5 Subjective estimate of how long a tooth will last

	Tooth loss unlikely within 10 years	Tooth loss likely within 2 years
Presence of caries	None/arrested	Frank caries with exposed soft, light colored dentin
Attachment/bone loss	None to moderate Grade A periodontitis	Very severe (>10 mm); progressive (Grade C)
Tooth mobility (Miller grade)	None to Grade 1	Grade 3
Furcation involvement	None to Glickman class I	Glickman class III, untreated
Probing depth	Low (<5 mm)	Very deep (>8 mm)
Bleeding/suppuration	None	Significant bleeding; suppuration
Root length	Long	Short
Occlusal trauma/fremitus	No	Yes

Note: For a a given tooth, the speed of tooth loss usually depends on caries activity and periodontal disease activity. Match the characteristics of a given tooth with each column. If the tooth does not fit the description in more than 2 categories in either column, the speed of tooth loss is likely intermediate.

Table 4.6 Subjective tooth prognosis categories by clinical meaning (adapted from McGuire et al.[5])

Category	What does it mean?
Excellent	No issue with tooth and surrounding tissue No treatment is needed
Good	Minor tooth/tissue condition posing risk for future disease Needs preventive treatment or minor restorative treatment
Fair	Clinically significant condition/disease, but treatment will likely restore health Any dental treatment is possible
Poor	Severe disease/condition. Treatment aims to preserve tooth "as is." Usually not suitable as abutment for fixed/removable partial dentures
Questionable	Tooth may be lost because of severity of condition Consider removing tooth if initial treatment fails to improve prognosis
Hopeless	Tooth will likely be lost regardless of treatment Consider removing tooth early in treatment

preparing the tooth as best as possible for the final restoration.

- ○ Once only sound tooth structure remains, and the tooth is prepared, the following dimensions suggest that a tooth is restorable:
  - At least 1.5-mm space to opposing occlusal surface at centric occlusion.
  - At least 5-mm preparation height from the preparation margin. Less height usually requires axial retention grooves for retention. Crown-lengthening procedures can assist in achieving this preparation length in some cases.
  - If the tooth needs root canal treatment, a rim of at least 1-mm height of sound tooth structure from the gingival margin.
  - Caries/restorative margins should not involve furcation entrances. Biologic shaping techniques may present a solution in some cases.
  - Root canal treated teeth are best avoided as abutments for fixe d and removable partial dentures as they are prone to fractures in these uses.

- *Strategic value*: Generally, 1st molars are of most importance to mastication, with minor contribution from 2nd molars and 2nd premolars. Canines and maxillary incisors are needed for occlusal guidance and esthetics. Contrary, diseased 3rd molars should be removed.
- *Endodontic status*: Prognosis diminishes with repeated root canal treatment attempts.
- *Tooth position/occlusal relationship*: Major malposition increases the risk of occlusal trauma and plaque accumulation and is difficult to correct in the presence of periodontal disease.
- Crown-to-root ratio needs to better than 1:1 for indirect restorations and abutments
- Long root, root trunk, and multiple roots provide increased periodontal ligament area and thus greater resistance against occlusal force and tooth loss from attachment loss.
- *Probing depth*: Deep pockets > 5 mm are difficult to maintain and worsen prognosis
- *Gingival inflammation*: Bleeding and suppuration likely indicate active disease, which leads to continued attachment and bone loss, resulting in eventual tooth loss.
- *Attachment/bone loss*: As discussed earlier, tooth loss risk increases with attachment loss.
- *Tooth mobility*: Mobile teeth have poorer prognosis.
- *Furcation involvement*: Prognosis worsens with furcation involvement,[4] although the latter can be managed with various procedures that allow long-term retention of some teeth with furcation involvement.
- *Soft tissue defects*: While the absence of keratinized gingiva may not increase the risk of recession with good oral hygiene, the presence of keratinized gingiva and normal architecture is preferred for indirect restorations.
- *Plaque levels*: High plaque levels pose a risk for disease progression.
- *Local factors*: The more local factors contribute to periodontal disease, the more treatment is needed to remove these factors. If it not possible to remove these factors, prognosis diminishes as there is a higher risk for disease recurrence.

Considering all these factors, it is possible to assign a tooth prognosis category and associated restorative usefulness as shown in ▶ Table 4.7.

In this scheme, each tooth is assessed for these categories, and individual tooth prognosis is determined by the worst scoring category (see McGuire & Nunn, for a decision tree on prognosis survival[5]). Prognosis can change with treatment, and often improves with periodontal treatment as pocket depths become reduced, and periodontal health improves.

4.4 Judging How Likely Periodontal Treatment Will Succeed

A prominent concern of patient is the question "will this work," especially if it requires a significant financial and time commitment. While periodontal treatment typically improves clinical measures such as probing depths, these are usually not significant for patients. Instead, from a patient perspective, success is a function of how well treatment is delivered, and how well treatment contributes to the prevention of tooth loss, and having a pain-free functional dentition that looks natural to the patient (▶ Fig. 4.5).

4.4.1 Factors that Lead to Successful Treatment Delivery

How well periodontal treatment is delivered is a function of technical competence and the manner treatment is delivered by the primary dentist, specialists, and office staff. For technical competence, key areas that contribute to the overall success of periodontal therapy are as follows:

- *Effective patient counseling*: Specific oral hygiene instruction tailored to patient needs; gentle, but consistent and well-informed advice on a healthy lifestyle including tobacco abstinence; and encouraging patients to work with their other healthcare providers for best overall health.
- *Restorative excellence*: Restorations should have proper embrasure profiles, anatomy, occlusion, emergence contours, and interproximal contacts. Margins need to be sealed and surfaces as smooth as possible. Implant placement needs to be aligned with restorative goals. Root canal therapy needs to be sound with complete cleaning and shaping, and good apical seal.
- *Proper occlusion*: The aim should be to achieve a mutually protective occlusion that distributes occlusal loads evenly and allows for easy, pain-free mastication.
- *Scaling and root planing excellence* produces clean root surfaces free of microbial contaminants without excessive tooth structure removal.
- *Surgical excellence*: Efficient incisions, surgical root surface cleaning, bone shaping, application of biologics, grafts and membranes, and suturing are the key elements that reduce the incidence of delayed healing, prolonged postoperative pain, and unresolved periodontal problems.

Table 4.7 Properties of teeth within each tooth prognosis category

	Excellent	Good	Fair	Poor	Questionable	Hopeless
Caries/loss of tooth structure	None	Stained pit/ fissure; Incipient	>5 mm crown height remaining	1–5 mm crown height remaining	No crown; subgingival caries	Caries to furcation or bone level
Strategic value	Needed for function and esthetics			No added value	Removal of tooth simplifies treatment	
Endodontic status	Healthy			Needs RCT	Needs endo. retreat	History of multiple retreats
Tooth position/occlusion	Within arch Normal tooth position Does not cause occlusal problem			Malposition Malocclusion		Severe extrusion/ malocclusion
Crown: root Root form	Much better than 1:1 Long root; long root trunk, multiple roots			About 1:1	Much worse than 1:1 Short, conical root	
Probing depth	<4 mm	<5 mm		5–10 mm		>10 mm
Gingival inflammation	None	Mild erythema/ isolated light bleeding		Bleeding/suppuration		
Attachment/bone loss	None None	Mild <10%	3–4 mm 10–30%	5–8 mm 30–60%	8–10 mm 60–90%	>10 mm > 90%
Tooth mobility	None			Grade I	Grade II	Grade III
Furcation involvement*	None		Class I	Class I-II Class IV	Class II	Class III
Soft tissue defect	*None	Isolated mild recession	Significant recession	Mucogingival defect	Generalized lack of keratinized gingiva	
Plaque level	None	Minimal		High Patient can remove plaque	High Patient attempts to improve	High Patient will not remove plaque
Local factors contributing to disease	None	Present, but no disease	Present, causes disease	Many local factors, significant disease	Difficult to remove local factor	Cannot eliminate local factor

For a given tooth, analyze all the listed factors and select the best matching column for each factor. Tooth prognosis is then determined by the most-right column matching with the tooth. *Without treatment. Furcation and soft tissue defects can be treated in some cases with a variety of methods (see chapter 7 and 8), which improves prognosis and predictability of restorative treatment.

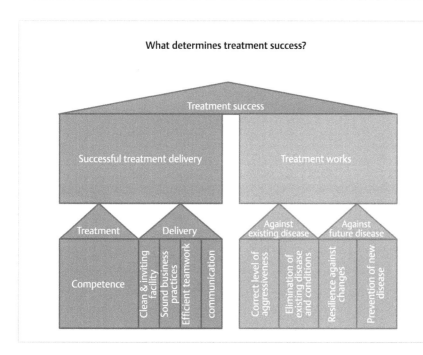

What determines treatment success?

Fig. 4.5 Treatment success is a function of successful treatment delivery and the treatment working against the disease for a specific patient. Treatment delivery is very much controllable through developing technical competence, sound business practices, efficient team work, good communication skills, and by providing treatment in a clean and inviting environment. The second factor that determines treatment success is if the proposed treatment works against the disease, regardless of who provides treatment. This depends on the proposed treatment controlling existing disease and preventing new disease. For control of existing disease, causes and contributing factors have to be eliminated at a speed or aggressiveness that matches that of the existing disease. Likewise, future disease needs to be prevented by eliminating risk factors for disease and providing treatment resilience against unforeseen challenges such as an accidental injury.

While technical competence is needed for treatment success, equally important is the way treatment is delivered. Successful treatment delivery is a function of the following:
- *Good communication skills*: To prevent disappointment and loss of trust, patients need to understand expectations, limitations, alternatives, and risks of treatment from the onset of therapy. For this, it must be ensured that everyone involved in a dental office must:
  ○ Project integrity, competence, fairness, and genuine concern.

○ Convey consistent and truthful information at every patient encounter.
○ Respect patient autonomy.
○ Respond to patient wishes and concerns.
- *Sound business practices*: This includes proper marketing, accounting, management, communications, record keeping, credentialing, staff training, and compliance with applicable laws and regulations. Sound business practices prevent unnecessary expenses and unpleasant surprises, and patients appreciate a well-run office.
- *Team work*: This includes working toward fulfilling the mission or goals of the practice, maximizing efficiency, supporting each team member's function, and preventing treatment errors.
- *Clean and inviting facility*: Patients will certainly notice dated, dirty, worn, or cluttered spaces in an office and assume poor quality treatment. First impressions matter and a clean and inviting office entrance can set a positive tone for the first appointment day.

While technical competence can be developed readily with continuing education and training, the softer skills of treatment delivery take more effort to develop. Some of these treatment-delivery skills can be learned through continuing education courses, and various business management and communication texts. Otherwise, professional consultants can help improve various aspects of a dental office, and self-reflection or a team approach can identify areas that can be improved.

4.4.2 Factors that Lead to Clinical Success

How well treatment contributes to the prevention of tooth loss and having a pain-free functional and natural-appearing dentition depends on two factors: ending existing disease and preventing new disease. This depends on the following:
- *Appropriate level of treatment aggressiveness:* Treatment speed and aggressiveness must match the patient's disease activity and treatment need in order to be effective. For instance, in a patient with destructive periodontal disease, professional tooth cleanings every 12 months is not effective in preventing disease progression as the disease-causing microbes will likely be re-established 3 months after cleaning the subgingival root surfaces.
- *Elimination of existing disease factors*: If all contributing factors to a patient's periodontal disease are not eliminated, the disease will likely continue and eventually cause tooth loss. Periodontal disease also complicates other dental treatment such as:
○ *Orthodontic treatment*: Tooth movement can exacerbate bone loss.
○ *Extractions*: Periodontal diseases increase the incidence of alveolar osteitis.
○ *Restorative procedures*: Gingival bleeding may lead to inaccurate impressions.
- *Treatment plan resilience*: The treatment plan needs to allow for future treatment options as teeth and restorations fail in the future. For example, clinical crown lengthening can save selected teeth, but at the cost of removing bone and reducing the height of alveolar bone. If the same tooth develops recurrent caries and becomes unrestorable after a decade, the now-reduced alveolar

bone may not be tall enough for the placement of a conventional dental implant.
- *Prevention of new disease*: The reason for premature failure of dental treatment is usually recurrent disease such as caries and periodontal disease. Consequently, it is important to educate the patient about preventive treatment and maintenance before and during treatment, and conduct frequent periodontal maintenance for patients with complex restorations.

4.4.3 Judging How Aggressive Treatment Should Be

In periodontal treatment, usually there are several treatment options ranging from aggressive removal of teeth to conservative maintenance of teeth. Situations that favor a more aggressive treatment including tooth removal at the beginning of initial therapy include the following (▶Fig. 4.6):
- *Caries experience*: In case of deep or widespread caries, gross caries removal and provisionalization should be performed prior to periodontal therapy in order to assess restorability and need for extractions. Then, any nonrestorable teeth should be removed immediately.
- *Severity of bone/attachment loss/pocketing*: Consider tooth removal with deep pocketing (>9 mm) or severe attachment/bone loss, as periodontal therapy is less predictable for these teeth.
- *Incorrigible local factors*: Consider removing the affected tooth as there is no other treatment.
- *Incorrigible severe systemic factors*: Tooth removal may be more effective and aid control of the systemic condition (i.e., Type II diabetes mellitus).
- *Consistently poor oral hygiene*: Consider tooth removal and complete denture therapy.
- *Periodontal disease poses a risk to the patient*: For patients where an abscessed tooth poses a major risk of infection such as in immunocompromised patients (i.e., planned chemotherapy, patients with organ transplants, and AIDS), patients about to start bisphosphonate therapy, patients with implanted medical devices, and patients with a history of infective bacterial endocarditis, removal of any abscess-prone teeth or diseased teeth should be considered prior to periodontal therapy.
- *Patient goals*: Occasionally, a patient's esthetic or functional needs may require sacrifice of selected teeth to allow fabrication of prosthesis. Typically, this is determined with a diagnostic wax-up on a mounted cast (or virtually with planning software), which will then identify teeth that are "in the way" of the desired restoration. If these teeth cannot be orthodontically moved or reshaped with a restoration including root canal treatment, then they need to be removed.

Situations where a conservative approach that focuses on the preservation of teeth is favored include the following:
- *Mild to moderate bone/attachment loss/pocketing*: Periodontal therapy is very predictable in these conditions and favors tooth retention.
- *Presence of modifiable contributing factors*: Conservative periodontal treatment is usually less expensive and traumatic compared to extractions and tooth replacement.

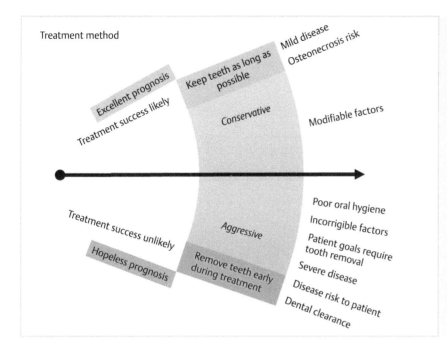

Fig. 4.6 For each patient, there are treatment options that are more conservative (keep teeth, less surgery) or more aggressive (remove teeth, move quickly to surgical treatments). The decision on whether to recommend more aggressive or more conservative treatment hinges on the risk of disease progression and patient treatment needs to be as shown here.

- *Young patients*: Even though a dental implant supported restoration can replace teeth, many implants develop periodontal problems in the long term, and given the lack of evidence-based methods for treatment of periimplantitis, it is still advisable to maintain teeth as long as possible.
- *Current and past use of medications related to osteonecrosis of the jaw (i.e., bisphosphonates)*: Extractions, pocket-reduction surgery, implant therapy, and associated bone grafting procedures pose a risk for osteonecrosis of the jaw as these procedures typically involve exposing large areas of bone to the oral environment. In these cases, periodontal therapy needs to aim at preventing tooth loss and the need for extractions through nonsurgical and preventive treatment.

4.4.4 Judging How likely Periodontal Treatment will Eliminate Periodontal Disease

Assuming that all factors related to treatment delivery are maximized for success, the likelihood of eliminating periodontal disease depends mostly on how well the contributing factors to periodontal disease can be removed. To answer this question, the contributing factors to the patient's periodontal disease should be listed, and assessed if they can be changed with the treatment. The likelihood of treatment success can then be estimated using the terminology defined by Drs Caton and Kwok[6]:

- *Favorable*: All contributing factors for a given tooth/patient can be removed with treatment. Comprehensive periodontal treatment can fully control periodontal disease and prevent future attachment/bone loss.
- *Questionable*: Some contributing factors for a given tooth/patient can be removed. Periodontal treatment can only partially control periodontal disease, and future attachment/bone loss may continue at a slower rate.

- *Unfavorable*: Most or all of the contributing factors for a given tooth/patient cannot be removed. Future attachment/bone loss is likely to continue at the current rate despite comprehensive treatment.
- *Hopeless*: This represents terminal periodontal disease where the severity of attachment loss likely will lead to tooth loss regardless of treatment. Periodontal therapy should not be attempted and teeth should be removed as part of initial treatment.

In general, the characteristics shown in ▶ Table 4.8 may present a guide that allows for a judgment on how likely periodontal treatment may succeed.

As with the other prognostic tables, this table works by matching patients with the columns, and the prognosis is determined by the right-most column matched by the patient. As with individual tooth prognosis, the likelihood of treatment success may change during treatment depending on treatment progress.

4.4.5 Judging Which Teeth Are Most Suitable for Restoration

Individual tooth prognosis or judging the likelihood of tooth loss correlates with the type of restorative treatment a tooth should receive.
- *Hopeless*: Consider removing the tooth instead of restoring it. Occasionally, it may be beneficial to temporarily restore such teeth, for instance, to aid occlusal record taking.
- *Questionable:* Avoid any restoration other than direct restorations.
- *Poor*: Direct restorations and maybe a single tooth inlay/onlay or crown if dentist and patient are satisfied with the tooth's long-term survival prognosis.
- *Fair-excellent*: Tooth can be abutment for fixed or removable partial dentures, crowns, and direct restorations.

Table 4.8 Likelihood of treatment success

Caton and Kwok categories	Favorable	Questionable	Unfavorable	Hopeless
Tobacco use	Nonsmokers Former smokers	Light smokers	Heavy smokers (>1 pack/day)	Heavy smokers
Diabetes	HbA1c < 7	HbA1c ~8–9	HbA1c > 10	HbA1c > 10
Other systemic factors	Healthy or mild systemic disease	DIGO-associated medications Poor overall health	IL-1 genotype Osteoporosis Poor nutrition Stress Obesity Alcohol abuse Immune defects	Severe immunosuppression/genetic defects causing periodontal disease
Initial probing depths	PD < 7 mm	PD 7–9 mm	PD > 9 mm on teeth other than 1st molars/ canines	PD > 9 mm on 1st molars and canines
Initial attachment/bone loss	< 30% of root length	>30% Crown : root = 1:1	Poor crown : root ratio on teeth other than 1st molar/canine	Near complete loss Poor crown : root ratio on all teeth
Plaque retentive factors	Can be removed	Partial removal possible	Cannot be removed on some teeth	Generally cannot be removed without removing teeth
Occlusal trauma/ parafunctional habits	None/can be stopped completely	Control possible with adjustment/ occlusal guard	Cannot be stopped	Severe and not controllable
Tooth mobility	None/grade I	Localized grade I/II, but not molar/canines	Generalized grade I/ II, but still has molars/ canines as possible abutment teeth	Grade II/III Canines + molars/no abutment teeth
Periodontal treatment success	Likely	Limited, may be able to keep teeth "as is," but may not be able to restore	Unlikely, may need extractions and partial dentures	Unlikely Extraction indicated Likely needs complete dentures

For fixed and removable partial dentures, abutment teeth need to have sufficient root surface area to provide support for the missing teeth, in general one root for each missing root. In addition, teeth need to be aligned properly so that a denture insertion path can be established. Tipping and rotation of teeth are problematic as they may prevent insertion or delivery of a denture, unless this can be corrected with odontoplasty, a survey crown, a telescoping restoration, or orthodontics. Although root canal treated teeth can be used as abutments for either fixed or removable partial dentures, vital teeth are less prone to root fractures and are preferred abutments whenever possible.

For removable partial dentures, a tissue-supported partial denture should be supported by at least a canine on both sides of the jaw. For a tooth-supported removable partial denture, the minimum support should come from a canine and molar abutment on both sides of the jaw.

4.4.6 Judging Resilience of the Treatment Plan

Patients can lose teeth or implants during maintenance phase as a result of accidents, tooth fractures, periodontal abscesses, failed restorations, and other mishaps. Since the unexpected can happen anytime, it is useful to make treatment plans more resilient against future failure. While the following list is incomplete and highly dependent on each patient and skill level, consider the following concepts:

- *Keeping teeth*: More procedures are possible to retain teeth than with implants, and well-maintained teeth preserve alveolar bone. A restored implant experiencing progressive bone loss is much more difficult to address than a tooth experiencing periodontal disease, and a failing implant is typically more difficult to replace with another implant compared to a failing tooth.
- Removable partial dentures are a flexible, cost-effective, and relatively noninvasive treatment option as only limited tooth preparation is usually required. In addition, if a tooth other than an abutment tooth fails, a tooth can easily be added to a partial denture in most situations.
- Short-span fixed partial dentures on teeth or implants are usually a better choice than long-span fixed partial dentures as they are simpler to fabricate and maintain. In addition, it is easier to remove and replace a shorter span partial denture than a costly long-span partial denture.
- *Crown-lengthening procedures*: These can rescue some teeth from being "not restorable" to "restorable" by surgically exposing more tooth structure after removing surrounding supporting bone. While beneficial in many cases, the reduction of bone height can prevent future implant placement in the posterior mandible once the crown-lengthened tooth fails in the future. Consider tooth removal and implant therapy over crown

lengthening, if the distance of the alveolar ridge to inferior alveolar (IA) nerve is less than 15 mm.
- *Number of implants*: If the patient can afford and if placed appropriately, increasing the number of implants placed in an edentulous jaw provides resilience against implant failure.

4.4.7 Judging the Likelihood of New Periodontal Disease

Patients may complain that they had periodontal surgery a decade ago, but it did not work since they developed new periodontal disease. Although periodontal surgery often simplifies periodontal maintenance through pocket reduction, it does not prevent periodontal disease in the long-term if there is no consistent periodontal maintenance program. The likelihood of periodontal disease redeveloping can be judged using the periodontal risk-assessment tools described in the section "judging the speed of periodontal disease progression," earlier in this chapter. In essence, characteristics of a patient who is unlikely to experience new periodontal disease progression are as follows:
- Maintains good overall health through good nutrition, exercise, preventive medicine, and compliance with medical treatment.
- Maintains good oral hygiene and achieves low supragingival plaque levels.
- Presents regularly for scheduled periodontal maintenance/prophylaxis as appropriate for periodontal disease risk.
- Reports and takes care of dental conditions as soon as they develop.

In contrast, the less a patient fits these characteristics, the more likely new periodontal disease will develop. Typically, patients who report new periodontal problems despite periodontal treatment have received treatment decades ago, and then quit regular periodontal maintenance for a few years either because of financial, relocation, or medical reasons.

4.5 Determining Which Teeth Should Be Removed

An important aspect of treatment planning for patients with severe caries or periodontal disease is to identify teeth that need to be removed at the onset of initial therapy. Removing teeth early in treatment quickly eliminates sources of infection and pain, simplifies periodontal therapy, and may be easier to accept for patients than later during therapy.

4.5.1 Identifying Teeth that Need to Be Removed

Teeth that need to be removed generally are those which have the following:
- "Hopeless" prognosis (with some exceptions).
- Low strategic value, especially if they threaten the survival of valuable teeth.
- Teeth interfere with dental treatment/special circumstances.

While hopeless teeth usually should be removed as soon as possible, there are some exceptions for hopeless teeth that are not acutely infected or painful:
- Patient understands reasons for tooth removal, but refuses the removal of a given tooth. The "informed refusal" should be well documented.
- Teeth need to be retained temporarily for diagnostic and restorative purposes such as maintaining an appropriate vertical dimension of occlusion until registration.
- Maintain space with a provisionalized, disease-free tooth for implant therapy until the patient is ready for it.
- Medical reasons contraindicate tooth removal until the medical condition is controlled (i.e., severe hypertension, recent myocardial infarct).

Determining Strategic Value

At times, individual tooth prognosis suggests equally questionable prognosis for two adjacent teeth, but it may be strategically useful to only remove one tooth based on strategic value, and attempt to preserve the other tooth.

For instance, in a given patient, teeth nos. 14 and 15 are made questionable by deep pocketing extending to Glickman Class II furcations involvement on the distal of no. 14 and mesial of no. 15, and both should be restored with an indirect restoration as they have large existing occlusal amalgam restorations. Both teeth have questionable prognosis and could be removed. However, retaining no. 14 would benefit the patient's chewing ability on the left side, since the patient has all teeth mesial to it. Removing only no. 15 may also improve prognosis of tooth no. 14, as it provides access for oral hygiene access to the furcation involvement of no. 14. Odontoplasty and a fluted crown can also make the furcation entrance more cleansable, and improve maintenance of the tooth for increased longevity.

Consequently, beyond tooth prognosis, strategic value needs to be considered for extraction decisions. Teeth can be ranked by strategic value as shown here from high to low:
- *Canines*: Canines are critical for occlusal function, and at a minimum a canine on either side could serve as abutment for a mostly tissue-supported removable partial denture.
- *First molars*: These teeth have the largest occlusal surface area and are most important for mastication. Combined with a canine on either side, this provides the minimum necessary support for a tooth-borne partial denture.
- *Second molars*: If first molars are missing, 2nd molars may serve as terminal abutment for a partial denture along with at least a canine on either side of the mouth.
- *Maxillary incisors*: Most patients require these for esthetics, and all maxillary incisors must be present for a normal appearance. If one or more maxillary incisors are considered for removal, and to be replaced with a removable partial denture, denture appearance is most acceptable if all incisors are removed and replaced at the same time.
- *Premolars, mandibular incisors*: Maxillary premolars contribute to esthetics in a minor way, and 2nd premolars participate in a small amount in occlusion. Occasionally, a premolar-based occlusion can be appropriate for some partially edentulous patients.

- *Third molars*: Not needed for most patients, and should be removed if not cleansable or if they show signs of any disease.

When faced with deciding to extract teeth of same prognosis, but different strategic value, consider holding off on extracting the tooth with higher strategic value and see if periodontal therapy improves prognosis.

4.5.2 Special Circumstances Where Tooth Removal Is Indicated

While the aforementioned guidelines generally apply to extraction decisions, there are special circumstances where it is imperative for the provider to understand that extractions can aid the survival of strategically important teeth. Typically, tooth removal should be considered even if the individual tooth prognosis is not "hopeless".

- Malposed teeth or impacted third molars can make it extremely difficult to maintain or cause pain for the patient. The angulation of the offending tooth creates a significant plaque and food trap, which then causes deep caries on the adjacent tooth rendering it nonfunctional and needing to be extracted. ▶ Fig. 4.7 depicts a third molar mesio-angularly tipped causing significant resorption of the second molar. In this case, since the second molar is irreversibly damaged, it will need to be sacrificed along with the third molar to maintain ideal health of the periodontium. If this situation had been recognized at a younger age, it may have been possible to preserve the second molar.
- Supraerupted teeth can warrant extractions if significant interference with a provider's prosthetic plan is anticipated.
- Severe periodontal disease rendering numerous teeth with extreme mobility can provide a dangerous risk to the patient if not identified correctly. For example, if a patient presents with poor oral hygiene and significant mobility in

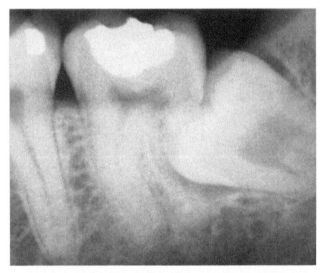

Fig. 4.7 A tipped-impacted 3rd molar is causing root resorption on the second molar. While these teeth may not show signs of periodontal disease other than radiographic findings, the only solution to this problem is removal of both teeth. (This image is provided courtesy of Dr. Jeffrey Elo.)

multiple localized areas, it would be prudent to extract the teeth that would be deemed with a hopeless prognosis. This would benefit the patient and provider by saving multiple appointments, and more important the risk of aspiration would be decreased.

- *Need for limited treatment*: Patient finances and existing oral hygiene play an important role in the treatment planning discussion on which teeth need to be retained or not. If a patient displays extremely poor oral hygiene and presents with a hopeless to poor prognosis of their dentition, it is critical to have a serious discussion with the patient on their long-term dental goals. A mutual understanding and agreement needs to be undertaken by both the provider and patient on extracting these teeth.
- Need for immediate disease removal as in patients awaiting organ transplants, head and neck radiation therapy, or chemotherapy. While uncommon, medical specialists may request patients to have any dental disease eradicated within a few weeks prior to certain cancer treatments and organ transplants. In this case, tooth removal of any tooth that has a prognosis less than "good" may be needed, even though these teeth could be treated restoratively or surgically under normal circumstances.

4.5.3 Sacrificing Teeth in Favor of Implant Therapy

Numerous parameters have to be taken into consideration when considering extracting a tooth and sacrificing it with a dental implant. In certain cases, patients display extreme reluctance in having a tooth extracted especially if it is their first extraction, and generally it is beneficial to the patient and sound practice to maintain teeth as long as possible. However, certain conditions render a tooth extremely challenging to restore without a dental implant, and extraction followed by implant therapy is preferred over preserving a tooth in the following situations:

- *Crown lengthening would complicate or prevent future implant therapy:* This usually happens for a tooth that has already been crowned and has recurrent caries that extends subgingivally on a posterior tooth. In this case, a crown-lengthening surgery is done to expose sounder tooth structure for a new crown preparation, but it will require the removal of alveolar bone. Since the restoration will likely fail again in several years due to recurrent caries, renewed crown lengthening cannot likely be done, since it will either expose the furcation or result in unacceptable crown-to-root ratio at that time. At the same time, the bone height will be reduced as a result of the original crown-lengthening surgery and any bone damage from the current dental infection. If the bone height toward the IA nerve or sinus floor is now too low, implant therapy is either difficult or impossible to achieve (▶ Fig. 4.8). Therefore, if crown-lengthening surgery is considered in the posterior mandible, one aim of the surgery should be to preserve at least 15 mm of alveolar ridge height from the IA nerve canal. If crown lengthening is considered in the posterior maxilla, the patient should be advised of the possible future need of sinus augmentation procedures if the predicted residual bone height is less than 15 mm after crown-lengthening surgery.

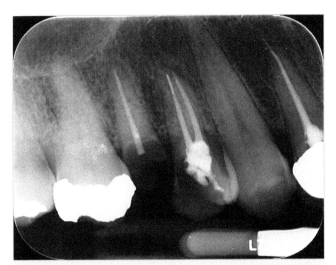

Fig. 4.8 Crown lengthening versus extraction and implant therapy. Teeth nos. 4 and 5 are carious with #4 lacking any coronal tooth structure, no. 5 is fractured on the distal aspect and caries are approaching alveolar bone. If you wanted to restore teeth nos. 4 and 5, root canal retreatment, placement of a core build-up, crown lengthening, and fabrication of a crown will be needed. However, crown lengthening would be risky because bone removal may expose the furcation entrance, possibly requiring odontoplasty, and results in a poor crown-to-root ratio. You also see that removal of bone would further reduce the low bone height to the sinus floor, which then may not be sufficient to allow implant placement. As consequence, implant therapy would require sinus floor augmentation, possibly delay implant placement, and increase the cost of treatment. In contrast, if the tooth was removed now and assuming the site would heal with no complications, the residual bone height may allow placement of an implant with at most minimal need for sinus augmentation, which would significantly reduce cost and time to tooth replacement. While in this case, extraction is the only realistic option, the decision between crown lengthening and tooth retention versus extraction and implant therapy is less than clear.

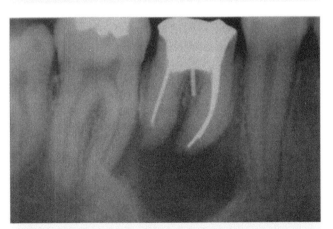

Fig. 4.10 Tooth no. 30 has had a root canal with a pin perforating the furcation roof. This tooth is nonrestorable, and has a large periapical lesion associated with the tooth. This tooth needs to be extracted and the lesion biopsied because of the size. Prior to implant therapy, this lesion must heal completely and form normal, healthy bone in sufficient amounts. (This image is provided courtesy of Dr. Jeff Elo.)

- *Failed root canal therapy that requires apicoectomy or cannot be retreated at all:* When root canal treatment fails, endodontic retreatment is usually the treatment of

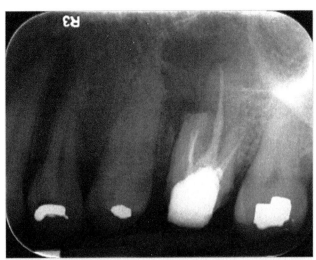

Fig. 4.9 Failed root canal treatment not resolvable with endodontic retreatment. Teeth nos. 13 and 14 have coronal fractures, recurrent caries, inadequate post length, and periapical lesions. The patient also complained of significant pain in the area. Apicoectomy is impractical in this case because of the proximity to the sinus.

choice to preserve the tooth. However, there are times when renewed cleaning and shaping of the root canal system from the crown end of the tooth will not work. This may be because of a separated file, transportation of the apical foramen, complex root apex anatomy, or simply the fact that renewed cleaning and shaping will result in too little remaining root structure (▶ Fig. 4.9). In this case, apicoectomy surgery, which removes the root apex and seals the remaining apical root canal ends, is considered. However, since this procedure usually requires drilling a dime-sized hole into the facial bone overlying the root apices, it usually leaves behind a bony defect at the apical end of the tooth. If the retreated tooth fails eventually, little residual alveolar ridge remains, and implant therapy may not be possible unless the site is managed with grafting, which adds to expense and surgical risks.

- *Severe xerostomia/extreme caries risk coupled with low periodontal risk:* In a patient with extreme caries risk posed by severe xerostomia or other conditions that cannot be controlled, the rate of caries progression is so fast that any restorative treatment based on teeth will fail. On the contrary, there have been case reports of successful oral rehabilitation of these patients with completely implant-supported prostheses, which cannot develop caries. Therefore, in a patient with extreme caries risk and good periodontal health associated with good oral hygiene, implant therapy should be considered.

Occasionally, tooth extraction is indicated without immediate plans for tooth replacement. Typically, these fall into two scenarios:

- Patient is not able to have tooth replacement done for various reasons (i.e., cannot meet financial and time needs currently).
- Tooth has associated pathology (i.e., periapical lesion) that needs to resolve prior to implant therapy. Large periapical lesions may take years to diminish in size, or may never resolve on their own (▶ Fig. 4.10).

Predicting the Quality of a Future Implant Site

For easy and predictable implant placement after extraction of a tooth, the extraction site should maintain or develop these characteristics: good bone density, sufficient ridge width in bucco-lingual and mesiodistal directions, sufficient bone height, good alignment of the center of the ridge with the center of the future restoration, and minimal height discrepancy between the edentulous ridge and the interproximal bone of the surrounding teeth.

The likelihood of getting these desirable characteristics depends on how the extraction was done and on wound healing of the site. The following factors will likely reduce the quality of the future implant site after extraction:

- *Low existing bone volume*: If an infection has destroyed most of the existing alveolar bone, or destroyed the buccal or lingual plate, it is uncertain how much bone will grow back after extraction. Often, there will only be partial bone regrowth, and the site will likely lack bone to place an implant at a correct position relative to the other teeth.
- *Excessive bone removal during extraction*: Excessive force and poor extraction technique can break the bone surrounding teeth and cause removal of alveolar bone along with the tooth. Needless to say, the lost bone will not grow back and result in diminished bone volume at the future implant site, especially if this is not managed with bone grafting, placement of a stiff, space-maintaining membrane, and primary closure.
- *Loss of buccal plate*: Bone facial to most teeth, and especially on the anterior maxilla, forms a paper-thin plate of bone, the buccal plate. This bone is readily damaged and removed during extraction, and often disappears or is missing prior to extraction. In addition, because tooth removal removes a significant portion of its blood supply, it tends to resorb during wound healing. In any case, loss of the buccal plate will result in a much narrower edentulous ridge in place of the missing tooth, and it will prevent implant placement unless expensive and time-intensive bone grafting procedures are performed, which aim to regenerate the lost bone.
- *Tobacco use*: Nicotine is a strong vasoconstrictor that can decrease vascularity in a socket site and prevent proper wound healing. Lack of proper wound healing likely results in reduced bone volume for implant placement.
- Medically compromised or older patients tend to have slower healing and less regrowth of bone in extraction sockets, resulting in poorer implant sites.
- Postoperative infections or alveolar osteitis prevent formation of bone and result in slow wound healing that favors bone resorption.

In contrasts, factors that improve extraction site healing, reduce bone loss and increase the chance of uncomplicated later implant placement are as follows:

- *"Atraumatic" technique*: While extraction always causes tissue trauma, the goal of the "atraumatic" technique is to minimize tissue damage and resulting bone loss. Unnecessary tissue trauma can be avoided with the following steps:
  - Plan the surgery and develop a sense for what local factors (i.e., root deformities, dense bone, curved roots, multiple roots, …) necessitate special extraction strategies.
  - Aim for reduced surgery time with efficient technique. The longer bone is exposed to air, the more postoperative pain and greater the amount of bone loss will be.
  - Avoid elevating soft tissue unless surgical access is required.
  - Section multi-rooted teeth before removal.
  - Remove dense cortical bone only from interseptal and interproximal areas if necessary.
  - Use little force effectively, and focus on gradual tooth elevation using periotomes and small elevators before using extraction forceps.
  - Remove the tooth with either specialized atraumatic tooth removal instruments, or use extraction forceps only to retrieve the tooth root with little force.
  - Avoid expanding the facial bone with the forceps.
  - Once the tooth is removed, thoroughly remove any soft tissue within the extraction socket to promote bleeding and wound healing.
- Place bone graft material or membranes designed for ridge preservation. Many studies, using a variety of bone graft materials and membranes, demonstrate reduced bone loss after extraction compared to not placing any material into the socket. Generally, ridge preservation should be performed for any site where a patient considers implant therapy and where the existing buccal plate is less than 2 mm in thickness, as these sites will lose at least a third of bone thickness without bone grafting.[7] In practice, this means that ridge preservation is mandatory for any maxillary anterior teeth that will be replaced with implants, and patients need to understand that even with bone grafting, additional bone grafting may be needed as a part of implant therapy.

4.5.4 Predicting the Difficulty Level of Tooth Removal

The quality of a future site depends in part on using an appropriate extraction technique that minimizes tissue damage. For treatment planning purposes, one has to choose from the following two extraction techniques:

- "Simple" tooth extraction using only elevators and extraction forceps.
- "Surgical" extraction involving scalpel incisions, flap elevation, and bone removal to aid tooth removal.

Choosing the wrong technique can result in lost chair time and productivity, increased risk of postoperative complications and loss of bone, and, most importantly, very significant patient pain and dissatisfaction with treatment.

Besides relying on clinical experience, the decision to choose either technique can be made by analyzing the tooth to be extracted and assessing difficulty:

- *Root anatomy*: Exodontia is extremely predictable if an appropriate root shape-matching instrument is used that will fully engage the tooth root along the natural extraction path dictated by the root shape and position. Roots that are conical will possess less of a challenge than roots that are curved or have dilacerations. Single-rooted teeth are less difficult to remove than multirooted teeth, which may benefit from sectioning and individual root removal. Roots with bulbous shape pose a special challenge and most likely cannot be removed with elevators and forceps alone (▶ Fig. 4.11).
- *Subgingival caries/restoration*: Restorative material or caries that extends subgingivally can significantly increase complexity of tooth removal, especially if the periodontal

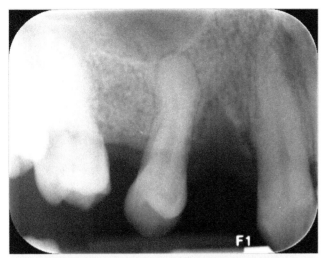

Fig. 4.11 This premolar presents a special challenge for simple tooth removal as it has a curved root, has an apical root bulge and a figure 8-shaped root, is slightly tipped, has no neighboring teeth, and lacks a good purchase point for elevation. In addition, it is close to the sinus floor, is surrounded by relatively dense bone around the root bulge, and has a cervical abfraction lesion visible clinically that posed a fracture risk during extraction. It was removed surgically with no complications.

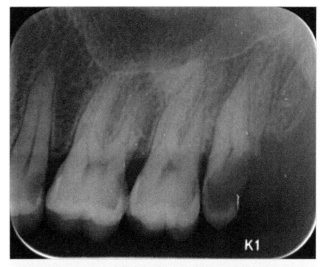

Fig. 4.12 Carious teeth make extraction difficult. Subgingival extent of this large carious lesion on the third molar makes it extremely difficult to remove this tooth since there is little sound tooth structure to engage, and there is little periodontal ligament space for insertion of the luxating or elevating instrument.

ligament (PDL) space is narrow. The caries or restorative material weakens the tooth and will likely cause the crown to break off when pressure is applied in this area with a forceps or elevator. This becomes likely if the PDL space is narrow, since it will be difficult finding a coronal purchase point on sound tooth structure that the elevator can grab to luxate the tooth out of the socket. The same problem also exists if caries extends into a furcation area, where application of extraction forceps will cause the tooth to break. An example of this is the carious third molar shown in ▶Fig. 4.12, which is extremely challenging to remove.

- Proximity of teeth to vital structures must be studied before attempting to remove a tooth. For posterior mandibular teeth, the main concern is the proximity of teeth to the IA nerve. Here, it is possible that surgery can push the tooth root into the IA nerve, or surgery trauma can directly damage the IA nerve, resulting in permanent numbness (paresthesia) or disturbed pain sensation in the mandible. Both complications in the maxilla or mandible are avoided by using a careful surgical technique that aims to minimize movement of the tooth toward the vital structure (▶Fig. 4.13a). In isolated maxillary teeth, the maxillary sinus can expand ("pneumatized") and surround the tooth roots of molars and premolars (▶Fig. 4.13b). Removing these teeth can also accidentally tear out a small amount of bone and sinus floor membrane, resulting in a channel between the oral cavity and sinus floor, which may never heal and close. Creating such oroantral fistula should be avoided since it is uncomfortable for the patient and requires additional surgical repair procedures. If a root tip is close to the sinus, there also is a possibility of pushing the root tip into the sinus where it can set up a chronic sinus infection, and root tips need to be removed surgically from the sinus.
- *Lone standing teeth:* Pose a unique challenge during exodontia due to the lack of any identifiable purchase point needed for significant luxation (▶Fig. 4.14). In most cases, when a

purchase point cannot be identified, a surgical method is needed to extract such teeth, as "simple" extraction techniques will simply cause bits of tooth structure fracturing off the remaining tooth without actually removing the tooth.
- *Root canal treatment:* Teeth previously treated with root canal treatment are more brittle than teeth with vital pulps, and are likely to break or crumble during extraction attempts (▶Fig. 4.15a). Consequently, surgical extraction should be anticipated for root canal treated teeth.
- *Lack of PDL space:* Lack of PDL space prevents insertion of periotomes, elevators, and luxators, which then places undue pressure on the tooth crown, which may then break off since it has been compromised by caries or restoration. Lack of PDL space (▶Fig. 4.15b) often requires surgical exposure of a tooth, and removal of cortical bone around the tooth for a better purchase point on the root.

4.5.5 Judging if Immediate Implant Placement is an Option

Traditionally, dental implants are placed in edentulous sites well after tooth extraction. For teeth that need to be removed and where replacement with a dental implant is desired, the usual treatment sequence is extraction with ridge preservation, an 8 to 12 week healing time, implant placement, and yet another 12 to 16 week healing time.

An alternative implant placement with a potentially much shorter time to tooth replacement is immediate implant therapy. Although highly technique sensitive and requiring considerable implant placement and restoration experience, if done well for the right site and patient, this procedure has several advantages over conventional implant placement. For immediate implant placement, an implant along with any bone grafting materials is placed immediately after tooth removal. Since this eliminates one surgery appointment, the patient will experience less pain overall and will have tooth replacement 2 to 3

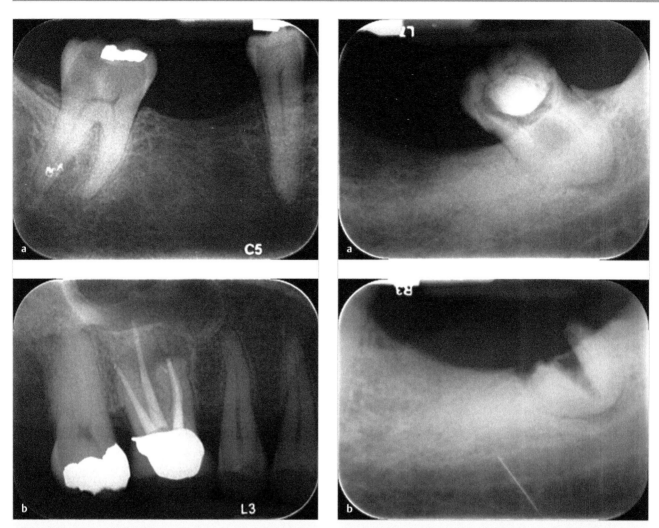

Fig. 4.13 Importance of vital structures in extraction decisions. (a) Tooth no. 31 has significant decay on the coronal aspect and is not restorable. Upon careful examination, we note that the root tips are in close proximity to the inferior alveolar nerve (IAN), and surgical extraction is needed. (b) Tooth no. 14 has a failing root canal with that was already treated with apicoectomy and continued evidence of infection at the root apices. Given the proximity of the palatal root to the sinus, a surgical extraction technique is indicated.

Fig. 4.14 The challenge of lone-standing teeth. (a) This molar presents multiple challenges to "simple" extraction techniques: lone-standing position, deep caries, large restoration, close proximity to the IA nerve, and lacking any significant PDL space. (b) A provider tried "simple" extraction techniques for 3 hours, fracturing off the crown and losing root structure to the bone level before giving up and referring the patient with significant trismus for tooth removal. The tooth was removed at the next appointment with little difficulty using appropriate surgical techniques, and a muscle relaxant to relieve the patient's trismus for improved access.

months sooner. Moreover, since there is always some bone loss any time the alveolar bone is exposed, having only one surgery limits the amount of bone loss and produces better esthetic outcomes since there is less gingival recession in the area. At the same time, the likelihood of successful implant restoration is the same as for conventional implant placement in the hands of experienced providers.

Here are the criteria needed for a site receiving immediate implants:

- Surgeon and patient are comfortable with the added risk of the procedure, and the possible need for bone and soft tissue grafting during and after the procedure.
- *The restorative dentist feels comfortable with using custom abutments and other advanced restorative procedures*: Immediate implants tend to be placed slightly lingual to engage bone, and more apical to compensate for a small amount of gingival recession that occurs with surgery.

- *Patient has low esthetic expectations*: Since there is a risk of recession, the patient needs to be aware of the risk. In addition, it is helpful if the lip margin, while smiling, does not show the gingival margin at the site.
- *Patient is not using tobacco*: Smoking is associated with more pain.
- *Patient is healthy*: Any condition decreasing wound healing ability and increasing the risk of infection makes it more likely that complications arise and the implant fails.
- No parafunctional habits such as bruxism.[8]
- Stable occlusion with good posterior support.
- *Thick gingival biotype*: Although immediate implant placement is possible in both, a thick biotype will be more forgiving and produce less tissue changes after surgery and implant restoration.[9]

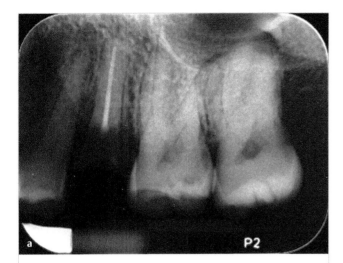

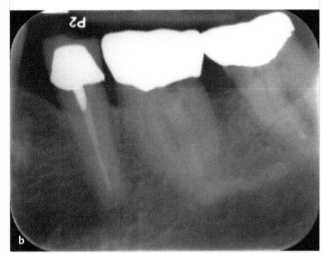

Fig. 4.15 Other factors making extractions more difficult. (a) Failed root canal. (b) Lack of PDL space.

- *Lack of infection*: Although it is possible to place immediate implants with equally good success rate into sites that had periapical infections, it adds a complication to treatment since the best protocol in cleaning these sites is yet unknown. The same is true for sites with periodontal infection, where immediate implant placement is possible with no long-term effect,[10] but it likely results in an implant that is more difficult to manage restoratively because of the previously existing bone and soft tissue loss.
- *"Atraumatic" extraction*: The more tissue trauma occurs during surgery, the more likely there will be recession and bone loss, which complicates restoration of the implant.
- *Intact tooth socket after extraction*: Although it is possible to place implants into extraction sockets that lack a buccal plate, it requires more management and is more risky.
- Enough bone to engage the implant with high stability. Usually, for anterior teeth that requires placement of a longer 13 to 16-mm implant that is placed into the disto-apical wall of the socket in a way that the implant platform occupies the cingulum area and there is 2-mm distance between the facial edge of the implant and the buccal bone surface. For

posterior teeth, this means that the implant has to either be longer than the tooth root by at least 4 mm or the implant needs to be placed into interseptal bone.

4.6 Benefits and Risks of Tooth Removal, Tooth Replacement, and Tooth Retention

Whenever tooth removal is considered, a "do nothing" treatment option that does not involve tooth removal needs to be explained to the patient. The importance of the "do nothing" option is that tooth removal is irreversible, and providing this option forces the dentist and the patient to consider all the risks and benefits of tooth removal. It is also important to point out that even "hopeless" teeth can be maintained for a significant amount of time and with little detriment to surrounding teeth.[11] For informed consent purposes, if tooth removal is indicated, the patient must receive treatment options ranging from preserving teeth to removing teeth and all applicable tooth replacement options, and explain for each option what procedures are required, how much time and money it will cost and the major benefits and risks of each option. This ensures that the patient has all the information needed to make an informed decision, and greatly reduces treatment doubts and anxieties on the side of the patient.

When discussing treatment plans with patients that involve tooth removal, the following risks and benefits should always be considered.

4.6.1 Preserving Teeth

Except for the most hopeless cases, preventing complete tooth loss is always preferred because of the damaging psychological effect of losing all teeth, diminished nutrition associated with dentures and the long-term possibility of not being able to wear dentures due to complete bone resorption. Similarly, the ideal goal should be to preserve all teeth as long as possible since tooth replacement carries the risk of damaging surrounding teeth as in denture abutments, and the possibility of periimplant disease with implant-supported prostheses.

Procedures

At a minimum, oral hygiene instruction, scaling and root planing procedures, frequent periodontal maintenance may need restorative, periodontal surgery, orthodontic, endodontic, and oral surgery procedures.

Cost and Time Commitment

Periodontal surgeries involve significant cost, but usually less than tooth replacement. While the cost of each surgical and restorative treatment can approach the cost of a home appliance such as a refrigerator, the out-of-pocket cost of periodontal maintenance visit is comparable to paying for a cell phone or cable service. Maintaining teeth requires a lifetime commitment to oral hygiene, healthy lifestyle, and frequent preventive dental care.

Benefits for the Patient

- *Proprioception*: The innervation in the periodontal ligament allows patients to feel food and efficiently chew it in the mouth.
- *Stimulation of bone*: Normal occlusal forces applied to teeth stimulate remodeling and maintenance of sound alveolar bone.
- *Defense against periodontal disease:* Even though periodontal disease develops around teeth, the periodontal ligament provides protection against periodontal disease as it allows immune cells migrating to the area. In addition, periodontal disease treatment around teeth is more predictable than around implants.
- *Maintains gingival position*: If teeth are removed, there will always be bone and soft tissue loss. This will make restoration more difficult, and make surrounding teeth appear longer.
- *Maintains normal face contours*: Keeping teeth prevents drifting of teeth into abnormal positions and bone loss. Both bone and teeth support the lower 1/3 of the face. Losing teeth leads to an "aged" appearance as the perioral region sinks inward and the vertical dimension collapses.
- *Maintains proper nutrition and quality of life*: Retention of teeth is associated with better nutrition and quality of life compared to those who lost teeth.[12]
- *Cost*: Removing many teeth at once, denture construction, and implant therapy are expensive compared to maintaining teeth.

Risks to a Patient with Severe or Uncontrolled Periodontal Disease

- *Risk of infections*: Periodontal maintenance patients can experience periodontal abscesses, and new periodontal disease may develop. Exposed root surfaces are prone to caries, which risks endodontic infections.
- *Lack of function*: Loose teeth may make chewing difficult and may be painful when biting on them. However, splinting can eliminate noticeable tooth mobility and improve function.
- *Systemic risk*: Uncontrolled periodontal disease may pose a risk to systemic health. Periodontal treatment may reduce the systemic risk for some conditions such as type 2 diabetes mellitus.
- Need for frequent periodontal maintenance to prevent tooth loss every 3 months or even more frequently.
- *Possible need for additional medications*: Management of periodontal disease may involve exposure to local delivery antimicrobials, biologics, and other novel medications that are being developed to treat periodontal disease, and a patient may need to take medications such as low-dose sub-antimicrobial tetracyclines to slow down periodontal disease activity for the rest of their lives.

4.6.2 Removing Teeth

Removing teeth is one of the surest, but also most radical, and irreversible treatments to eliminate periodontal disease.

Procedures

Surgical removal of teeth, with local anesthesia and possibly some level of sedation depending on patient needs, often requires tooth replacement to restore function and appearance, and tooth replacement may be done with dental implant placement and restoration; fixed, removable partial dentures, or with a removable complete denture.

Cost and Time Commitment

High cost at the beginning for extractions and temporary ("interim") denture to replace missing teeth during healing; but cost is often partially or fully covered by most forms of dental insurance. Full mouth extraction and complete denture therapy, if not subsidized by insurance, is comparable in a dental school clinic setting to the cost of a large TV set. There may be additional high costs for implant therapy, if this is desired by the patient. It requires a number of dental visits for extractions and denture construction, but usually is complete within 6 months to a year. Patients may require frequent preventive dental care depending on the number of teeth or implants present and the complexity of the restorative treatment. However, in completely edentulous patients, only annual evaluation is required once the final dentures have been delivered, and replacement of dentures should be anticipated about every 5 years.

Benefits

- Eliminates periodontal disease and caries as the disease process of both depends on the presence of a tooth surface.
- *Efficient treatment*: Extractions take little time.
- *May have improved appearance*: Prostheses may achieve better appearance than natural teeth, especially with complete dentures that can replace teeth and gingival tissues.
- *Less maintenance required for complete dentures*: Maintenance is limited to periodic inspection of the oral mucosa and cleaning of the denture once or twice yearly. Typically, dentures should be replaced with a new denture every five years.

Risks

- Irreversible.
- Decreased chewing force with removable dentures. This effect is most pronounced with completely tissue-supported dentures where chewing force is limited by the ability of the remaining keratinized tissue to withstand pressure created by the dentures. In addition, chewing efficiency is decreased since denture teeth often have flat anatomy to allow for a balanced occlusal scheme at the expense of occlusal surfaces being able to cut through food.
- Continued loss of bone. Eventually, this may lead to alveolar ridge anatomy that can no longer support dentures.
- Shifting of teeth and collapse of vertical dimension resulting in "aged" appearance.
- Increased chance of tooth loss. Loss of teeth leads to occlusal changes because of gradual tooth position changes, and

increased occlusal load on remaining teeth which are then more prone to fracture.

- Possible need for tooth replacement. Increased tooth loss risk translates into increased chance of needing tooth replacement. Tooth replacement is expensive, and requires either preparation of adjacent teeth for support or extensive surgical treatment as part of implant therapy.

If removing teeth, tooth replacement usually needs to be considered. The major risks and benefits of implant therapy, tooth-supported fixed partial dentures, and removable dentures are as follows.

4.6.3 Implant-supported Tooth Replacement

For patients who have lost teeth, implant therapy presents a chance of regaining almost tooth-like function and appearance, but at significant cost and time commitment.

Procedures

Requires diagnostic work-up using detailed radiographic surveys and scans; require implant-placement surgery and possible second-stage surgery. It may also require extensive bone grafting and soft tissue grafting surgery prior to implant placement or as part of the implant surgery; require restoration of the implant with any fixed, removable, or hybrid fixed-removable appliances.

Cost and Time Commitment

Implant therapy is likely the most expensive dental treatment. Diagnostic work-up costs are followed by very expensive surgical treatment and restorative treatment. Treatment costs may approach the cost of a luxury car with the most extensive oral rehabilitation cases. Implant therapy requires many visits and a lifetime commitment to good oral hygiene, healthy lifestyle, and frequent preventive dental care.

Benefits

- From a patient's perspective, implant supported restorations typically feel and function most like natural teeth compared to dentures and bridges. However, it is very difficult to match the esthetics of a natural tooth because of the metal component of most implants, the round diameter of an implant compared to the irregular cross-section of teeth, and the lack of a cementoenamel junction and gingival fiber attachment.
- *Preserves existing teeth, bone*: Implant placement provides mechanical stimulation of bone and thus maintains it to some degree.
- Restores chewing ability compared to having an edentulous site.

Risks

- Typically, most expensive treatment.
- May require expensive soft and hard tissue grafting procedures, which often needs to be done by specialists, and also

require significant amount of healing time. For a posterior maxilla site needing lateral window sinus augmentation, it may take 1 to 2 years to replace a failed molar with an implant because of the time required for bone formation and integration of the implant into the new bone.

- Surgical and restorative complications.
- Risk of periimplant disease and implant failure.
- May not achieve the same appearance as natural teeth. Implant crowns tend to be more opaque because of the need to mask the typical metal abutment and framework. White Zirconia and gold-colored abutments have been developed for improved appearance, but they are also more technique sensitive and still may not fully replicate translucent teeth. In addition, there is always a loss of interdental papilla height with implant therapy, which requires slightly longer interproximal contacts for masking. As a consequence, implant crowns tend also to be slightly bulkier than the tooth they are replacing.
- Requires good oral hygiene and frequent maintenance for long-term success.

4.6.4 Tooth-supported Fixed Partial Dentures

Fixed partial dentures can usually only be done when few teeth are missing, and if the edentulous site is surrounded by teeth that can serve as fixed denture abutments. While it is possible to create cantilevered fixed partial dentures that rely on support only on one side, their predictable use is limited to few situations where a strong tooth is used as abutment and there is no occlusal force placed on the cantilevered pontic. In general, Ante's law must be followed in selection of abutment teeth, meaning that there needs to be at least as many tooth roots on the abutment teeth as there are on the teeth to be replaced. In addition, abutment teeth need to have good crown-to-root ratio, strong bony support, a large root surface, and a sound crown that can support the abutment crown. Ideally, root canal treated teeth should be avoided to serve as abutment because of their possible fracture risk. Implant therapy should be considered if the edentulous site is surrounded by unrestored teeth in order to preserve healthy tooth structure.

Procedures

Fixed partial denture treatment requires the preparation of surrounding teeth and routine restorative procedures such as impression taking, frame-work try-in, cementation, and occlusal adjustment. Treatment may require root canal treatment and placement of cores, although this may increase the risk of future abutment failure.

Cost and Time Commitment

Fixed partial denture therapy can be very expensive, in cost similar to major home appliances, and provides for fast tooth replacement usually in a matter of weeks or few months.

Benefits

- Fixed tooth replacement.

- *No bone/soft tissue surgery needed usually*: Ridge augmentation procedures can improve the pontic site and provide a more natural appearance.
- Ovate pontic design may achieve tooth-like appearance.

Risks

- *Only possible for short spans and if there are enough abutment teeth*: While long-span fixed partial dentures are possible, they are more difficult to produce, which increases the chance of treatment failure.
- Compromises surrounding teeth used for preparation as surrounding teeth need to support higher occlusal loads.
- Continued bone loss in pontic site.
- Prosthetic complications (porcelain chipping) may not be repairable without removing the entire unit.
- Requires frequent maintenance.

4.6.5 Removable Partial/Complete Dentures

Tooth replacement with removable partial dentures has the most basic requirements. Partial dentures require selection of abutment teeth much the same way as for fixed partial dentures (see above), except that abutment failure sometimes can be compensated with modification of the partial denture. Complete dentures require presence of keratinized tissue in the denture-supporting areas, and a decent amount of alveolar ridge height with no significant undercuts and muscle attachments that allows for denture stability and support. Generally, stable, retentive, and well-accepted maxillary complete dentures can be made for most patients. In contrast, mandibular complete dentures tend to present retention and stability problems for many patients with resorbed ridges, and basic implant therapy with two implants placed in the canine regions should be considered to add denture retention for those patients.

Procedures

Basic removable denture procedures involving rest preparation into abutment teeth, impressions, framework and denture try-in visits, delivery, and denture adjustment. Some patients may also need fabrication of surveyed crowns to fit the denture or other restorative treatment to improve abutments. Implant surgery may be considered for some complete denture patients.

Cost and Time Commitment

There may be significant cost at the beginning of treatment if denture therapy is not subsidized by insurance, and out-of-pocket cost for a set of removable dentures can be similar to a major home appliance. Both partial and complete denture fabrication require multiple visits at first, but treatment usually is complete within a few weeks or months.

Benefits

- Least-invasive tooth replacement.
- Usually, cheapest tooth replacement option.
- Complete dentures allow good esthetic appearance.

Risks

- May need to relearn chewing, speaking.
- Decreased chewing ability.
- Large and bulky appliance.
- Limited use for multiple tooth replacement.
- Unsightly clasps.
- Requires frequent maintenance.

4.7 Essential Takeaways

- A prognosis is a prediction on how quickly a patient's periodontal condition will deteriorate and how well treatment might prevent further tissue destruction.
- *Individual tooth prognosis depends on multiple factors*: Caries/restorability, strategic value, endodontic status, occlusion, crown-to-root ratio, root morphology, probing depths, etc.; these factors guide in the selection of abutment teeth and help to decide which teeth should be sacrificed for overall health.
- Prognosis can change depending on the success of treatment. Because periodontal disease is episodic, it needs to be reevaluated periodically. The patient's disease risk determines the recall frequency.
- When deciding to remove teeth, careful assessment is needed to determine the strategic value and the complexity of the procedure. A tooth can be removed with routine elevation and forceps delivery or via flap surgically. The goal is to preserve and maintain bony support for future consideration.
- It is important to carefully weigh the risks and benefits of maintaining teeth versus replacing teeth with dental implants or prosthetic appliances. Patient expectations and wishes should be considered and respected. Informed consent is paramount.
- Periodontal disease is sporadic, so it is important to plan and allow flexibility in future treatment.

4.8 Review Questions

For the following questions consider this case.

A 69-year old female presents to you complaining about pain in the upper left quadrant and a "bump that comes and goes" in the same area (pointing to no. 15). The teeth in the area are sensitive to hot or cold, and to eating anything. The pain started about 6 months ago, and she obtained amoxicillin from an urgent care center, which made the pain go away for a few months.

The patient has a history of hypertension, and takes Lisinopril for it. Otherwise, she does not know of any medical conditions and sees a physician regularly. Blood pressure is 128/83 mm Hg, and pulse is a steady 75/min.

Extraoral exam reveals no abnormal findings other than slightly more tender palpation of the cervical lymph nodes on the left side. Intraoral exam reveals no findings other than periodontal disease as shown in the periodontal chart (no mobility was found; furcation involvement was suspected, but not clearly identified), and possible endodontic conditions in the upper left quadrant.

Pulp vitality tests were done, and produced the following results:

- *No. 13*: Cold response–normal, palpation–normal, percussion–normal.
- *No. 14*: Cold response–exaggerated, but short-lived; palpation–normal, percussion–normal.
- *No. 15*: Cold response–exaggerated, but short-lived; palpation–causes dull pain, percussion–painful.
- *No. 16:* Cold response–exaggerated, but short-lived; cannot palpate as there is too little space; normal response percussion.

Here are the relevant clinical photographs (▶Fig. 4.16) and radiographs (▶Fig. 4.17).

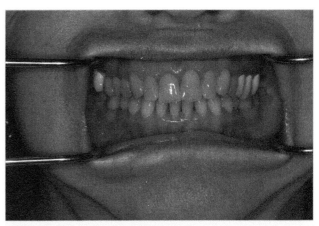

Fig. 4.16 Facial view of review case.

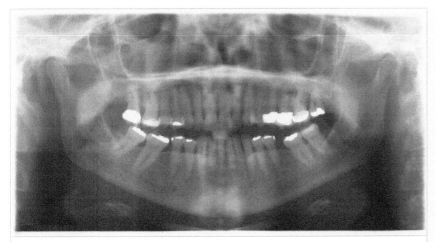

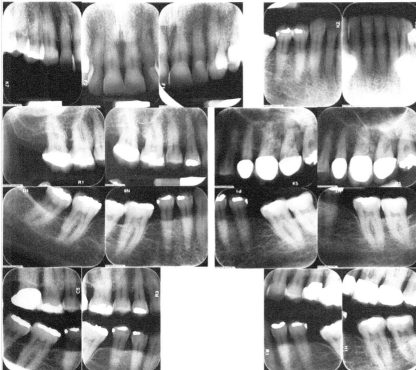

Fig. 4.17 Radiographs of review case.

Findings in the periodontal chart are as follows:

Facial		1	2	3	4	5	6	7	8	9	10	11	12	13	14	15	16
	PD	323	322	213	312	212	212	111	222	222	112	212	314	324	525	537	635
	BOP													1	1 1	111	
Lingual	PD	354	533	323	323	312	212	211	211	213	222	222	214	425	624	5127	745
	BOP	11	1	1 1	1 1	1	1		111	111					111	111	111
Lingual		32	31	30	29	28	27	26	25	24	23	22	21	20	19	18	17
	PD	345	524		333	322	222	111	111	212	212	212	223	222		226	534
	BOP						111	111	111	111	111	111					
Facial	PD	324	423		112	212	211	111	112	112	112	112	212	212		334	533
	BOP	111	1		1	1 1					1						

Abbreviations: BOP, bleeding on probing (1); CAL, clinical attachment level; Furc, furcation involvement (Glickman class); GR, gingival recession; MGJ, position of mucogingival junction from margin; Mobil, tooth mobility (Miller grade); PD, probing depths; PLQ, plaque level (0 = none, 5 = heavy).

Learning objective: Judge how likely a patient will lose teeth.

1. This patient's disease activity level is indicative of
   A. Patients with rapid disease progression
   B. Patients with average disease progression
   C. Patients resistant to periodontal disease

2. What is the likelihood of the patient losing teeth?
   A. Very likely will lose most or all teeth
   B. Likely will lose at least some teeth
   C. Unlikely to lose teeth in the near future
   D. Very unlikely to ever lose teeth

3. What is the prognosis for tooth no. 15?
   A. Excellent or good
   B. Fair
   C. Poor
   D. Questionable or hopeless

4. Scaling and root planing has been completed, and pocket reduction has been achieved to 5 mm or less except for tooth no. 15 and the third molars, which have been removed. There are four sites left with 5-mm pockets and about 30% show gingival bleeding. What is the most appropriate recall interval?
   A. 3–4 months
   B. 4–6 months
   C. 6–12 months
   D. 12–24 months

Learning objective: Judge how likely periodontal treatment will succeed.

5. Given the patient's initial presentation, conditions are _____ for saving all the patient's teeth with periodontal treatment.
   A. Favorable
   B. Questionable
   C. Unfavorable/hopeless

6. Scaling and root planing has been completed, and pocket reduction has been achieved to 5 mm or less except for tooth no. 15 and the third molars, which have been removed. There are four sites left with 5-mm pockets and about 30% show gingival bleeding. Given these conditions, conditions are now _____ for saving all the patient's teeth with continued periodontal treatment.
   A. Favorable
   B. Questionable
   C. Unfavorable/hopeless

7. The patient would like to replace the missing tooth no. 19, and you run through the different treatment options in your mind. If you planned a fixed partial denture, which of the following conditions of tooth no. 18 make it a less than ideal fixed partial denture abutment?
   A. Mesial tipping
   B. Occlusal amalgam
   C. Crown-to-root ratio
   D. Root shape

Learning objective: Determine which teeth should be removed.

8. No restorative treatment is planned for the right side. For the lower right quadrant, how many teeth should you consider removing?
   A. None 1
   B. 2
   C. 3 or more

9. For which of the following conditions should you consider sacrificing a tooth for dental implant placement?
   A. Tooth has 6-mm pocket with minor amount of bone loss
   B. Tooth has caries on mesial, distal, and occlusal surface reaching into dentin
   C. Tooth has severe caries due to xerostomia and despite good oral hygiene
   D. Tooth has discolored enamel from excess natural fluoride

10. Evaluate the following statements about tooth no. 15 in this case.

Statement 1: The restorative status of no. 15 is of little consequence for extraction planning.

Statement 2: The no. 15 site will produce a poor implant site with after extraction with ridge preservation.

A. Both statements are true
B. Both statements are false
C. The first statement is true, the second is false
D. The first statement is false, the second is true

11. Generally, which of the following are essential to improving the likelihood of implant placement for replacing a nonrestorable tooth no. 8?
A. Gentle extraction technique
B. Bone grafting and/or membrane placement
C. A and B
D. None of the above

Learning objective: Weigh benefits and risks of tooth removal, toot replacement, and tooth preservation

12. Evaluate the following statements comparing benefits of tooth replacement methods.

Statement 1: Implant therapy is typically a quick and cost-effective method for replacing lost teeth.

Statement 2: Removable partial dentures require less tooth preparation than fixed partial dentures.
A. Both statements are true
B. Both statements are false
C. The first statement is true, the second is false
D. The first statement is false, the second is true

4.9 Answers

1. **B.** The patient experiences mild to locally severe bone loss, and given the patient's age the disease progression is not overly aggressive. There are definitely signs of significant disease, so the patient is also not resistant.

2. **B.** It is unlikely that the patient will lose all teeth since most teeth have minimal bone loss at age 69. However, there is at least one tooth with near complete bone loss (no. 15), and probably she will lose that in the near future. While it is possible to maintain hopeless teeth, she has a recurring periodontal abscess at no. 15, which is continuing to destroy bone, so C and D are unlikely answers.

3. **E.** Using the classification system outlined in this chapter the deep furcation involvement and deep pocketing produce at least "questionable" if not "hopeless" prognosis. Number 15 has multiple problems that are very difficult if not at all possible to address: pocketing up to 12 mm, which makes it highly unlikely that all calculus can ever be removed. Deep furcation involvement from all sides, which makes it possible that there is complete, class III furcation involvement, which is impossible to maintain in this maxillary tooth. Less than 90% bone loss, which explains the mobility.

4. **B.** The patient has a medium risk of periodontal disease progression based on the subjective assessment presented here (▶Table 4.7) or as calculated by Lang's periodontal risk assessment tool. Therefore, the recall interval should not be longer than 6 months, ruling out answers **C** and **D**. While more frequent recall intervals, as in answer **A**, will not worsen the disease, they also will be not more useful

in preventing disease progression and needlessly cost the patient money and time.

5. **C.** Given the patient's initial condition, it is unlikely that you can save all the patient's teeth because tooth no. 15 has near complete bone loss and very deep pockets. Using ▶Table 4.8 and the Caton-Kwok terminology, conditions for complete treatment success in saving teeth are at probably "hopeless."

6. **A.** Now that all significant periodontal disease has been eliminated, the chance of keeping the remaining teeth is very likely or "favorable" (see ▶Table 4.8). The key point of this question is that prognosis can change over time, and usually improves with periodontal treatment as areas that are difficult to maintain are eliminated.

7. **A.** The problem here is that the tooth is tipped mesially, which prevents insertion of a partial denture framework unless you are willing to significantly remove mesial tooth structure, and possibly perform root canal therapy and a core buildup. Alternatively, orthodontic uprighting is possible, and very difficult with molars. The occlusal amalgam is not a concern as it would be removed during tooth preparation. The crown-to-root ratio and root shape are very supportive of the tooth serving as abutment, as the crown is much shorter than the roots embedded in the bone, and the roots are long and curved, which provides lots of bony support.

8. **A.** None. Even though nos. 31 and 32 are tipped mesially, their prognosis is not hopeless while they have strategic value as occluding surface and do not interfere with restorative treatment as none is planned.

9. **C.** Implant-supported restorations will not get caries, and as long as periodontal disease can be prevented, this is a good option. **A** can be treated with standard periodontal therapy, **B** can be treated with a direct or indirect restoration depending on size, and **D** can be likely treated with a veneer instead.

10. **D.** The crown of no. 15 may come off during extraction, and makes extraction more challenging as you have little sound tooth structure for an elevator or forceps to engage. While it is possible that this tooth elevates easily because of the lack of supporting bone, you should be ready to perform a surgical extraction exposing more tooth structure in case the crown comes off. Since there is so much bone loss, it is quite likely that even despite ridge preservation, you will have little bone regrowth and a poor implant site with much reduced bone height.

11. **C.** For anterior maxilla sites, the buccal plate is usually very thin, and ridge preservation should always be done if implant therapy is anticipated. This means that the nonrestorable tooth has to be gently removed and the socket filled with graft material and/or be protected with a membrane.

12. **D.** Implant therapy is usually the most expensive and lengthy treatment compared to fixed and removable partial denture therapy since it requires surgery and prolonged healing time after surgery. The rest preparations required for removable partial dentures are much smaller than the tooth preparation required fixed partial dentures.

4.10 Evidence-based Activities

- Obtain the studies published by Dr. McGuire on tooth prognosis, and trace the development of the prognosis system from initial idea to statistical validation. Judge how well this system would apply to a general practice.
- Most periodontal prognosis systems were developed by periodontists in private practice. Pretend to be a general dentist, and decide what your prognosis system would look like. How would you validate your system?
- Obtain the commentary by Drs. Kwok and Caton on prognosis, and review the various existing prognosis systems. Which categories do you think is the easiest/hardest to assign and why?

References

[1] Neely AL, Holford TR, Löe H, Anerud A, Boysen H. The natural history of periodontal disease in humans: risk factors for tooth loss in caries-free subjects receiving no oral health care. J Clin Periodontol 2005;32(9):984–993

[2] Kassebaum NJ, Bernabé E, Dahiya M, Bhandari B, Murray CJ, Marcenes W. Global burden of severe tooth loss: A systematic review and meta-analysis. J Dent Res 2014;93(7, Suppl):20S–28S

[3] Lang NP, Tonetti MS. Periodontal risk assessment (PRA) for patients in supportive periodontal therapy (SPT). Oral Health Prev Dent 2003;1(1):7–16

[4] Pihlstrom BL. Periodontal risk assessment, diagnosis and treatment planning. Periodontol 2000 2001;25:37–58

[5] Nunn ME, Fan J, Su X, Levine RA, Lee HJ, McGuire MK. Development of prognostic indicators using classification and regression trees for survival. Periodontol 2000 2012;58(1):134–142

[6] Kwok V, Caton JG. Commentary: prognosis revisited—a system for assigning periodontal prognosis. J Periodontol 2007;78(11):2063–2071

[7] Cardaropoli D, Tamagnone L, Roffredo A, Gaveglio L. Relationship between the buccal bone plate thickness and the healing of postextraction sockets with/without ridge preservation. Int J Periodontics Restorative Dent 2014;34(2):211–217

[8] Al-Sabbagh M, Kutkut A. Immediate implant placement: surgical techniques for prevention and management of complications. Dent Clin North Am 2015;59(1):73–95

[9] Kinaia BM, Ambrosio F, Lamble M, Hope K, Shah M, Neely AL. Soft tissue changes around immediately placed implants: a systematic review and meta-analyses with at least 12 months of follow-up after functional loading. J Periodontol 2017;88(9):876–886

[10] Crespi R, Capparè P, Gherlone E. Immediate loading of dental implants placed in periodontally infected and non-infected sites: a 4-year follow-up clinical study. J Periodontol 2010;81(8):1140–1146

[11] Machtei EE, Hirsch I. Retention of hopeless teeth: the effect on the adjacent proximal bone following periodontal surgery. J Periodontol 2007;78(12):2246–2252

[12] Musacchio E, Perissinotto E, Binotto P, et al. Tooth loss in the elderly and its association with nutritional status, socio-economic and lifestyle factors. Acta Odontol Scand 2007;65(2):78–86

5 Controlling Gingival Inflammation

Abstract

Generally, dental treatment begins with pain management, if needed, and progresses through acute disease control, definite treatment, and maintenance phases. The acute disease control phase consists of biopsy and initial management of suspicious oral lesions, removal of hopeless teeth, initial root canal treatments, caries control, and initial treatment of periodontal disease. Initial periodontal disease treatment aims to control periodontal inflammation, which is a prerequisite for most restorative procedures and often the first treatment step in patient care. This chapter addresses how periodontal inflammation can be controlled nonsurgically with **scaling** and **root planing** (SRP) procedures, **adjuncts**, oral hygiene methods, and tobacco cessation counseling. These methods are also applied in the maintenance phase in order to prevent periodontal inflammation and tooth loss.

Keywords: initial treatment, oral hygiene, tobacco counseling

5.1 Learning Objectives

- Given clinical findings, develop a comprehensive periodontal treatment plan that aims to reduce periondontal inflammation.
- Describe how to perform efficient and effective scaling and root planing (SRP).
- Describe the benefits and risks of adjunctive agents used during SRP.
- Given a patient's oral hygiene needs, develop personalized oral hygiene instructions.
- Develop a strategy to assist a patient with tobacco cessation.

5.2 Case

A 30-year old healthy Hispanic male presented complaining of "hurting gums" and "cavities" (see ► Fig. 5.1 and ► Fig. 5.2 for initial presentation). He saw a dentist 2 years before this visit, but did not remember what was done. He stated that he brushes regularly twice daily with a manual brush and fluoridated toothpaste, but does not floss "since it makes his gums bleed." Oral examination showed no pathology other than slight marginal and moderate papillary erythema, accompanied by generalized gingival bleeding, deep pocketing, and heavy calculus. **Idiopathic osteosclerosis** was found in some areas of the mandible during the radiographic exam. More significantly, mild generalized bone loss was found along with occlusal caries at some posterior teeth.

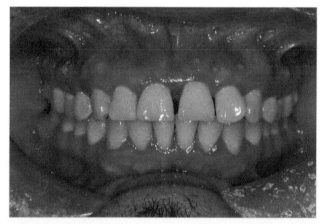

Fig. 5.1 Facial view.

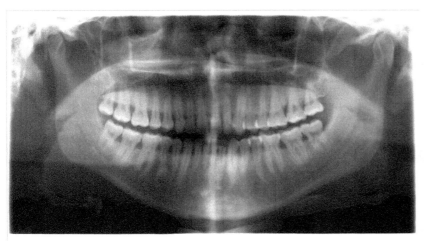

Fig. 5.2 X-ray series radiographs at initial visit and 2 years later.

At Initial Exam

2 Years After Exam

Initial findings in the periodontal chart are as follows:

Maxilla		1	2	3	4	5	6	7	8	9	10	11	12	13	14	15	16
	PD	555	636	637	737	735	536	636	636	635	636	746	637	738	737	747	745
	BOP	111	111	111	111	111	111	111	111	111	111	111	111	111	111	111	111
	CAL	1	2	2	2	2	2	2	2	2	2	2	2	2	2	2	2
	GR																
	MGJ	333	555	578	999	999	999	999	999	999	999	999	999	999	999	999	444
	Furc																
	PLQ	1	1	1	1	1	1	1	1	1	1	1	1	1	1	1	1
Maxilla lingual	PD	656	745	745	856	535	636	645	526	635	545	535	536	645	646	668	868
	BOP	111	111	111	111	111	111	111	111	111	111	111	111	111	111	111	111
	CAL																
	GR																
	Furc																
	Mobil																
	PLQ	1	1	1	1	1	1	1	1	1	1	1	1	1	1	1	1
Mandible lingual		32	31	30	29	28	27	26	25	24	23	22	21	20	19	18	17
	PD	758	547	536	635	534	534	445	533	434	435	535	666	646	648	847	767
	BOP		111	111	111	111			1		1		111				111
	CAL																
	GR																
	MGJ	999	999	999	999	888	777	777	777	777	777	777	888	999	999	999	999
	Furc																
	PLQ	1	1	1	1	1	1	1	1	1	1	1	1	1	1	1	1

Mandible facial	PD	756	645	637	736	534	545	434	635	636	535	636	635	635	437	636	665
	BOP																
	CAL	2	2	2	2	1	1		1	2	1	2	2	2	2	2	2
	GR																
	MGJ	456	867	878	879	999	989	989	989	989	989	999	998	998	888	888	543
	Furc																
	Mobil																
	PLQ	1	1	1	1	1	1	1	1	1	1	1	1	1	1	1	1

Abbreviations: BOP, bleeding on probing (1), suppuration (2); CAL, clinical attachment level; Furc, furcation involvement (Glickman class); GR, gingival recession; MGJ, position of mucogingival junction from margin; Mobil, tooth mobility (Miller grade); PD, probing depths; PLQ, plaque level (0 = none, 5 = heavy).

Oral hygiene instruction was provided for using interproximal brushes. All teeth were thoroughly scaled and root planed, followed by sulcular irrigation with chlorhexidine gluconate. Any carious lesions were restored. This resulted in gradual reduction of pocketing and inflammation over time, with only one 5-mm pocket remaining after 2 years. The patient's condition appears stable as there was no additional radiographic bone loss since the patient was seen initially (see ▶ Fig. 5.2 "2 year" radiographs).

Probing depths after 2 years are as follows:

Facial		1	2	3	4	5	6	7	8	9	10	11	12	13	14	15	16
	PD		324	424	313	213	313	212	212	312	213	213	213	323	324	324	
	BOP																
Lingual	PD		324	414	323	323	312	111	223	323	212	213	212	323	334	433	
	BOP																
Lingual		32	31	30	29	28	27	26	25	24	23	22	21	20	19	18	17
	PD		325	323	323	312	312	212	212	211	212	223	323	323	424	334	
	BOP		1														
Facial	PD																
	BOP		323	323	312	312	312	212	111	111	212	212	223	313	323	323	

What can be learned from this case?

The key to successful management of periodontal disease is to remove irritating factors causing or contributing to gingival inflammation. In this case, the patient's periodontal disease can be described in the dimensions given in ▶ Table 5.1.

The dimensions of the periodontal disease described in this case match best with a mild periodontitis (Stage II, Grade B)-type scenario based on the presence of moderate inflammation and generalized signs of mild attachment (1–2 mm)/ bone loss (within coronal third of root length). The presence of few local contributing factors (plaque and calculus) and the absence of specific microbial and systemic contributing factors provide a plausible explanation for the observed disease severity. Removal of plaque and calculus did generally restore periodontal health (except at one site), generally demonstrating effective treatment and complete removal of factors that lead to periodontal disease on most teeth.

The single residual pocket at tooth no. 31 is a concern since bleeding on probing and pocketing predicts potential for future attachment loss, and further treatment is needed. It is likely that this site contains residual subgingival plaque associated with either remnant calculus or another contributing factor such as the mild tipping of this tooth, shallow root concavity, or food impaction leading to enhanced inflammation there.

Table 5.1 Periodontal disease characteristics of case

Dimension	Description	Evidence
Severity of inflammation	Produces erythema and gingival bleeding/bleeding on probing	"Slight to moderate erythema," history of gingival bleeding, clinical record of "Bleed/S"
Depth of inflammation	Involves gingiva, periodontal ligament, and crestal bone	1–2 mm clinical attachment level, mild bone loss within coronal third of root
Extent of inflammation	Generalized	Signs of periodontal disease near all teeth
Local factors	Plaque and calculus	"PLQ" charting, radiographic calculus
Microbial factors	No specific microbial infection	Not described other than presence of plaque
Systemic factors	None	None described in case, relatively young age (30)

5.3 Controlling Periodontal Inflammation

Common periodontal disease is caused by a disease-causing microbial community within the periodontal sulcus, and periodontal treatment aims to remove and prevent the establishment of a disease-causing microbial community. Initial periodontal disease and periodontal maintenance therefore involves the following:

- Mechanical removal of plaque and calculus, which removes and disrupts the original disease-causing microbial community.
- Removal or control of factors that promote periodontal disease or tissue injury.
- Oral hygiene instruction and other preventive dental treatment that prevents the growth of a disease-causing microbial community.

Initial treatment planning therefore involves taking up the problem list of systemic factors and local factors collected during periodontal assessment and correlating these factors with the following treatments:

For systemic factors, treatment usually involves consultation and collaboration with a physician or medical specialists (▶ Table 5.2a). Dentists can and should provide at least limited

Table 5.2 (a) Systemic factors and corresponding treatment

Specific factor	Factor	Treatment
Amphetamines	Medication associated with gingival overgrowth	Consult with physician and explore potential of using different replacement medication (unlikely in most cases)
Calcium channel blockers		
Cyclosporine, tacrolimus, and sirolimus		
Dilantin/phenytoin		
Phenobarbital		
Valproic acid		
Anti-HIV medications (some) and gray discoloration	Medications associated with gingival discoloration	
Minocycline and gray gingival discoloration		
Estrogen replacement	Estrogen replacement	
Xerostomic medications and actual xerostomia	Xerostomia-inducing medication	
Medication known to cause lichenoid reaction and actual lichenoid lesions	Lichenoid reaction-inducing medication	
AIDS	Immunosuppressive medication	Consult with physician; Palliative treatment until medical treatment is done
Leukemia/lymphoma		
Chemotherapy		
Radiation therapy and oral mucositis	Radiation induced mucositis	
Cancer (including oral cancer)	Cancer	Referral to appropriate provider
Pregnancy and hormonal changes	Hormonal changes	Focus on preventive treatment
Sexually transmitted disease and oral ulcers/growths	Sexually transmitted disease (STD)	Referral to physician for further management
Stroke and decreased manual dexterity	Manual dexterity issue	Adjust treatment as appropriate for communication ability; modify oral hygiene tools (i.e., create large handle)
Dementia/Alzheimer and decreased manual dexterity		
Rh./osteoarthritis and decreased manual dexterity		Modify oral hygiene tools (i.e., create large handle; caregiver training; antiseptic mouthwash)
Decreased manual dexterity		
Rheumatoid arthritis	Rheumatoid arthritis	Consult with physician; empower patient to address medical issue
Diabetes mellitus	Diabetes mellitus	
Obesity	Obesity	Refer to physician; encourage healthy lifestyle
Poor nutrition	Nutrition	
Genetic conditions	Genetic conditions	Consult with physician if needed; For severe genetic conditions, treatment may only be palliative; discourage tobacco use with IL-1 genotype
IL-1 genotype		
Autoimmune diseases	Autoimmune	Refer to physician
Tobacco use	Self-medication	Ask and assist patient in quitting; refer to appropriate specialist/counseling/self-help group
Recreational drug use		
Alcohol use		

Table 5.2 (b) Local factors and corresponding nonsurgical treatment during initial treatment

Specific factor	Factor	Treatment
Plaque	Plaque	Oral hygiene instruction
Calculus	Calculus	Scaling or SRP
Specific microbial infection	Microbes	Prescribe appropriate agent
Caries	Caries	Check restorability and restore
Endodontic infection	Endodontic infection	Root canal treatment
Nonrestorable teeth (i.e., root tips)	Nonrestorable teeth	Extract (may be surgical)
Open contact/diastema and food impaction	Defective restoration	Replace defective restoration
Open margin		
Overhanging restoration		
Rough restorative surface/fractured restoration/coronal fracture		
Bulky/over contoured restoration		
Subgingival margin and gingival inflammation	Symptomatic subgingival margin	Consult with periodontist; may need crown-lengthening surgery
Deep pocketing and gingival inflammation	Deep pocketing and gingival inflammation	Initially: see plaque/calculus May need periodontal surgery
Furcation involvement and gingival inflammation	Furcation involvement	
Tooth mobility	Tooth mobility	Check occlusion—see Chapter 9
Recession and other mucogingival defects	Mucogingival conditions	Initially: see plaque/calculus May need periodontal surgery
Implant conditions	Implant conditions	Consult with periodontist
Crowding, orthodontic appliances	Tooth position issue	Consult with orthodontist
Rotated/tipped teeth		
Severe Angle Class II, III		
Excessive overjet/overbite		
Marginal discrepancy/infra/supraerupted teeth		
Enamel ridges and enamel projections	Anatomic abnormalities	If minor, odontoplasty If severe, consider extraction
Root surface concavities		
Enamel pearls		
Cervical enamel projections		
Dentin projections, ridges		
Unusual root/tooth anatomy		
Partially impacted 3rd molars (and other teeth)	Impacted teeth	Remove third molars. May need oral maxillofacial surgery consult
Cemental tears	Cemental tears	If infected, extract tooth
Occlusal trauma	Occlusal trauma	Occlusal analysis and adjustment
Bruxism	Parafunctional habit	Fabricate occlusal guard. Consult with appropriate specialist
Clenching		
Nail-biting		Assist patient in quitting destructive habit
Pipe chewing		
Piercings		Have patient remove piercing
Other parafunctional habits		Refer to appropriate specialist

tobacco cessation and nutrition counseling since they interact with patients more often than physicians. There are appropriate Current Dental Terminology (CDT) codes dentists can use for insurance reimbursement. Patients should also be referred to a physician for these counseling services as medications and referrals to dietitians and other specialists may be covered through medical insurance if prescribed by a physician.

Consequently, initial periodontal treatment typically follows the following dental treatment steps:
- If present, manage acute pain or infection with appropriate analgesic or antibiotic, and treat the affected tooth/teeth either by extraction or initial root canal therapy.
- If present, refer or perform biopsy and management of any suspicious oral lesions found during the exam.

- If present, check the restorability of questionable teeth. Extract any nonrestorable teeth or hopeless teeth. Consider ridge preservation if the patient considers implant therapy to replace missing teeth.
- Provide oral hygiene instruction.
- Provide other preventive procedures (i.e., topical fluoride, nutritional counseling, tobacco cessation counseling) if applicable.
- Remove calculus with one of the following procedures depending on the case:
  - Healthy/Mild gingivitis: Prophylaxis.
  - Gingivitis with heavy calculus: Scaling.
  - Periodontitis: Scaling and root planing.
  - Healthy, but reduced periodontium: Maintenance.
- Any direct restorative procedures and interim prostheses.
- If needed, occlusal analysis and adjustment.
- Reassess the periodontal condition and decide if periodontal surgery/referral to a periodontist is needed. Generally, the goal is to perform the first eight steps within 3 months.
- If periodontal disease is resolved, continue with definite treatment such as orthodontic therapy and indirect restorations, including definite prostheses. Implant therapy and associated restorations are generally performed last, and an occlusal guard, if needed, is fabricated after completion of all restorations.
- Once treatment is complete, the patient is periodically evaluated and the patient's condition is maintained with procedures based on initial diagnosis (▶ Fig. 5.2), such as:
  - *Healthy/Gingivitis*: Prophylaxis and other preventive treatment as needed every 6 to 12 months depending on the risk of new periodontal disease and caries.
  - *Periodontitis*: Periodontal maintenance and other preventive treatment as needed every 3 to 6 months depending on the risk of new periodontal disease and caries.

5.3.1 Insurance Coding

For patients using dental insurance or government-subsidized dental care programs, use of proper treatment codes and documentation is important for claim acceptance. For example, useful **ADA CDT procedure** codes and typical documentation needs in the US are shown in ▶ Table 5.3.

Table 5.3 Common CDT codes that may be used for initial periodontal therapy in general practice

Procedure	Code	Plan per	Documentation/reimbursement limits
Exams			
Debridement	D4355	Visit	Prior to exam; photos/radiograph showing calculus
Comprehensive (initial)	D0150	Visit	No more than once every 2 years
Periodontal	D0180	Visit	Periodontal chart/chart notes describing disease Usually used by periodontists as initial exam
Periodic	D0120	Visit	May be limited to once/year
Extractions			
Routine (simple)	D7140	Tooth	Radiograph showing entire tooth
Surgical (involves flap or sutures)	D7210	Tooth	Radiograph showing entire tooth, chart note Should be <30% of extractions by general dentist
Ridge preservation	D7953	Tooth	In addition to extraction code
Preventive services			
Oral hygiene instruction	D1330	Visit	
Tobacco-cessation counseling	D1320	Visit	Chart note indicating need
Nutrition counseling	D1310	Visit	Chart note indicating need
Topical fluoride varnish	D1206	Visit	Chart note indicating caries risk factors; may have age limit
Calculus/plaque removal			
Prophylaxis (adult)	D1110	Visit	>13 years; 2 per year
Prophylaxis (child)	D1120	Visit	<14 years; 2 per year
Scaling	D4346	Visit	Reimbursed usually as prophylaxis (limit 2/year)
SRP Requires complete periodontal chart, full set radiographs, diagnosis, and treatment plan	D4341	Quadrant	>3 teeth; 4+ mm PD; once every 2 years
	D4342	Quadrant	<4 teeth; 4+ mm PD; once every 2 years
Maintenance	D4910	Visit	May be reimbursed as prophylaxis (limit 2/year) Do not alternate with prophylaxis
SRP adjuncts			
Local delivery antimicrobials	D4381	Tooth	4+ mm probing depth; cannot be used for initial **SRP**; limit once/2 years; agent must be FDA-approved; if used, no longer allows reimbursement for osseous surgery in same quadrant for 2 years
Subgingival irrigation	D4921	Quadrant	4+ mm probing depth; may not be reimbursed
Periodontal medication delivery trays	D5994	Arch	4+ mm probing depth; may not be reimbursed

As can be seen from this table, coding of nonsurgical procedures may be complex, and reimbursement requirements may be different between insurers. For practices focused on serving patients utilizing 3rd party payment schemes, it may be advisable to appoint a staff member to oversee procedure coding and manage insurance claims.

5.4 Scaling and Root Planing Procedures

Even though there are four different procedures for calculus and plaque removal, the technique is similar for prophylaxis, scaling, root planing, and periodontal maintenance. The difference between these techniques is mostly a matter of time, effort, desired outcome, and the need to decontaminate exposed root surfaces. Regardless of the procedure, all require similar precautions in patients with certain medical conditions.

5.4.1 Medical Conditions that Require Precautionary Measures

Prior to SRP, it is important to ask the patient about any changes in their overall and oral health since the last appointment, and address these concerns prior to SRP. Particularly, attention should be placed on the status of medical conditions that could trigger a medical emergency while SRP, such as diabetes mellitus, asthma, cardiovascular disease and allergies, and conditions that may pose an infection risk from aerosolized bacteria (▶ Table 5.4).

5.4.2 Setup and Patient Preparation

For maximum effectiveness, the operatory should be set up neatly with universal precautions in place and a clutter-free operatory. The following steps may help increase appointment efficiency and reduce triggers of dental anxiety:
- Utilize pre-procedural NSAIDs (i.e., 2 × 200 mg Ibuprofen or 500-mg Acetaminophen 1 hour prior) for deep SRP procedures for decreased soreness after treatment.
- Sharpen instruments prior to the appointment to minimize sharpening time during the appointment.
- Set up instruments in order of use (i.e., mirror, probe, anesthetic syringe, scaler, curettes from anterior to posterior, calculus explorer, gauze, sharpening stone), and have polishing cup and ultrasonic scaler ready.
- Tape opaque bag to operatory side for discreet disposal of blood-stained gauze.
- Cover instruments with the patient bib prior to the patient being seated.

5.4.3 Appointment Structure

Generally, the appointment structure for prophylaxis, maintenance, and SRP appointments is the same. Typically, a recall appointment with a periodic exam and prophylaxis procedure should take slightly less than 1 hour in a private practice, with about 15 minutes of actual scaling/polishing in a healthy patient. SRP appointment should usually take about 1 hour per quadrant depending on difficulty, and a recall appointment for a patient on periodontal maintenance may take about 1½ hours or less. In any of these procedures, the appointment steps are usually as follows:
- Check/update of medical history. Document changes/adjust treatment, if needed.

Table 5.4 Medical conditions that require caution with scaling and root planing techniques

Condition	Risk mitigation
High risk of infectious bacterial endocarditis	Prescribe antibiotic prophylaxis according to current American Heart Association guidelines. Consult if needed
Total joint replacement	Minimal risk and may not need antibiotic coverage. Consult with patient's orthopedic surgeon
HIV/AIDS	Low risk of HIV transmission. May have postoperative infection risk. Consider antibiotic prophylaxis if CD4 T-cell count is low or symptomatic for AIDS.
Chronic leukemias; chemotherapy	Consider antibiotic prophylaxis. Consult with patient's oncologist.
Diabetes mellitus	Consider antibiotic prophylaxis if prone to infections due to poor glycemic control. Assess hypoglycemia risk, and consider in-office blood glucose measurement. Have glucose source available. Assess if cardiovascular or renal disease pose local anesthesia risk
Cardiovascular disease	Assess myocardial infarct risk. Weigh benefit of epinephrine for pain control versus cardiovascular risk
Cardiac pacemaker (and other implanted electronic devices)	Avoid magnetostrictive ultrasonic scalers unless implanted device is known to be shielded. Consult with cardiologist or check with manufacturer of device
Asthma	Assess asthma attack risk. Have patient bring inhaler if available. Aerosol created by ultrasonic may trigger asthma attack
Infectious disease (i.e., flu, cold, active tuberculosis; other diseases transmissible by airborne droplets)	If possible, delay treatment until infection is over for respiratory infections. Use antiseptic rinse prior to SRP. Use high volume suction tip if using ultrasonic/air abrasion device
Bleeding disorder and anticoagulants	Consult with patient's hematologist for bleeding disorder, or physician who prescribed anticoagulant. Usually, continue anticoagulant therapy. Apply hemostatic measures and avoid unnecessary tissue trauma

- *Dental exam:* Evaluates extra/intraoral check for soft tissue lesions; **TMJ** conditions; occlusal condition; caries; failing restorations and periodontal disease (including at least charting of pockets/ gingival bleeding). See Chapter 2, for exam techniques.
- If a new disease is present, obtain appropriate radiographs and evaluate them.
- Disclose plaque, provide specific oral hygiene instruction.
- Perform scaling. Root plane where needed. Commonly, ultrasonic instrumentation is used to remove the majority of calculus first, and followed by hand instrumentation to produce smooth root surfaces.
- Polish teeth.
- Apply fluoride or other preventive treatment (i.e., counseling) based on risk.
- Set up next appointment and arrange payment for next procedures.

It is possible to perform oral hygiene instruction after the polishing step, but it reduces the educational value as the patient cannot see any shortcomings of the current oral hygiene regimen. Likewise, it is possible to perform the dental exam (steps 2 to 3) after SRP so that caries and restorative conditions are more readily visible. The downside is that this does not allow assessment of oral hygiene prior to scaling, and it is useful to be aware of dental conditions that impact SRP prior to performing the procedure.

These dental conditions are listed here, along with management considerations (▶Table 5.5).

5.4.4 Local Anesthesia

Providing effective pain control for SRP increases appointment efficiency and builds patient confidence. Consider the following suggestions:
- Choose appropriate local anesthesia method:
  - Gingiva sensitive to instrumentation (i.e., probing) and shallow pockets: Topical anesthetic applied to gingival margin is sufficient.
  - Sensitive gingiva with deeper pockets (4 to 6 mm): **Oraquix** is sufficient.
  - Deep pockets (5+ mm): Local infiltration anesthesia near mucogingival junction.
  - Sensitive teeth/dentinal hypersensitivity: Local infiltration (maxilla), inferior alveolar nerve block (mandible).
- Topical anesthesia agents work best if applied undisturbed for as long as feasible.
- When providing local anesthesia, recline patient and keep syringe out of the patient's sight until injection. Use distraction methods (i.e., pulling on the lip/cheek) just prior to needle insertion to minimize "needle stick" sensation and avoid touching periosteum. Slow, gentle injection technique with pre-warmed anesthetic or buffering solutions can decrease unpleasant burning sensation of local anesthesia.

5.4.5 Ultrasonic Scaling and Root Planing

Ultrasonic instrumentation is a key to fast and efficient SRP appointment in the hands of an experienced operator. In the hands of a novice operator, however, it may not be effective and lead to the formation of burnished calculus, which is more difficult to remove. Consider the following principles:
- *Tip selection*: Use thick, shorter (standard size) tips for supragingival calculus and moderate pockets (4 to 5 mm). Use finer, longer (perio) tips for subgingival SRP. Diamond-coated tips are used for tenacious calculus but also can easily gauge the root surface. For implants, specialized implant inserts should be used, which are often made of titanium.
- Waterlines of the ultrasonic device should be purged before use, and magnetostrictive insert handles be filled with water prior to inserting the magnetostrictive insert. Magnetostrictive inserts should be handled with care to prevent damage.
- Power should be adjusted appropriately to the tip size as recommended by the manufacturer. Typically, "standard-size" tips require 60 to 80% power and "perio" tips 30 to 40% power.
- Water flow should be adjusted to produce a thick water spray around the instrument tip when the unit is activated. If the instrument handle becomes hot, there is too little water flow.

Table 5.5 Oral conditions that complicate scaling and root planing techniques

Condition	Solutions
Sensitive root surfaces, and dentinal hypersensitivity	Provide local anesthesia. Avoid excessive instrumentation. Apply desensitizing agents after treatment
Cervical caries and demineralization	Avoid instrumentation of cavitation. Careful plaque and calculus removal on unaffected surfaces. Consider remineralization techniques, and restore caries as soon as feasible
Crowding	Use sickle scaler tip supragingivally. Fine-tipped ultrasonics, and worn, but sharp curettes work subgingivally
Implants	Use implant-safe scalers and curettes (i.e., titanium based). Emphasize on oral hygiene
Fixed partial dentures and crown margins	Use horizontal strokes with curettes. Do not use ultrasonics at the restorative margin. Emphasize on good interproximal oral hygiene
Orthodontics	Use fine-tipped ultrasonic instrumentations away from bracket base. Stress oral hygiene with interproximal brushes and oral irrigation
Shallow sulcus (probing depth less than 3 mm)	Do not instrument subgingivally

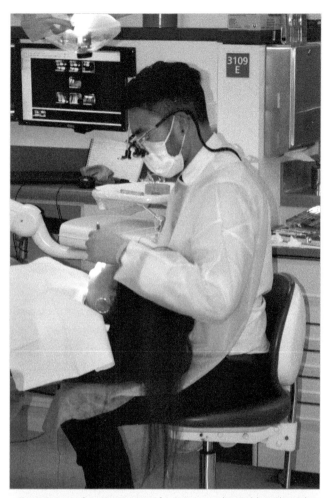

Fig. 5.3 Typical seating position for SRP procedure. Although rarely achievable in perfection, the aim is to achieve a posture as close as possible to ideal resting position to minimize fatigue.

- Operator positioning and finger support are the same as for hand instruments.
- The ultrasonic tip should never be pointed at a root surface to avoid pitting.
- Movement (▶ Fig. 5.3):
  - *Magnetostrictive (i.e., Cavitron)*: Brush the side of the instrument tip gently back and forth over the root surface in various directions (▶ Video 5.1).
  - *Piezoelectric (i.e., Acteon Satelec)*: Subjectively will feel less aggressive, and requires drawing it over the root surface for effectiveness in finer, overlapping strokes parallel to the root surface (▶ Video 5.2).

Using Ultrasonics Alone for Scaling and Root Planing

An experienced clinician can achieve effective SRP with ultrasonics that is at least equal, if not better, in effectiveness than manual instrumentation, and there is an electron microscopy study showing no statistical difference in surface texture after root planing with either method.[1] However, this requires multiple sets of ultrasonic instrument tips and mastery of using

these. A "blended approach," in which powered scalers followed by hand instruments, is likely the most practical method in most settings.

Magnetostrictive versus Piezoelectric Ultrasonic Scalers

Historically, there used to exist air-driven SRP devices that produced high pitched, audible (thus, "sonic") vibrations for calculus removal. These have been replaced by devices producing much higher vibration frequencies that are near and above audible limits (thus, "ultrasonic"). There are two broad categories of ultrasonic devices, based on the mechanism on how the vibration is produced: magnetostrictive and piezoelectric. Differences between these devices are compared below (▶ Table 5.6).

5.4.6 Hand Scaling and Root Planing

Other than for the novice operator, ultrasonic instrumentation should be performed prior to hand instrumentation, to remove the majority of calculus deposits. For hand instrumentation efficiency, there are the following areas of concern: patient/operator positioning, finger positioning, instrumentation, SRP technique, and instrument sharpness.

Patient/Operator Positioning

Poor operator posture during SRP procedures can lead to operator fatigue, muscle cramping, and chronic neck and lower back pain. Poor patient positioning makes SRP more difficult. For operator positioning, the goal is to achieve a seating position that is as relaxed and self-centered as possible (▶ Fig. 5.3):
- Feet flat on the ground.
- Thighs parallel to the ground.
- Good lumbar support.
- Upper back straight.
- Upper arms resting on the sides of your chest.

The goal of patient positioning is to allow direct vision as much as possible, which is often achievable for all teeth except the lingual side of maxillary incisors (▶ Video 5.3):
- *Mandibular teeth*: Recline patient moderately, mandibular plane parallel to the floor.
- *Maxillary teeth*: Fully recline patient. Use headrest to support neck and tilt head posteriorly. Maxillary plan is about 10 degrees tipped relative to vertical:
- *Anterior teeth*: Sit behind the patient.
- *Posterior teeth*: Sit beside the patient.
- *Lingual sides of posterior teeth adjacent to you, buccal sides of teeth on far side of arch*: Tip patient head toward you.
- *Buccal sides of posterior teeth adjacent to you, lingual sides of teeth on far side of arch*: Tip patient head away from you.
- For the distobuccal area of 2nd or 3rd maxillary molars, have patient move jaw sideways away from the tooth, and insert mouth mirror so that the back side of the mirror faces toward vestibule/mandibular raphe.
- Lingual of maxillary incisors usually requires indirect vision.
- Lingual of mandibular incisors usually benefits from having patient tip chin toward chest.

Table 5.6 Differences between magnetostrictive and piezoelectric devices

Mechanism	Magnetostrictive	Piezoelectric
Handpiece	Contains electric coil producing magnetic field that induces insert motion	Contains ceramic disks that contract when electricity is applied
Insert (see ▶ Fig. 5.5)	Tip is attached to a bundle of thin metallic sheets	Tip only
Tip motion	Ellipsoidal/▶ Fig. 5.5	Linear
Advantages	• Subjectively produces more effective calculus removal • More forgiving in technique	• Gentler feel to patients • Potential for smoother root surface finish • Unlikely to interfere with pacemaker • Some devices provide sterile irrigation
Disadvantages	• Cannot sterilize handpiece • Insert is easily damaged	• More difficult to use effectively

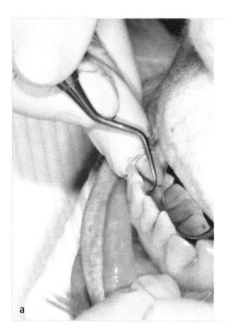
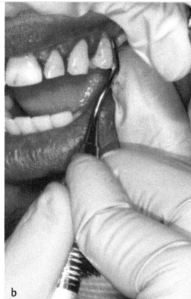

Fig. 5.4 (a, b) Finger rests. The goal is to create a stable fulcrum point, which allows for maximizing SRP force and efficiency. Ideally, the resting finger should be as close as possible to the instrumented surface, regardless of location or instrument.

Finger Positioning

For efficient SRP, the instrument should be grasped with a modified pen grasp and a good finger rest established nearby (▶ Fig. 5.4). Selection of a proper finger rest is important to achieve maximum SRP power with little effort as it will serve as a fulcrum point. The finger rest should be as close as possible to the area that is instrumented, and usually rank in this order of desirability (▶ Video 5.4):

• Adjacent tooth surface.
• Anterior tooth (requires extending instrument, and reduces fulcrum effect).
• Tooth on opposing arch (also is less stable as patient's jaw might move).
• Chin/subnasal area (even further away from the tooth, and is soft surface).
• Cheek (worst area for finger rest as it is not supported by hard structure).

5.4.7 Instrumentation

If treatment is not provided by a novice operator, the majority of plaque and calculus should be removed with ultrasonics prior to hand instrumentation for maximum efficiency (▶ Fig. 5.5).

Universal Scaler Use

Next, any supragingival calculus should be removed with a universal scaler, focusing around line angles, cingula, and interproximal contacts (▶ Fig. 5.6). Any of the three sharp cutting edges of the sickle scaler can be used to dislodge calculus from tooth surfaces, and the pointed tip can be used to clean tooth surfaces around the interproximal points and in any grooves on the tooth surface (▶ Fig. 5.6, ▶ Video 5.5). For the most efficient calculus removal, the cutting edge of a scaler should engage calculus on a tooth surface with an angle of about 85 degrees toward the tooth surface. A scaler should not be used for subgingival scaling.

Gracey Curette Use

Sulci that are shallow, bordered by healthy appearing gingiva, and devoid of deposits should not be instrumented as this may cause gingival recession. Site-specific Gracey curettes are ideally suited for removing subgingival deposits in pockets (▶ Fig. 5.7, ▶ Fig. 5.8). Generally, the goal is to minimize flipping instrument sides and instrument changes for maximum speed, and a methodical approach to ensure all root surfaces are instrumented.

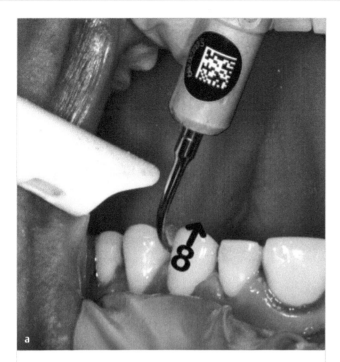

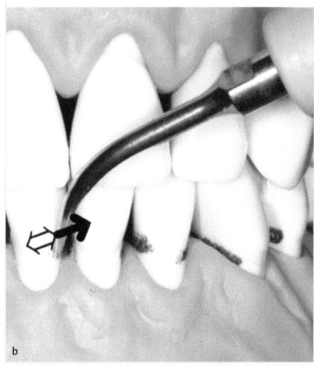

Fig. 5.5 Using ultrasonic instrumentation with magnetostrictive or piezoelectric handpieces. For any machine, use the manufacturer recommended power setting and sufficient water flow to produce a dense spray from the vibrating tip. Also, make sure to flush the handpiece thoroughly before use. **(a)** Magnetostrictive unit (i.e., Cavitron): make sure to insert the magnetostrictive insert into a completely water-filled handpiece. Gently move the side of the instrument tip repeatedly over any calculus ledges or areas of staining, making sure not to wedge the tip into any crevices or staying too long at one spot. As the tip moves in a figure 8 motion, it will rapidly remove calculus in any direction. **(b)** Piezoelectric: gently move side of tip across deposits with many overlapping strokes. The tip moves in a linear fashion so that it will feel less aggressive than a magnetostrictive tip to the patient and requires closer overlapping strokes than the magnetostrictive tip.

Site-specific Gracey Curettes

One basic approach is to begin with a basic Gracey 1/2, 5/6 or 7/8 curette and use it to instrument all incisors and canines, followed by the lingual and facial surfaces of posterior teeth as much as they are accessible. For each tooth, one side of the curette is used to instrument the distobuccal quarter and mesiolingual quarter of the root surface for about three teeth at a time, followed by the other side of the instrument for the remaining tooth surfaces (▶ Video 5.6).

The interproximal surfaces of posterior teeth, especially molars, is usually not reachable by a basic Gracey curette and a more complex instrument is needed. For the mesial surfaces, a Gracey 11/12 curette should be used and a 13/14 for distal surfaces (▶ Fig. 5.9, ▶ Video 5.7).

5.4.8 Technique

Regardless of the area, the curette blade should be inserted as flat as possible against the tooth, with the intended cutting edge closest to the sulcus floor. The pocket depth of the site will correlate with how deep the blade has to be inserted, and the blade should be used to feel for calculus during blade insertion. As a guide for insertion depth, the blade of a standard Gracey curette typically is about 0.9-mm wide, 4-mm long, and the terminal shank is about 11-mm long.

Calculus usually presents as a hard, rough-edged "ledge" on the tooth surface, whereas the sulcus floor has a rubbery consistency. Often, calculus is found just apical to the cementoenamel junction (CEJ), which will feel like an outward step in the tooth surface toward the glassy smooth enamel. Burnished calculus is found sometimes after incomplete SRP, and presents as a smooth, round "bump" on a root surface.

Once calculus is identified, tip the handle away from the tooth until an angle of about 70 to 80 degrees from the blade to the tooth surface is reached, and the blade "bites" into the calculus (▶ Fig. 5.8). Pull the blade out of the sulcus while pressing it against the root surface using forearm muscles, which will shave a bit of calculus from the root surface, and repeat the same motion until the root surface feels glassy smooth. The typical SRP motion is a vertical apico-coronal movement along the long axis of the tooth, keeping the blade tangential to the cross section of the tooth (▶ Fig. 5.7a).

While this works well on buccal and lingual surfaces, it cannot be done on interproximal surfaces with a contact point. In these cases, an oblique stroke is needed to reach under the contact point (▶ Fig. 5.7b). In some instances, such as SRP, the root surface apical to a crown margin, or a furcation entrance, it is useful to use the tip of the blade as a "scoop," and move it horizontally along the tooth surface (▶ Fig. 5.7c). This can also be useful in SRP the distal most surface of the terminal molar with a 13/14 Gracey.

Care should be taken around restorative margins, where curettes should be moved parallel to the restorative margin. Care should also be taken to avoid instrumenting caries, glass ionomer, and provisional restorations.

When to Sharpen

Instrument sharpening should be performed whenever root planing effectiveness decreases as evidenced by the reduced ability to remove calculus, higher finger pressure needed to remove calculus, the lack of "biting" of the instrument into

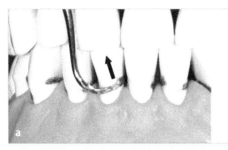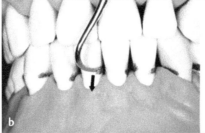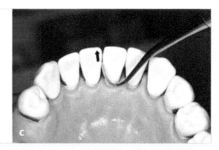

Fig. 5.6 Sickle scaler stroke directions. Pull stroke using sides (**a**), push stroke using third cutting edge (**b**), interproximal cleaning (**c**), and generally, feel for calculus with the scaler tip, place it under the calculus ledge, and chip or shave off the calculus from the edges of the deposit using any of these stroke techniques, depending which one provides the best access at the moment.

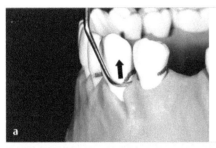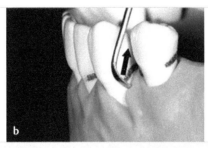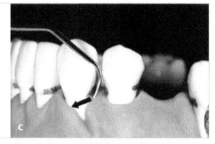

Fig. 5.7 Curette stroke directions. Gracey curettes can be used with (**a**) vertical, (**b**) oblique, and (**c**) horizontal stroke directions. The vertical stroke tends to be used most often, whereas the oblique and horizontal stroke directions are useful for line angles and interproximal surfaces of posterior teeth. The horizontal stroke direction is useful when SRP root surfaces apical to crown margins. As with the scaler, the general technique involves detecting the calculus deposit with the tip, placing the instrument cutting edge apical to the deposit, and gradually shaving the deposit off the tooth using any of the above stroke techniques, working from the edges of the deposit.

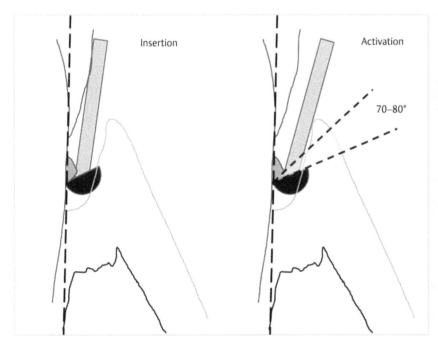

Fig. 5.8 Engaging calculus with a Gracey curette: the Gracey curette is first inserted with the cutting edge toward the tooth surface, feeling for calculus and letting the cutting edge rest just below the area of calculus. The instrument is then activated by moving the terminal shank slightly away from the tooth, so that the cutting edge is angled 70 to 80 degrees away from the tooth surface, and then pulled across the tooth surface, essentially shaving off calculus and contaminated cementum.

a test stick, or a rounded cutting edge that shows as a white reflective line on the blade edge (▸Fig. 5.10, ▸Video 5.8). In our experience, limited instrument sharpening is needed about every eight teeth, and sooner in the presence of tenacious calculus, overhanging restorations or a worn-down curette.

Calculus Check

After SRP has been performed, cleanliness should be checked by visual inspection or a fine probe such as the 11/12 Old Dominion University Explorer, checking for a smooth surface that does not produce audible or tactile "clicks." Care should be taken to inspect the following areas as these typically retain calculus after SRP by inexperienced operators: line angles of all teeth, CEJ (if pronounced), distalmost surfaces, mesial root concavities of maxillary 1st molars, mesial, and distal root concavities of mandibular incisors, and furcation entrances (especially if narrow, V-shaped, or containing ridges and concavities).

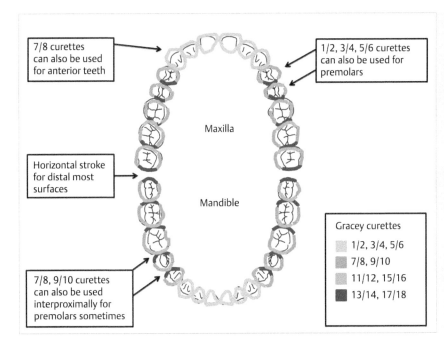

7/8 curettes can also be used for anterior teeth

1/2, 3/4, 5/6 curettes can also be used for premolars

Horizontal stroke for distal most surfaces

7/8, 9/10 curettes can also be used interproximally for premolars sometimes

Maxilla

Mandible

Gracey curettes
- 1/2, 3/4, 5/6
- 7/8, 9/10
- 11/12, 15/16
- 13/14, 17/18

Fig. 5.9 Use chart of curettes. While Gracey curettes are designed for best use in the indicated locations, it is often possible to extend the usage range depending on patient's mouth opening, tooth anatomy, and other factors. For example, it may be possible with some experience to scale and root plane nearly all surfaces with the Gracey 7/8 curette with a patient with average mouth and tooth anatomy, and use the Gracey 11/12 and Gracey 13/14 to reach the interproximal molar surfaces that cannot be reached with the Gracey 7/8 curette.

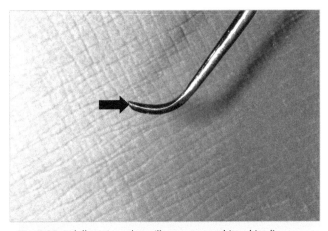

Fig. 5.10 A dull cutting edge will appear as a white, shiny line separating the blade and outer surface of the curette. If sharp, this will not be visible.

- Wet ceramic sharpening stone, or place a drop of mineral oil on an Arkansas or India sharpening stone.
- Identify the cutting edge.
- Securely grasp of the instrument.
- Keep the cutting edge in contact with the sharpening stone (▶ Fig. 5.11).
- Even pull blade across sharpening stone several times. Avoid pressing against the tip.
- Check for sharpness visually or with a plastic test stick, where a sharp instrument will "bite" into the soft plastic surface. Visually, a dull edge will reflect light, resulting in appearance of a bright white line separating the blade from the external surface of the instrument (▶ Fig. 5.10) when the blade is rotated. A sharp edge will not reflect light.

Hand Instrument Sharpening

Dull instruments require greater force and time for continued calculus removal. Dull instruments also burnish calculus instead of removing it, creating smooth, round, compacted "bumps" of calculus on root surfaces that are hard to detect and harder to remove. Dull instruments also tend to slip, causing gingival tears and patient pain.

This can be avoided by periodic instrument sharpening, and instruments can be sharpened with rotary ceramic stones, sharpening machines, or commonly through manual sharpening. The most efficient way of sharpening periodontal instruments is through using sharpening machines, and a designated staff member should perform this task before instrument sterilization. For manual sharpening, the goal is to maintain a cutting edge that contains an internal angle of about 70 degrees, and the clock method[2] is an easy method to obtain these angles. Keys for successful and safe sharpening are the following steps:

5.4.9 Stain Removal and Coronal Polishing

Heavy staining can be effectively removed with air abrasion, but can also be removed with careful ultrasonic or hand scaling, and on flat, exposed surfaces with fine pumice or abrasive polishing paste applied with a rotary brush. When calculus removal is complete, tooth surfaces should be gently polished with a rubber cup and polishing paste. The rubber cup needs to be applied lightly and moved quickly across the tooth surface to avoid pain and pulpal damage, and should not be inserted deeply into the gingiva to avoid laceration and gingival recession.

Care should be taken to avoid pushing polishing paste into deep pockets, and to avoid polishing restoration surfaces with standard polishing pastes. Instead, restorative surfaces should be polished with dedicated polishing disks and points to avoid scratching and dulling of these surfaces. Rotary polishing brushes can be very effective for removal of heavy stains such as chlorhexidine or tobacco staining, and are useful for cleaning orthodontic appliances. However, polishing brushes can readily pierce and lacerate gingival tissues and should not be used near the gingival margin.

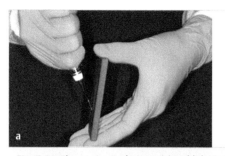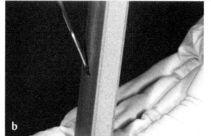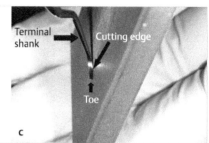

Fig. 5.11 Sharpening technique. (**a**) Hold the instrument to be sharpened with a firm grip, and since this instrument is a Gracey 7/8 curette sharpened by a right-handed operator, the instrument is held at 11 AM and the sharpening stone at 1 PM position. (**b**) The key is to maintain a straight cutting edge, with the cutting edge in contact with the sharpening stone. (**c**) Once stone and instrument are lined up properly, a few strokes with the sharpening stone will restore the cutting edge. At the end, the toe of the instrument should be inspected to ensure a round shape, and metal shavings should be removed from the instrument with gauze.

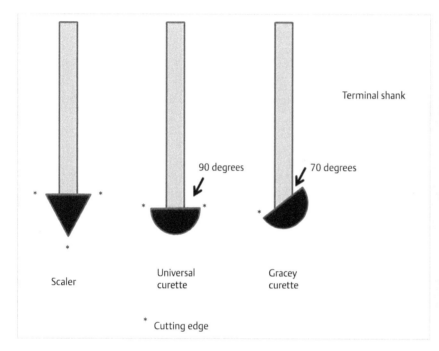

Fig. 5.12 Scalers have three possible cutting edges, universal curettes two and Gracey curettes just one cutting edge. Given the slanted blade, Gracey curettes can be inserted easier into a pocket and are suitable for delicate tissues. The blade surface of a Gracey curette is angled 70 degrees in relation to the terminal shank, whereas the blade of a universal curette is angled at 90 degrees in relation to the terminal shank. For both types of curettes, the internal angle of the blade cross section at the cutting edge is typically about 70 degrees.

5.4.10 Hand Instrument Variants

Beyond the basic variations of scalers, universal curettes, and Gracey curettes (▶ Fig. 5.12), manufacturers often provide variations of Gracey curettes for specialized uses (see ▶ Table 5.7), and other instruments that may be useful for selected patients. For instance, since stainless steel is harder than titanium, stainless steel scalers should not be used on titanium implant surfaces. Instead, titanium instruments should be used. Plastic curettes are not advisable as they are bulky and tend to leave microscopic plastic particles on rough implant surfaces. Furcations present a challenge since furcation entrances often are slightly smaller than the width of a curette blade if furcations cannot be instrumented with a regular curette, or a fine ultrasonic tip, spoon-shaped DeMarco furcation curettes, or a diamond-coated Nabers probe can be used to remove calculus from narrow furcations. Thick, tenacious calculus, or even restorative overhangs can be removed using calculus files such as the Hirschfeld type. On large exposed convex root surfaces, the McCall 17/18 curette can be useful with its curved blade similar in curvature to a Nabers probe.

5.5 Glassy Smooth versus Satin Finish as Desired Root Planing Outcome

There is a debate whether a root surface after completed root planing should be "glassy smooth" or "satin smooth," as attempting to achieve "glassy smooth" on all root surfaces may result in excessive dentin removal. In time, this will result in "rifling" of the root surface, or create large round, smooth root surface concavities under the CEJ producing an appearance similar to an apple core. However, it is difficult to distinguish between a "satin smooth" finish and a contaminated surface that has a slight sandpaper finish caused by residual smear layer with embedded calculus. Therefore, for students, it may be easier to aim for "glassy smooth" as desired outcome.

5.5.1 Other Devices

While manual and ultrasonic methods are the typical methods used for cleaning root surfaces, there are other methods that

Table 5.7 Gracey curette variations

Variant	Example names	Use
Increased metal hardness	"Ever Edge" (Hu-Friedy). Other manufacturers simply provide hardest metal grade for all instruments (American Eagle, Hartzell)	The higher the hardness, the longer the cutting edge will stay sharp, i.e., less sharpening
Increased shank rigidity	"Rigid" and "Extra-rigid" (Hu-Friedy)	Instrument bends less while SRP. Potentially, more aggressive as higher force can be applied to cutting edge, and used for moderate to heavy calculus
Shorter Blade length	Mini (Hu-Friedy, others)	Easier to use on small roots such as mandibular incisors
Thinner blade cross section (about ½ diameter)	Micro (Hu-Friedy, Nordent)	Small spaces and deep pockets
Longer terminal shank (about 3 mm)	After-Five Mini-Five "Long" (Nordent)	Increased reach into deep pockets. Variant with shorter blade length is called Mini-Five
Angle variants in shank design	1/2 vs. 5/6, 3/4 vs. 7/8 vs. 9/10, 11/12 vs. 15/16, 13/15 vs. 17/18	More accentuated shank allows deeper interproximal reach and into pockets with less interference from opposing teeth

Names of curette variations may differ between manufacturers, and some manufacturers may only carry one type of metal or shank design.

have been developed over time. These alternative methods are generally not permitted on licensing exams, and are usually used for special circumstances. The methods are as follows:

- *Chemical calculus removal using acids (i.e., citric acid) or caustic agents (i.e., antiformin)*: A historical method, that is no longer used given the potential for uncontrolled tissue damage and lack of clinical effectiveness. Citric acid, other mild acids, and Ethylenediaminetetraacetic acid (EDTA) are sometimes used by clinicians for "root conditioning," where it is believed that these agents produce a root surface more conducive for regenerative surgical procedures.
- *Rotary instrumentation using diamond burs*: Generally not used for nonsurgical periodontal treatment given the potential for excessive tooth structure removal. However, this method may be used during surgical periodontal treatment as part of odontoplasty procedures.
- *Surgical lasers*: These can effectively remove calculus, disinfect root surfaces, and produce a smooth root surface with clinical outcomes comparable to conventional SRP with Er:YAG lasers. However, such lasers are expensive, and incorrect use can produce root damage, delayed healing, and severe injury.
- *Air polishing*: Such devices (▶Fig. 5.13) focus a stream of particles on a surface, which is slowly abraded by the impact of these particles. Air abrasion is useful for removing external tooth staining, and treatment of contaminated implant surfaces with glycine particles. Disadvantages of this method are: potential for tissue emphysema, poor taste, discomfort, and the excessive dust produced by this method.
  - *Use*: An air abrasion unit is similarly used as an ultrasonic unit, except that the tip is brought close, but not in contact with the root surface. The tip is swept across the root surface in an "airbrushing" motion, with the goal to remove all visible root surface contamination. To avoid excessive dust creation, the tip should only be activated inside the mouth near a high-speed evacuation tip. In addition, wet gauze strip placed on the lip or gingival margin can trap excess powder.
- Periodontal endoscopy (i.e., Perioscope) uses an endoscopic camera to visualize subgingival calculus so that it can be

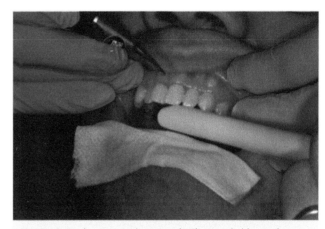

Fig. 5.13 Air abrasion used on a tooth. The tip is held away from the root surface and a strip of wet gauze placed over the lip to catch overspray and abrasion material. It is essential to high-speed suction to avoid release of large amounts of dust.

removed with other methods. This can produce very thorough calculus removal on single-rooted teeth, but the clinical outcome in general is similar to meticulously executed SRP.

5.6 Scaling and Root Planing Adjuncts

Much research has been performed on SRP adjuncts that may improve clinical outcomes. In general, these approaches include using biologics such as enamel matrix derivative; probiotic agents applied after SRP; surgical lasers; low-level laser irradiation and photodynamic therapy; host-modulatory agents such as subantimicrobial dose tetracyclines; and local antiseptic or antimicrobial agents.

5.6.1 Surgical Lasers

Surgical Er:YAG and Nd:YAG infrared lasers can remove calculus, create a smooth root surface, and disinfect root surfaces through focal delivery of high-energy doses at specific wavelengths. Clinically, there is much anecdotal evidence of these lasers producing large pocket reduction and clinical attachment gain as adjunct to SRP combined with occlusal adjustment. There is also limited histologic evidence of regeneration in some cases.[3] While there is limited histologic evidence and clinical trial data suggesting effectiveness of Nd:YAG and Er;YAG lasers, questions remain on case selection and what constitutes an optimal laser protocol.[3] If laser therapy is effective, the advantages would include minimal pain, low invasiveness, and patient acceptance compared to surgical periodontal treatments. The disadvantage of this technology is the significant added cost, and the need for laser precaution steps to avoid patient and operator injury. The general indication for this technology seems to be the elimination of deep pockets, but it is unclear at this point which sites and patients would benefit the most from this technology.

5.6.2 Low-level Laser Irradiation and Photodynamic Therapy

While surgical lasers are effective as cutting instrument, low-energy density visible and near-infrared laser light may produce biologic effects on tissue. For example, low-powered red/near infrared diode lasers have been shown to stimulating fibroblast growth and suppressing neutrophil numbers in areas of inflammation. Adding low-energy laser irradiation to SRP can improve in bleeding on probing scores, pocket depths, and plaque indexes,[4] but these effects are quite small.

In photodynamic therapy, a photosensitizer (i.e., Toluidine blue [PerioWave], Indocyanine Green [Perio Green]) is applied to a periodontal pocket after SRP, and the photosensitizer activated by low-level laser light. During activation, this photosensitizer dye absorbs energy and transfers it to oxygen molecules nearby, creating singlet state oxygen. Singlet state oxygen is very reactive, and oxidizes nearby proteins, thus causing damage to bacteria in the periodontal pocket, which may favor pocket reduction. Two clinical trials demonstrated an additional probing depth reduction of about 0.5 mm compared to SRP alone. No specific indication is known for either technique.

5.6.3 Host Modulation Agents

Another approach in attempting to coax local tissue in producing better clinical outcomes is to manipulate host molecular mechanisms of wound healing. So far, research has investigated the potential of the following agents as adjuncts to periodontal therapy: anti-inflammatory agents such as NSAIDs including Aspirin, polyunsaturated fatty acids,[5] and lipoxins; locally applied bisphosphonates, and teriparatide, a bone-forming drug. However, none of these agents have regulatory clearance as adjunct for SRP at this time.

Subantimicrobial doxycycline (PerioStat) is the only host modulation agent available for clinical use, and is specifically used to slow attachment loss. Doxycycline interferes with matrix metalloproteinases, which generally break down collagen fibers and extracellular matrix as part of normal connective tissue turn over and attachment loss during periodontal disease. At the low dose (20 mg per day) prescribed, there is no antimicrobial activity, and no development of antimicrobial resistance. Several clinical trials demonstrate significant, up to 0.5 to 1 mm of additional pocket depth gain after SRP if combined with subantimicrobial doxycycline compared to placebo.[6] Typically, this medication is used long term in periodontal maintenance patients who either have severe attachment loss or are at the risk of losing attachment.

5.6.4 Local Antimicrobial Agents

Local delivery antimicrobials can be effective in killing subgingival bacteria as they achieve very high concentrations of antimicrobial agent at the site of periodontal infection, and reduce the chance of systemic side effects. Generally, indications for local delivery antimicrobials include localized, residual pocketing (PD ≥ 5 mm) and inflammation after conventional SRP, especially if surgical treatment is not feasible. Local delivery antimicrobials produce on average 0.2 to 0.5-mm pocket reduction compared to **SRP** alone, which produces 1 to 2-mm pocket reduction on average.[7] Clinical improvement is unlikely if plaque-retentive factors such as defective restorations or calculus are not removed. Clinical improvement tends to be less than that seen with surgical treatment, especially if bony defects or furcation involvements are present. Currently, the most commonly available agents are as follows.

Doxycycline Hyclate (Atridox)

Atridox is supplied in an envelope containing two syringes, one containing a solution of doxycycline hyclate, and the other the delivery gel. The syringes are connected and the contents are mixed by pushing the plungers back and forth, and once mixed, the gel is applied into pockets after thorough SRP using a cannula connected to the filled syringe. The gel solidifies once injected into the pocket, and a plastic instrument is useful to push the material back into the pocket if it adheres to the syringe tip. An advantage of Atridox is that the amount of material supplied in one envelope is often sufficient for the entire mouth.

Minocycline Hydrochloride (Arrestin) Microspheres

Arrestin consists of a kit with specialized syringe, and cartridge/delivery tip containing a small amount of yellow powder. For delivery, the cartridge is loaded into the Arrestin syringe, and the tip of the syringe-loaded cartridge inserted into a pocket that has been thoroughly scaled and root planed. Light pressure on the syringe will push the powder into the pocket, and there is enough material to last for 1 to 2 pockets (▶Fig. 5.14). An advantage of this agent is the easy delivery method.

Chlorhexidine Gel (Periochi)

Periochip comes in a package containing a single chip that can only be used for one site. The chip is rather rigid. It usually requires small cotton forceps to insert the chip into a fairly deep (>5 mm) and wide pocket (>4 mm) next to a flat tooth surface.

For all agents, the pocket may be sealed with a drop of cyanoacrylate tissue adhesive such as Periacryl-Glustitch, carefully applied to the pocket entrance. For any of these agents, the CDT code D4381 can be used for treatment planning for each

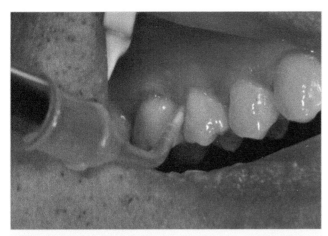

Fig. 5.14 One of the local antimicrobial delivery systems. Arrestin powder (yellow tip content) loaded in the Arrestin syringe is inserted into a pocket.

site, and should be bundled together with SRP, for the involved quadrants. Coverage by dental insurances varies, with some carriers not reimbursing it and others limiting it to two sites per quadrant refractory to SRP.

5.6.5 Subgingival Oral Irrigation

Some clinicians believe that irrigating periodontal pockets after SRP with an antiseptic agent (i.e., Chlorhexidine gluconate and Povidone iodine) maximizes clinical results by flushing out loose calculus and killing dislodged bacteria. Commonly, this is done by flushing the pockets after SRP with a cannula or Mono-jet syringe, containing the antiseptic solution of choice. To avoid soft tissue injury, the cannula should not be forced into the pocket and only gentle irrigation pressure should be applied.

The clinical benefit of this procedure is uncertain as for either chlorhexidine or povidone iodine the procedure results in the significant reduction of bacterial reduction right after the procedure, but questionable long-term clinical improvement with possible additional pocket reduction of up to 0.2 mm on average. Subgingival oral irrigation is used as part of the "soft tissue management" concept, which is critiqued for delaying necessary surgical periodontal treatment and as money-making scheme at the expense of patients.

Appropriate insurance codes (i.e., CDT codes D9630 or D4921) can be used for reimbursement purposes, but dental insurance rarely provides reimbursement, and some providers simply perform subgingival irrigation.

5.7 Oral Hygiene Instruction

Oral hygiene, in the context of periodontal treatment, does little for active disease control, but is important for prevention and long-term treatment success. Oral hygiene instruction has little effect on the existing subgingival microflora and does not arrest chronic periodontitis by itself. Improving oral hygiene, however, reduces gingival inflammation, and good oral hygiene is associated with better clinical outcomes for nonsurgical and surgical periodontal therapy including regenerative therapy and implant therapy.

In order to be effective, oral hygiene must be tailored to a patient's needs, abilities, learning styles, and treatment goals. Elements of effective oral hygiene instructions include the following:

- Plaque visualization with disclosing agents or other methods, so that a patient can see problem areas where plaque accumulates on their own.
- Explanation that is appropriate to a patient's background, and allows the patient to recognize the relationships between plaque, existing disease, patient concerns, and treatment goals.
- Demonstration of appropriate hygiene methods that a patient can perform on their own. Demonstration should include good visuals such as models or instructional videos for patients who are visual learners, thorough and clear explanation for auditory learners and demonstrating the hygiene method in the patient's mouth for kinesthetic learners. It may be useful to focus on one hygiene aspect per visit, such as interproximal cleaning between molars, which likely is more effective than providing too many instructions.
- Repetition of the demonstrated methods by the patient to ensure a patient can perform taught oral hygiene methods.
- Documentation of plaque levels and specific oral hygiene instruction.

Oral hygiene instruction may benefit from using motivational interviewing techniques that were originally developed for alcohol abuse counseling. In this technique, the dentist guides and facilitates the patient toward developing improved oral hygiene by letting the patient explore and discover why they want to improve oral hygiene (▶Table 5.8, ▶Video 5.9). This technique requires reflective listening skills, empathy, and a nonconfrontational style to affect behavior changes. There is recent evidence that motivational interviewing can improve dentist-patient communication, case acceptance,[8] and effectiveness of plaque removal.

5.7.1 Plaque Disclosing

For patient education and assessing compliance with past oral hygiene instructions, plaque disclosing (i.e., Young Dental Manufacturing's Trace, GUM RedCote, Sultan Disclosing Solution) can be useful. Plaque-disclosing agents contain a red dye (i.e., FD&C red no. 3, D&C no. 28, Fuchsine, Erythrosine) that binds to plaque and resists rinsing, thus making plaque-covered tooth surfaces visible. Two-toned plaque-disclosing solutions differentially stain thicker areas of plaque, thus showing new, thin plaque in one color and older, thicker plaque in a different color. The following technique works well with plaque-disclosing liquids, and minimizes the soapy taste of these solutions, reduces unsightly temporary soft tissue staining, and reduces the chance of permanent staining of clothing:

- Have patient wear bib, and recline patient.
- Rinse mouth with water syringe and remove excess liquid with saliva aspirator.
- Dip cotton tip applicator in a cup containing a small amount of disclosing solution (just enough to soak cotton tip).
- Per quadrant, apply cotton tip applicator to tooth surfaces, especially toward the gingival margin.

Table 5.8 Motivational interviewing techniques

Example	Technique
"I heard you earlier expressing concern about the unsightly metal edge of the crown that did not used to be there when the crown was placed"	*Reflective listening affirms patient's main concern*
"Now, using the mirror I gave you, can you describe the color and shape of the gum tissue in the area?"	*Open-ended question, develops discrepancy in patient's attitude toward gum disease*
"...You see that is more red and swollen than the gum tissue away from the tooth"	*Summarizes patient's observation*
"That is inflammation that causes you to loose gum tissue. Now why do you think your gums are inflamed?"	*Reflection, support patient discovery and ability to come to conclusion on his/her own*
"That is right"	*Affirm patient's conclusion if not too far-fetched and consistent with oral hygiene goal*
"Now what do you think you can do to stop this inflammation and prevent losing more gum tissue?"	*Enable patient to come up with solution to change*
"Ok, then can you do this starting today?"	*Get commitment; check if patient is ready to make this step*

- Per quadrant, rinse off tooth surface with water syringe and high-speed suction tip.
- Check and have the patient see with hand mirror red-purple patches of plaque. Plaque disclosing solutions will also highlight tooth surface cracks and margins of restorations.

5.7.2 Mechanical Plaque-Removal Methods

Mechanical plaque-removal methods usually fall into two categories based on plaque accumulation area: facial/lingual and interproximal. This can be treated as follows (▶ Fig. 5.15).

Tooth Brushing Methods for Facial and Lingual Surfaces

There are four general brushing methods: scrubbing technique, variations of the Bass method, variations of the Stillman method, the Charter technique, and the Fones' technique. The characteristics, indications, advantages, and disadvantages are shown in (▶ Table 5.9, ▶ Fig. 5.16).

In general, a patient's individual brushing method is acceptable as long as it is effective and avoids tissue injury, as there is little evidence suggesting the superiority of one brushing method over another.[9] For patients with persistent plaque buildup and gingival inflammation, the goal is to improve a patient's ability to perform brushing and increase efficiency. If a patient has trouble in achieving good plaque control with a manual brush, better plaque control can be achieved by having the patient switch to a rotary oscillating electric toothbrush. The large handle of an electric toothbrush makes it also easier to grip for patients with reduced dexterity. If a patient cannot obtain an electric toothbrush, inserting a manual brush into a tennis ball or foam tube can also assist arthritic or otherwise handicapped patients.

Tooth Brushing Methods for Interproximal Surfaces

For most patients with periodontal disease, the problem with oral hygiene is interproximal cleaning. Many interproximal hygiene aides exist, but generally dental floss is the preferred method for healthy dentition whereas interproximal brushes are the preferred method for teeth affected by periodontitis. The indications are as follows:

- No exposure of root surfaces, good manual dexterity—floss:
  - While unwaxed floss may be more effective in removing plaque, waxed, and shred-resistant floss made of cotton or synthetic material (i.e., polytetrafluoroethylene) may be easier to use for a patient.
- Pontics of fixed partial dentures and orthodontic appliances—super floss or floss threader.
- *Exposed interproximal root surfaces, furcation tunnels, diastemas, and open contacts—interproximal brushes*:
  - Sizing of the interproximal brush should be small enough to fit the interproximal space, and large enough to reach the root surfaces on both sides while inserting the brush from both sides of the embrasure.
- Narrow interproximal spaces and furcation entrances—interdental stimulator for plaque removal.
- Slight diastema/open contacts—dental tape.
- Implants, periodontal maintenance—add oral irrigator in addition to other interproximal cleaning methods.[10]
  - Start with low water pressure, and slowly increase to comfort.
- Poor manual dexterity:
  - Toothpicks.
  - Interproximal brushes mounted on a long handle.
  - Hummingbird Electric flosser.

5.7.3 Dentifrices/Toothpaste

From a periodontal perspective, dentifrices are not critical to oral hygiene, but dentifrices and prerinses can be used to increase the effectiveness of brushing as surfactants help loosen up biofilm. While any toothpaste that aids plaque removal without excessive abrasiveness is acceptable for most patients, recommendations for a specific toothpaste can be made depending on desired effect and specific ingredients, which are as follows:

- Antigingivitis and plaque effects:
  - *Triclosan*: Direct anti-inflammatory effects by inhibiting gingival prostaglandin and leukotriene synthesis, along with antimicrobial properties. It is also controversial as triclosan is toxic to marine life, may have estrogen-like effects in humans and is suspected to promote antimicrobial resistance.
  - Other antiseptic agents such as amine alcohols, essential oils, and other herbal products, bisguanides (chlorhexidine), quarternary ammonium compounds (cetylpyridinium

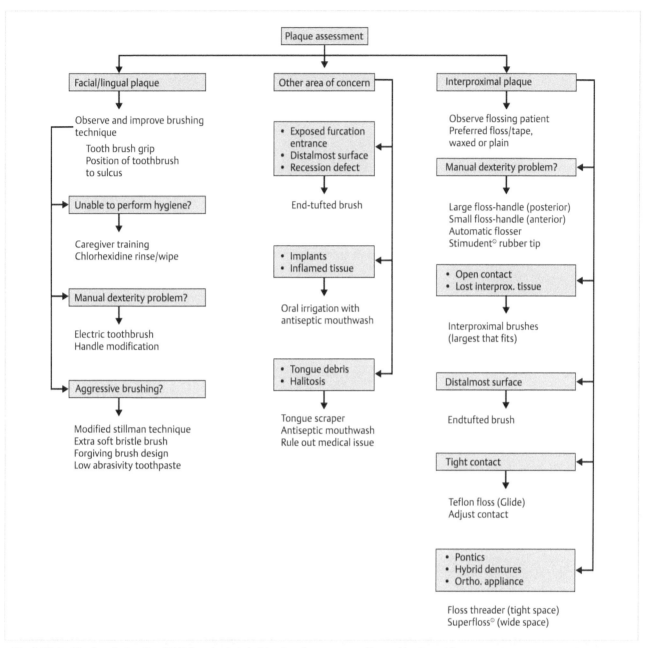

Fig. 5.15 Oral hygiene instruction (OHI) flowchart. A decision tree for recommending oral hygiene aids.

Table 5.9 Tooth brushing methods/techniques

Method/technique	Characteristic	Indication	Advantages	Disadvantages
Scrubbing	Horizontal brushing across tooth surfaces		Most commonly performed by patients, easy method	May not remove plaque at gingival margin. Potential for tooth abrasion and gingiva damage with hard brush and dentifrice
Fones	Circular motion over teeth. For facial surfaces, hold teeth together	Primary dentition	Easy to learn and understood ("big circles"). Works well with small teeth, and requires little dexterity	Not as effective as other methods for healthy adults
Modified Bass	Bristles point into sulcus. Short vibrating strokes	Healthy adults Orthodontic appliances	Effective marginal plaque removal and disease prevention	Requires good manual dexterity, patient motivation
Modified Stillman	Bristles placed on gingiva, rotated toward tooth surface	Adults with facial/gingival recession	Minimizes gingival trauma	Slow, may not be as effective in removing plaque if vestibule is shallow
Charter	Bristles aimed toward interproximal contact points	During healing after pocket reduction surgery	Avoids healing flap edges interproximally	Difficult to perform if vestibule is shallow

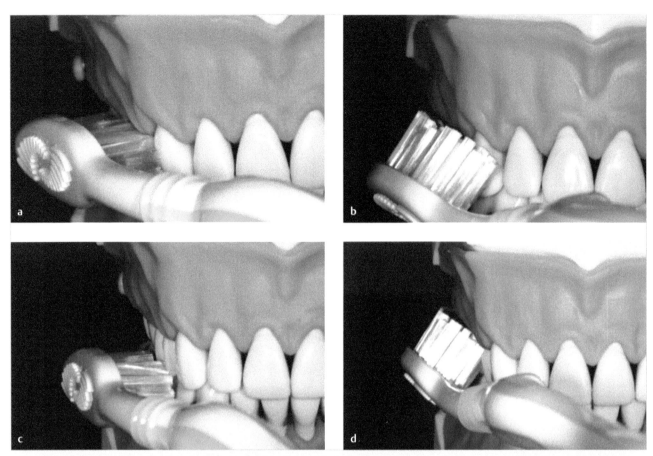

Fig. 5.16 (a–d) Comparison of bush positions during tooth brushing techniques. For the Charter's technique, bristles are pointing at the interproximal contacts, and the side of the toothbrush is resting on the gingiva. The toothbrush is then jiggled for each set of interproximal contacts, and this technique has been suggested for patients who had pocket-reduction surgery and are missing interproximal tissue. For the Fones' technique, the toothbrush is held perpendicular to the tooth surfaces and moved in a circular fashion. The technique was developed for children, and is useful for adults with limited manual or mental abilities. The Bass techniques have in common that the toothbrush bristles are aimed into the sulcus. For the modified Bass technique, the toothbrush is then jiggled for each tooth surface, and it may achieve good plaque control in adults with good manual skills. The Stillman techniques use a similar toothbrush position. For the modified Stillman technique, the bristles are placed on the gingiva first, and then rotated toward the occlusal surfaces. This is a gentle brushing technique useful for patients exhibiting gingival recession and cervical tooth erosions, and patients can be instructed to "brush the gums toward the teeth."

chloride), and various metal salts (zinc, stannous, silver salts containing fluoride, or aminofluoride). These agents assist in reducing plaque, and have varying effects on gingival inflammation.
- Reduction in dentinal hypersensitivity:
  - Potassium salts that inactive pulpal nerve fibers.
  - Dentinal tubule occluding agents such as oxalate salts (as mouth rinse or desensitizing agent),[11] strontium salts, and calcium sodium phosphosilicates.
  - Arginine/calcium phosphate compounds.
- *Calculus reduction (antitartar)*: Reduces the formation of calculus after scaling.
  - Pyrophosphate salts or hexametaphosphate salts that disrupt crystal formation within plaque and thus reduce supragingival calculus formation.
- "Whitening" or "Smoker's" toothpastes:
  - *Silica or silicon dioxide abrasives*: Erode surface deposits.
  - Oxidatives, chelators, and surfactants that help solubilize deposits.
  - Optical agents that increase the reflection of short wavelengths for increased "whiteness".

- Main concern with whitening pastes is the potential for tooth erosion, especially when combined with consumption of acidic beverages.

5.7.4 Mouthrinses/Mouthwash

Mouthrinses can be used to aid plaque removal, reduce gingivitis or halitosis, supply fluoride, and relief symptoms of xerostomia. For periodontal treatment, useful mouthwashes contain antimicrobial ingredients promoting plaque reduction and anti-inflammatory effects. The advantages and disadvantages of these mouthwashes are as follows:
- *Chlorhexidine gluconate (012% in 3M Peridex, Colgate PeriGuard or alcohol-free GUM Paroex)*: Well-established reduction in plaque and gingival inflammation. Bisguanide binds to tooth surfaces, producing a lasting antiseptic effect (substantivity). Disadvantage is brown tooth and tongue staining with long-term use (>2 weeks), and possible wound healing delay as chlorhexidine inhibits fibroblast growth.
- *Essential oil mixture of Thymol, Eucalyptol, Methol, and Salicylic acid (i.e., Listerine and generic formulations)*: Similar antiplaque

and antigingivitis effect as chlorhexidine, and widely available.[12] A disadvantage is the typical high alcohol content (20 to 25%), which may present an issue for recovering alcohol users, and present a possible, but not evident oral cancer risk.

- *Cetylpyridinium chloride and other quarternary ammonium compound (i.e., Scope)*: Reduces plaque and inflammation, but somewhat less than chlorhexidine and essential oils. Contains less or no alcohol than most chlorhexidine and essential oil-based rinses.
- *Triclosan*: Directly reduces plaque and gingival inflammation, but is also controversial as possible environmental hazard (see above).

There are also several noncommercial mouthwash alternatives:
- *"Oil-pulling" with sesame oil*: Derived from Vedic medicine and popular with some patients interested in nontraditional medicine. Here, a small amount of sesame oil is placed in the mouth, and forcefully swished around the mouth for about 15 minutes. Limited scientific evidence suggests that this method reduces plaque and gingival inflammation, and the method is likely impractical for most patients.
- *Hydrogen peroxide (1.5%, 1:1 dilution of generic 3% solutions)*: Kills catalase-negative bacteria and bleaches teeth. Disadvantage is possible carcinogenic potential, inconsistent evidence for plaque reduction, and potential for tissue damage with long-term use.
- *Sodium hypochlorite (0.05 to 0.25%, diluted from 5% household bleach)*: Very effective broad-spectrum antimicrobial that produces significant plaque and gingivitis reduction. Disadvantages are the potential for chemical burns and clothing damage from handling undiluted bleach, and the strong chlorine taste.

5.8 Tobacco-cessation Counseling

Tobacco use is one of the most significant contributing factors to severe periodontal disease. Tobacco use also makes it more likely that periodontal or implant therapy fails, and leads to a higher risk of future periodontal disease, oral cancer, and other significant health conditions. Dental healthcare providers are uniquely positioned to recognize the effects of tobacco on oral tissues at an early stage given the frequent interaction with patients. Since dental healthcare providers see patients more frequently than physicians, tobacco-cessation counseling is also more likely to be effective.

5.8.1 Consequences of Tobacco Use

Tobacco use leads to numerous, well-researched risks to overall health.

Systemic Disease Risks

Tobacco contains numerous potential carcinogens either naturally present in tobacco leaves (i.e., radioactive Polonium) or created by the burn process (i.e., polyaromatic hydrocarbons that acts as intercalating agents in DNA). All forms of tobacco use are linked to various cancers, with the method of tobacco use determining the most common cancer location. For example, cigarette smoking is linked to cancers in tissues coming into contact with cigarette smoke, or metabolizing/excreting tobacco content such as oral cavity, pharynx, larynx, lung, esophagus, stomach, pancreas, bladder, kidney, and cervix. Cigars produce larger smoke particles than cigarettes, and are inhaled less deeply into the lung, so the cancer focus is shifted toward the oral cavity.

Irritants from cigarette smoke also favor the development of emphysema and bronchitis, and increase the chance of contracting pneumonia.

Various tobacco substances, such as evaporated/dissolved nicotine from the tobacco leaves and carbon monoxide created by the slow-burn process, are irritants to blood vessels and immune cells. Consequently, tobacco use is associated with heart disease, myocardial infarcts, aneurysms, greater chance of infections, poor wound healing, reduced fertility, impotence, and various birth complications including still births.

Oral Disease Risks

Since tobacco use reduces the effectiveness of the immune response, it also allows more likely the development of severe periodontal disease and peri-implant diseases. Cancers are more likely to develop in areas of the mouth that are most likely to come into contact with tobacco. For smokers, this are the lips, tongue, palate gingiva, floor of the mouth, and buccal mucosa that may **develop pre-cancerous lesions**, **squamous cell carcinoma**, or **verrucous carcinoma**. For smokeless tobacco, this tends to be the buccal vestibule where tobacco is placed.

Tobacco use also leads to **halitosis** and dark brown tooth staining, as well as reduced taste sensation. Since smokeless tobacco often contains sugar, and nicotine reduces saliva formation, smokeless tobacco uses are more likely to develop root caries, especially mandibular posterior teeth.

5.8.2 Counseling Tobacco Users

Generally, most tobacco users understand at least some adverse effects caused by tobacco use and have a desire to quit. Many have also tried quitting before as they understand the benefits of quitting, but have relapsed into the habit for various reasons.

Therefore, the focus of successful counseling is less about providing information and instructions, but more about support and encouragement. The role of the tobacco cessation counselor is to let the patient be in charge, check on well-being of the patient, suggest strategies to overcome cravings, and provide continuous motivation in the form of explaining the rewards of quitting and demonstrating any progress in health that has been made. For tobacco cessation counseling, it is helpful to have various patient brochures and handouts available that list health risks, financial costs of tobacco, quitting strategies, and benefits of quitting. These can often be obtained for free or at low cost from dental associations, state organizations (i.e., California Smoker Helpline, 1–800-NO-BUTTS), and health associations (i.e., National Lung Association).

Generally, each counseling session follows the following pattern, the 5 A's (▶ Video 5.10):
- *Ask*: "Do you currently use tobacco?" If no, praise patient and move on to other treatment. If yes, determine what type of tobacco the patient uses, how much, when, and what triggers need for tobacco.

- *Advise*: "As your dentist/…, I need to advise you that using tobacco causes [oral condition – demonstrate in patient's mouth]." Explain and link oral signs of tobacco use in a non-judgmental manner. At a minimum, suggest referral to a professional tobacco cessation counseling service at this time.
- *Assess*: "I would like to know from you how willing you are to quit tobacco. Please tell me on a scale from 0, not interested at all, to 10, I want to quit now, how willing you are to quit."
  - *If the answer is less than 7, confirm that the patient is not willing to quit*: "It seems you are not ready to quit now, am I right." If the answer is "yes" at this point, politely respect this decision and offer assistance if needed, by saying: "Of course, even if you are not ready to quit, I would like you to think about quitting. I will give you some information to read, and I will ask you the next time if you have changed your mind. When you are ready to quit, I can help you, and you can also get help from many free services such as [name of a local/national tobacco quitting service]." If the answer is "no," have patient grade their interest in quitting again.
  - *If the answer is 7 or more, confirm that the patient is interested in quitting again*: "Great. It seems like you are ready to try to quit tobacco now, am I right?" If the answer is "yes," move to the next step. If the answer is "no," have patient grade their interest again.
- *Assist*: "Let's set a quit date. Are you ready to quit right now?"
  - *If yes, provide initial assistance in quitting*: "Great. Let's start by having you get rid of anything that may prompt you to [smoke/use tobacco]. If you have any tobacco products with you, let's throw them away now. Toss away any tobacco products that are in your car, your workplace and at home. Put away [ashtrays, pipes, e-cigs, …—any tobacco paraphernalia that a patient may have based on tobacco use]. As an idea, write down why you want to quit, and post it at the usual places at home where you normally [smoke, vape, chew tobacco, …]. I am going to give you some information to read that may help you quit."
  - *If no, encourage setting a quit date*: "That is ok, too. Most people are not ready to quit right away. It is a good idea, though, to set a date to get yourself ready for quitting, and each day make a change that helps you quit tobacco. For example, set a day that means something to you, like your birthday or anniversary, within the next 4 weeks, and everyday do something that helps you quit. This could be cutting down [one cigarette/pouch/vape each day, putting away ashtrays, …]. Tell others that you want to quit. Write down why you want to quit and post that at the places you usually use tobacco. On the quit day, toss all tobacco products and put way [ashtrays, … other tobacco paraphernalia]. I am going to give you some information that can help you quit as well."
  - *If you have prescription privileges, offer pharmacological assistance*: "Sometimes it helps to quit if you take medications that block the urge to smoke, or help your body withdraw from nicotine. I can suggest and prescribe medications for this, or you can talk to your physician about these medications. The most important thing, though, is to motivate yourself to quit, and I can suggest some strategies for that as well. Is this something you would be interested in?" If yes, prescribe medications and suggest strategies.

Suggest referral for additional help: "I have a list of tobacco cessation counseling services that can help you, and many are free."

Would you like to know more?" If yes, provide the information. If no, provide some information anyway: "That is ok, I am going to give you some information just in case you would like extra help [provide brochure]. Also, if you need help or have further questions, just give us a call here."
- *Arrange a follow-up*: "It is a good idea to check on you and see how you are doing with quitting, since it will more than double the chance of quitting. When would you like me to check on you?"
  - *If the patient provides a date*: "Great. When is a good time to call, and what number should we call?"
  - *If the patient is hesitant to provide a date*: "If you are not sure, I can check with you at the next visit and see how you are doing. Remember, as long as you try you will succeed eventually."

5.8.3 Encouraging Quitting

For tobacco users hesitant to try quitting, the "5 Rs" can be helpful. At each visit, discuss the following:
- *Relevance*: At each patient visit, provide a single bit of patient-specific information that drives home the relevance of quitting to the patient. Present this in a nonjudgmental way, and make sure to link it to the patient's chief complaint or significant oral conditions. When appropriate, linking quitting to family well-being (i.e., exposure of children to second-hand smoke) can be a potent motivator for quitting.
- *Risk*: At each patient visit, highlight a risk of continued tobacco use that is most relevant to the patient. This could be:
  - *Immediate risks*: Shortness of breath, persistent cough, infertility, asthma, bad breath, stained teeth, diminished taste, burn marks on clothes, and cigarette smell.
  - *Long-term risk*: Oral cancer, lung cancer, stroke, heart attacks, losing teeth, lack of dental treatment success, infection risk, poor wound healing, and fire hazard at home.
  - *Risk to others*: Increased cancer risk for spouse, increased asthma risk for children, children will likely develop tobacco habit, and increased risk of sudden infant death syndrome.
- *Rewards*: At each visit, identify one potential benefit of quitting that is relevant to patient.
  - *Improved health*: Better fitness, physical performance, and appearance.
  - *Quality of life:* Food tastes better, better smell, healthier family, and money saving.
  - *Well-being*: Confidence, good example for children, and less worry about tobacco risks.
- *Roadblocks*: Discuss past quitting attempts, and reasons not to try to quit. Address or provide strategy to overcome roadblocks:
  - *Withdrawal symptoms*: Provide pharmacologic aids.
  - *Fear of failure*: Assure patient and provide close follow-up for motivation.
  - *Weight gain*: Suggest exercise, nutrition counseling. Using Buproprion or Nicotine gum during the quitting attempt may reduce weight gain.
  - *Lack of support*: Use counseling service. Join a support group.
  - *Cravings*: Suggest strategies to overcome cravings. Cravings only last for a few minutes, and activities can overcome these moments.

○ *Enjoyment of tobacco*: Provide Varenicline prescription to block "reward" sensation.

○ *Depression*: Group sessions in support groups can help along with psychological counseling. Clinical depression needs treatment by psychiatrist.

• *Repetition*: Explain that quitting tobacco takes numerous times to succeed. On average, smokers need to quit 9 to 12 times in order to be successful.

○ Reinforcing relevance, risks, rewards, and discussing roadblocks persistently most likely will induce interest in quitting eventually. Alternatively, it may cause noncompliant patients to drop out of treatment.

5.8.4 Pharmacologic Agents for Tobacco Cessation

While not essential to tobacco cessation, pharmacologic agents generally improve the likelihood of successful tobacco cessation. Generally, there are three agents that dentists may prescribe: Nicotine-replacement products, Buproprion (Zyban), and Varenicline (Chantix).

Nicotine Replacements

Generally, nicotine replacement should be coordinated with a physician if a patient has a history of cardiovascular disease, gastric ulcers, diabetes, depression, asthma, or sodium-restricted diet. Nicotine-replacement therapy may not need a prescription, and is most commonly used as the first pharmacologic agent to assist quitting. For nicotine-replacement therapy to be effective, tobacco users must quit before taking the first dose of nicotine. The following nicotine forms are available:

• *Nicotine patches*: They are available without prescription, and provide a constant supply of nicotine replaced for patients who normally use tobacco throughout the day. Patches are easy to use, and usually prevent morning cravings for tobacco. A disadvantage of patches is that it does not provide the "mouth feel" of a cigarette, and applying the patch at bedtime may disturb sleep. For cigarette use, dosing depends on the number of cigarettes smoked per day:

○ *Heavy smoker (10+ cigarettes or ½ pack/day)*: Week 1 to 6: 21-mg patch once a day. Week 7 to 8: 14-mg patch once a day. Week 9 to 10: 7-mg patch once a day.

○ *Light smoker (<10 cigarettes/day)*: Week 1 to 6: 14-mg patch once a day. Week 7 to 8: 7-mg patch once a day.

• *Nicotine gums*: They are available without prescriptions, and provide a patient more control over nicotine supply along with a replacement mouth habit. The gums are quite hard compared to chewing gum, and need to be deliberately chewed for 10 to 20 times until a sharp, peppery taste is felt. Once this sensation sets in, the gum needs to be held in the cheek for about 5 minutes. When the taste subsides, the gum needs to be chewed again to release more nicotine. Nicotine gums may be effective in reducing weight gain during quitting, but are difficult to use with dentures. Dosing depends on the number of cigarettes smoked per day:

○ *Heavy smoker (25+ cigarettes/day:* 4-mg gums. Week 1 to 6: one piece every 1 to 2 hours. Week 7 to 9: 1 piece every 2 to 4 hours. Week 10 to 12: one piece every 4 to 8 hours.

○ *Light smoker (<25 cigarettes/day)*: 2-mg gums. Week 1 to 6: one piece every 1 to 2 hours. Week 7 to 9: one piece every 2 to 4 hours. Week 10 to 12: one piece every 4 to 8 hours.

• *Nicotine lozenges*: These are available without prescription, and have advantages similar to nicotine gum. Dosing depends on cigarette habit, and the patient needs to slowly reduce the number of lozenges used per day from 12 to 20 lozenges/day to 3 lozenges/day over 12 weeks:

○ Cigarette within half an hour of waking up: 4 mg.

○ Cigarette later than half an hour after waking up: 2 mg.

• *Nicotine nasal spray (Nicotrol NS; 10 mg/mL; 1 spray per nostril)*: It needs a prescription and may produce nasal irritation. However, it may be more appropriate for patients who used to smoke in bursts, and heavy smokers. Start dose is 2 to 4 sprays/hour (maximum 80 sprays/day), and patient keeps tally of doses. Every day, the patient reduces the sprays by two sprays until they quit.

• Nicotine inhaler (Nicotrol Inhaler) is a cigarette-like inhaler, which is easy to use and handles similar to a cigarette. The inhaler may not supply enough nicotine to be effective for heavy smokers, and creates a whistle sound when used. The start dose is 6 to 16 cartridges/day, and the patient uses one cartridge less every week until they quit.

5.8.5 Other Agents

While nicotine-replacement therapy can be sufficient for quitting, heavy tobacco users or those with a long history of unsuccessful quitting attempts, may benefit from other agents.

Buproprion (Zyban)

Buproprion is an antidepressant acting on dopaminergic pathways in the brain, and reduces tobacco craving. It is useful to supplement nicotine replacement therapy, but should not be prescribed if a patient has epilepsy, eating disorders, undergoes alcohol/drug addiction therapy, or already uses buproprion or monoamineoxidase inhibitors for the treatment of depression. Buproprion can also induce mood changes, vivid dreams, or suicidal thoughts in some patients, and a close follow-up is needed if buproprion is prescribed.

For tobacco cessation, a prescription of buproprion 150 mg is given while the patient still uses tobacco, and the patient is instructed to take one tablet in the morning on the first 3 days. After 3 days, the dose is increased to one tablet every 12 hours, and the patient instructed to quit within 2 weeks. After quitting, buproprion is continued for 7 to 12 weeks to maintain abstinence, and the dose tapered to one tablet in the last week.

Varenicline (Chantix)

Varenicline blocks nicotine receptors responsible for the "reward" sensation of tobacco use, and removes a major incentive to continued smoking. It cannot be used with nicotine-replacement therapy, and commonly produces some side effects. The most common side effect is nausea, and it may produce unusual dreams. Rarely, in some patients it can cause mood changes or suicidal thoughts. It is easy to use, as the medication is supplied in a blister pack that provides instructions when to take it. For the first month, a "starter" pack is prescribed that contains 0.5 to

1-mg tablets, and for subsequent months, the "continuing" pack is prescribed for as long as needed. If nausea develops with the starter pack, taking half a tablet can help avoid nausea. Typically, the patient can use tobacco when beginning Varenicline and is encouraged to quit tobacco use completely within 3 months.

5.9 Essential Takeaways

- Plaque is the etiologic agent of periodontal disease. Local factors (calculus, defective restorations, tooth malposition, etc.) and systemic and medical conditions (smoking, diabetes, pregnancy, etc.) influence and contribute to disease severity.

Controlling inflammation begins with oral hygiene instruction (OHI) for biofilm removal. Initial therapy of SRP aims to produce a smooth, clean, hard surface.

- A combined use of power and hand instruments in a "blended approach" is recommended. Various ultrasonic insert tips are available and are chosen due to access and efficacy. Hand instruments need to be sharpened for safety and efficiency.
- Adjuncts to SRP are available and can be useful. Efficaciousness still relies on meticulously cleaned, uncontaminated root surfaces.
- Individualized patient home care is vital for success (not all patients need to floss). One size does not fit all.

- Tobacco use has numerous adverse overall and oral health risks.
  - Tobacco cessation counseling should consist at least of "ask" about tobacco use and "advise" about tobacco risks, with possible "assess" willingness to quit, "assist" in quitting, and "arrange" follow-up for quitting.
- Pharmacologic agents such as nicotine-replacement agents can assist tobacco cessation.

5.10 Review Questions

Consider the following case for the practice questions below:

A 43-year-old patient with a history of gastric reflux and tobacco use presents to you complaining of "bleeding gums." He reports taking omeprazole once daily, antacids as needed and he states that he has smoked for about 15 years a pack a day. He smokes regularly throughout the day as he gets bored easily and gives him something to do. His last regular dental visit was 3 years ago for a "cleaning" and he states that he brushes his teeth with a soft brush using a scrubbing motion, and uses floss "sometimes" when food gets stuck between his teeth. He lost his maxillary left first molar a month ago as he developed a severe toothache, and had the tooth removed at a community dental clinic providing free emergency dental care. Consider the following areas representative of the entire mouth (see ▶ Fig. 5.17 for clinical appearance and ▶ Fig. 5.18 for radiographs).

11	12	13	14	15	Tooth	22	21	20	19	18
513	424	425		523	PD (facial)	424	324	424	545	423
*	* *	* *		*	BOP (facial)	* *			* * *	
524	434	434		634	PD (lingual)	435	325	535	554	534
*	* *	*		* *	BOP (lingual)		*		* * *	* * *
1	1	2		2	Highest CAL	2	2	2	3	1
					Furcation (lingual)				1	
					Furcation (buccal)				1	
		1			Tooth mobility					

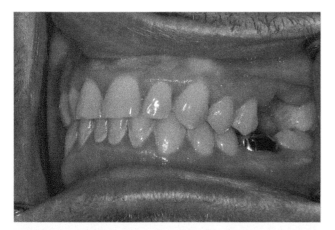

Fig. 5.17 Facial view.

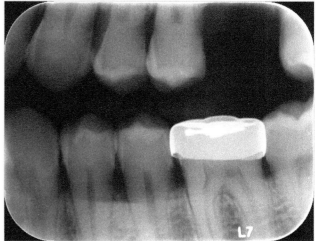

Fig. 5.18 Bitewing radiograph of left premolar/1st molar region.

Learning Objective: Given clinical findings, develop a comprehensive periodontal treatment plan that aims to reduce periodontal inflammation.

1. Evaluate the following statements:

Statement 1: Tobacco use is associated with increased severity of periodontal disease.

Statement 2: In this patient, tobacco-cessation counseling should be provided.

    A. Both statements are true
    B. Both statements are false
    C. The first statement is true, the second is false
    D. The first statement is false, the second is true

2. In this patient, the appropriate initial, nonsurgical periodontal treatment procedure for the mandibular left quadrant is
    A. Maintenance
    B. Prophylaxis
    C. SRP, 1 to 3 teeth
    D. SRP, 4+ teeth

3. Please evaluate the following statement:

Stainless steel crown as used in this case is not acceptable as permanent treatment, because it cannot be scaled and root planed without specialized instrumentation.

    A. Both the statement and the reason are correct and related
    B. Both the statement and the reason are correct, but NOT related
    C. The statement is correct, but the reason is NOT
    D. The statement is NOT correct, but the reason is correct
    E. NEITHER the statement NOR the reason is CORRECT

Learning Objective: Describe methods to increase the efficiency and effectiveness of scaling and root planing (SRP).

4. Please evaluate the following statements:

Statement 1: Ultrasonic instrumentation cannot be used in this patient.

Statement 2: For best root surface smoothness, hand instrumentation should be used prior to ultrasonic instrumentation.

    A. Both statements are true
    B. Both statements are false
    C. The first statement is true, the second is false
    D. The first statement is false, the second is true

5. Which of the following Gracey curettes is specifically designed for use on the lingual surface of the mandibular second left premolar?
    A. 1/2
    B. 7/8
    C. 11/12
    D. 13/14

6. The problem caused by dull curettes includes all of the following EXCEPT one. Which one is the EXCEPTION?
    A. Burnished calculus
    B. Increased operator fatigue
    C. More instrument wear
    D. Potential for tissue damage

7. All of the following strategies can increase SRP efficiency EXCEPT one. Which one is the EXCEPTION?
    A. Proper ergonomics including finger rests
    B. Sharp instruments
    C. Switch instruments frequently
    D. Ultrasonic instrumentation
    E. Variations of curettes (i.e., Everedge, rigid, …)

Learning Objective: Describe the benefits and risks of adjunctive agents used during SRP.

8. Typically, Er:YAG and Nd:YAG lasers are used for …
    A. As adjunct to SRP
    B. By themselves to replace conventional SRP instrumentation
    C. Exclusively for soft tissue surgery
    D. Rarely since diode lasers replaced them as cheaper alternative

9. Please evaluate the following statements:

Statement 1: Arrestin consists of a chlorhexidine-containing gel chip.

Statement 2: Locally delivered antimicrobials produce an additional average pocket reduction of about 1 to 2 mm compared to SRP alone.

    A. Both statements are true
    B. Both statements are false
    C. The first statement is true, the second is false
    D. The first statement is false, the second is true

Learning Objective: Given a patient's oral hygiene needs, develop personalized oral hygiene instructions.

10. Given that this patient works as a watch repair person, the most appropriate interproximal cleaning aid for the no. 22 to 23 area is:
    A. Endtufted brush
    B. Floss
    C. Interproximal brush
    D. Superfloss

11. Consider the following cause and effect statement:

This patient's brushing technique is useful for any patient with gingival recession, since a soft brush and toothpaste with low abrasivity likely prevent tissue damage.

    A. Both the statement and the reason are correct and related
    B. Both the statement and the reason are correct, but NOT related
    C. The statement is correct, but the reason is NOT
    D. The statement is NOT correct, but the reason is correct
    E. NEITHER the statement NOR the reason is CORRECT

12. Please evaluate the following statements:

Statement 1: The most common side effect of chlorhexidine is tooth staining.

Statement 2: Chlorhexidine binds to tooth surfaces and provides lingering antiseptic activity.

    A. Both statements are true
    B. Both statements are false
    C. The first statement is true, the second is false
    D. The first statement is false, the second is true

13. Based on the history, what specifically may help this patient to quit tobacco?
    A. Varenicline (Chantix)
    B. Attending a support group
    C. Exercise
    D. Strategies against boredom

14. Which of the following pharmacologic aids would be useful for a first-time quit attempt in this patient seeking an over-the-counter medication?
    A. Nicotine patch 21 mg
    B. Nicotine gum 2 mg
    C. Nicotine nasal spray
    D. Nicotine inhaler

5.11 Answers

1. **A.** Tobacco use has long been associated with increased severity and extent of chronic periodontitis, and given the risk of oral health posed by tobacco, you need to address this by educating smokers about adverse oral health effects and encourage the tobacco-using patient to quit.

2. **D.** The patient has significant pocketing and evidence of calculus (see radiographs) on more than three teeth, and shows signs of periodontitis (attachment loss and radiographic bone loss). In order to remove calculus in the presence of periodontitis, you need to perform SRP. Since at least four teeth have deep pockets and calculus, you should use the "4+ teeth" SRP code for treatment planning.

3. **C.** Stainless steel crowns should not be used in adult patients as permanent restoration for a variety of reasons, such as lack of proper contours, poor fit, risk of recurrent caries, lack of proper occlusal contacts, and concerns about restoration and tooth longevity. While difficult to scale and root plane because of the overhanging metal and poor contours of the restoration, it is possible to scale these with conventional hand instruments, mostly by using horizontal tip movement parallel to the crown margin.

4. **B.** The patient does not have medical conditions that preclude use of ultrasonics, and you can choose to instrument tooth no. 19 only with hand instruments, so the first statement is false. The second statement is false since ultrasonics produce a rougher surface than hand instrumentation, so in order to get the smoothest surface possible use hand instruments last.

5. **B.** The 1/2 Gracey curette is used for anterior teeth. 11/12 is designed for mesial surfaces of posterior teeth, and the 13/14 for distal surfaces of posterior teeth.

6. **C.** A dull instrument tends to burnish calculus into the root surface, and since it is less efficient in calculus removal, it takes more effort to remove calculus and causes more operator fatigue. Also, since the instrument is dull, it will tend to slip off the tooth surface unexpectedly and tear through the surrounding soft tissue.

7. **C.** Every time you need to switch an instrument, time passes for putting the used instrument back on to the tray, searching and picking up a new instrument, assessing its sharpness, sharpening it, and adjusting your focus back on the tooth surface you were working

on. Therefore, for best efficiency, you want to avoid switching instruments unless necessary.

8. **A.** Er:YAG and Nd:YAG are surgical lasers that can cut hard tissue, and are used for periodontal treatment as adjunct to SRP. While it is possible to use these lasers as monotherapy, it may be difficult and slow as much of SRP depends on tactile detection of calculus, which cannot be done with a laser tip.

9. **D.** The active ingredient in Arrestin is minocycline. Chlorhexidine is found as an active ingredient in the Periochip. The average pocket reduction seen with local antimicrobial delivery studies is few tenths of a millimeter.

10. **B.** Given the patient's profession, manual dexterity can be assumed and it poses no limitation. Since the interproximal space between nos. 22 and 23 is tight and mostly filled with soft tissue, floss is the most appropriate oral hygiene aid for this site.

11. **D.** While a soft brush and toothpaste with low abrasivity are useful to prevent tissue damage, a vigorous scrubbing technique is associated with gingival recession and not recommended here.

12. **A.** Chlorhexidine mouthrinses are generally safe to use, but cause brown tooth staining over time since chlorhexidine binds to oral surfaces including teeth.

13. **D.** According to the case, the patient smokes whenever he gets bored. So, a quitting strategy must provide him with a strategy to prevent boredom, such as starting a hobby, or suggesting an alternative to smoking such as using a relaxation ball or fidgeting toy to keep his hands busy. Exercise and support groups are usually helpful in general, but not specifically in this case. Varenicline may or may not be effective in this case as smoking is used by this patient to overcome boredom, and not necessarily for enjoyment.

14. **A.** The patient is a heavy smoker (1 pack/day), and therefore would need 21-mg nicotine patches. 2-mg nicotine gums are used for light smokers, and the inhaler and nasal spray requires a prescription.

5.12 Evidence-based Activities

- Perform a literature search and judge if patients using electric toothbrushes achieve better plaque control than patients using manual brushes.
- Perform a literature search and determine if long-term use of antiseptic mouthwashes (i.e., chlorhexidine and essential oils) produces a clinically significant reduction in gingival inflammation. Debate if any mouthwash is superior to others.
- Go to the University of Texas Health Science Center School of Dentistry at San Antonio's library of critically appraised topics (CAT) at https://cats.uthscsa.edu/ and search for a review on lasers and periodontal treatment. Read any CAT you can find, and debate if the conclusion is still correct based on current literature.
- Create a CAT on the merit of full mouth disinfection (or any other topic for which a CAT is not available) following the outline provided by Sauve S, et al. in "The critically appraised topic: a practical approach to learning critical appraisal" (Ann R Coll Physicians Surg Can. 1995; 28:396–398).

References

[1] Marda P, Prakash S, Devaraj CG, Vastardis S. A comparison of root surface instrumentation using manual, ultrasonic and rotary instruments: an in vitro study using scanning electron microscopy. Indian J Dent Res 2012;23(2):164–170

[2] It's About Time to Get on the Cutting Edge. Chicago, Illinois: Hu-Friedy; 2009

[3] Mizutani K, Aoki A, Coluzzi D et al. Lasers in minimally invasive periodontal and peri-implant therapy. Periodontol. 2000 2016;71(1):185–212

[4] Cappuyns I, Cionca N, Wick P, Giannopoulou C, Mombelli A. Treatment of residual pockets with photodynamic therapy, diode laser, or deep scaling. A randomized, split-mouth controlled clinical trial. Lasers Med Sci 2012;27(5):979–986

[5] Sculley DV. Periodontal disease: modulation of the inflammatory cascade by dietary n-3 polyunsaturated fatty acids. J Periodontal Res 2014;49(3):277–281

[6] Deo V, Gupta S, Bhongade ML, Jaiswal R. Evaluation of subantimicrobial dose doxycycline as an adjunct to scaling and root planing in chronic periodontitis patients with diabetes: a randomized, placebo-controlled clinical trial. J Contemp Dent Pract 2010;11(3):009–016

[7] Garrett S, Adams DF, Bogle G, et al. The effect of locally delivered controlled-release doxycycline or scaling and root planing on periodontal maintenance patients over 9 months. J Periodontol 2000;71(1):22–30

[8] Curry-Chiu ME, Catley D, Voelker MA, Bray KK. Dental hygienists' experiences with motivational interviewing: a qualitative study. J Dent Educ 2015;79(8):897–906

[9] Wainwright J, Sheiham A. An analysis of methods of toothbrushing recommended by dental associations, toothpaste and toothbrush companies and in dental texts. Br Dent J 2014;217(3):E5

[10] Goyal CR, Lyle DM, Qaqish JG, Schuller R. Evaluation of the plaque removal efficacy of a water flosser compared to string floss in adults after a single use. J Clin Dent 2013;24(2):37–42

[11] Sharma D, McGuire JA, Amini P. Randomized trial of the clinical efficacy of a potassium oxalate-containing mouthrinse in rapid relief of dentin sensitivity. J Clin Dent 2013;24(2):62–67

[12] Van der Weijden FA, Van der Sluijs E, Ciancio SG, Slot DE. Can Chemical Mouthwash Agents Achieve Plaque/Gingivitis Control? Dent Clin North Am 2015;59(4):799–829

6 Reducing Pockets

Abstract

For patients with more significant periodontal disease, there typically are residual deep pockets remaining after nonsurgical periodontal treatment. While it is possible that repeat scaling and root planing and other nonsurgical methods will further reduce pocketing, for most of these patients, surgical pocket reduction is needed. This chapter will describe why pocketing can persist after quality nonsurgical treatment, and how to prepare a treatment plan and perform these surgeries. The same techniques are also used for crown-lengthening surgery, which is used to prevent complications from restorations impinging on supracrestal attached tissues.

Keywords: pocket reduction, surgical treatment, crown lengthening

6.1 Learning Objectives

- Recognize indications for pocket-reduction surgery.
- Develop a surgical treatment plan for reducing periodontal pockets.
- Describe surgical pocket-reduction techniques.
- Identify when crown-lengthening procedures are needed.

6.2 Case

A 63-year old South Asian male presented to us asking for a "tooth cleaning" since he has not received dental care for about 10 years. He had a history of hypertension, but that abated with diet change and relaxation techniques, and a history of type 2 diabetes mellitus, which is controlled with 5-mg Glucotrol XL (Glipizide) once daily. He reported that he is not required by his physician to measure his glucose at home, but gets it tested regularly through his physician's office. He also brought in a printout showing the values measured last month: serum glucose 102 mg/dL; HbA1c 6.2%.

Although he had not seen a dentist for many years, he does not have any specific tooth-related complaint other than "feeling the need for a cleaning." He brushes his teeth twice a day with a hard brush and flosses twice a day. When asked about the tooth wear and suspected parafunctional habit, he replied that his previous dentist thought he grinds his teeth at night.

Extraoral exam findings revealed no abnormal findings for the facial skin, lymph nodes, thyroid gland, cranial nerves, salivary glands, masticatory muscles, and temporomandibular joint other than reduced hearing on the left side. Intraorally, no mucosal pathology was apparent other than periodontal disease and a small, 2-mm diameter white round nodule at the height of the occlusal plane on the left lateral border of the tongue. Teeth had worn occlusal surfaces and small abfraction lesions, but were otherwise in good repair.

Blood pressure was 124/83 mm Hg and pulse 70/min.

Initial findings in the periodontal chart were as follows (see ▶Fig. 6.1 for clinical presentation and ▶Fig. 6.2 for radiographs).

Maxilla facial		1	2	3	4	5	6	7	8	9	10	11	12	13	14	15	16
	PD	325		434	323	323	313	323	322			223	323	323	983		
	BOP								1			1			11		
	CAL	5		7	5	5	5	5	8			4	4	4	10		
	GR			333	121	232	122	233	554			211	101	101	112		
	MGJ	554		334	434	354	555	555	444			444	444	533	222		
	Furc			1													
	PLQ	0	0	0	0	0	0	0	0			0	0	0	0		
Maxilla lingual	PD	449		446	424	624	433	333	333			223	323	324	635		
	BOP	11				1						1	1		111		
	CAL	9		8	4	6	4	5	8			4	5	5	9		
	GR			342	12	21		112	354			22	22	21	264		
	Furc			2											2 1		
	Mobil			3					1						3		
	PLQ	1		1	1	1	1	1	1			1	1	1	1		
Mandible lingual		32	31	30	29	28	27	26	25	24	23	22	21	20	19	18	17
	PD	746	437	435	323	322	222	222	222	222	223	322	323	424	667	663	
	BOP		1												1		
	CAL	7	7	5	3	3	3	5	5	5	5	3	4	4	8	8	
	GR			11			1	123	233	232	232		1		121	122	
	MGJ	1	667	656	655	444	333	333	433	344	433	444	555	656	666	667	
	Furc			1											1		
	PLQ	2	3	3		1	1	1	1	1	1				1	1	

Mandible facial															
PD	524	426	425	323	323	323	342	322	223	332	233	323	323	626	657
BOP		1												1	11
CAL	5	7	6	4	3	3	5	5	5	6	3	4	3	6	7
GR		241	121	11	1	1	11	222	222	232	1	2		1	21
MGJ	334	324	324	444	434	435	444	444	444	444	444	433	545	545	444
Furc		1												1	
Mobil							1	1	1						1
PLQ	2										1				111

Abbreviations: BOP, bleeding on probing (1), suppuration (2); CAL, clinical attachment level; Furc, furcation involvement (Glickman class); GR, gingival recession; MGJ, position of mucogingival junction from margin; Mobil, tooth mobility (Miller grade); PD, probing depths; PLQ, plaque level (0 = none, 5 = heavy).

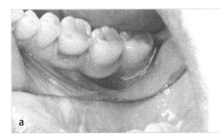
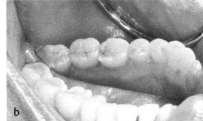

Fig. 6.1 (a, b) Initial presentation of lower right quadrant representative of all mandibular teeth.

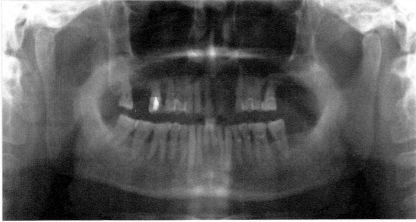
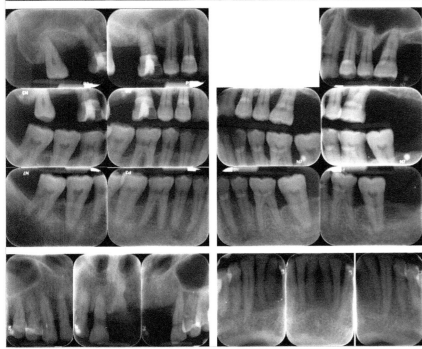

Fig. 6.2 Radiographs taken as part of initial exam.

Teeth nos. 1, 3, and 14 were considered hopeless and removed soon after the initial exam. The patient received scaling and root planing (SRP) in all quadrants and was instructed to use a gentle brushing technique using a soft brush. In addition, the patient was instructed on how to use interproximal brushes. This resulted in some pocket reduction, but there were still residual deep pockets between mandibular molars.

Pocket depths after SRP are as follows:

Facial		1	2	3	4	5	6	7	8	9	10	11	12	13	14	15	16
	PD				223	323	323	323	322			223	322	333			
	BOP				1	1											
Lingual	PD				223	523	322	322	322			222	323	322			
	BOP													1			
Lingual		32	31	30	29	28	27	26	25	24	23	22	21	20	19	18	17
	PD	733	435	325	323	222	332	222	222	212	122	213	324	323	647	532	
	BOP																
Facial	PD	1	11	1			1		1	1					1	11	
	BOP	423	426	324	323	322	323	342	222	223	422	223	323	314	627	542	

Partial osseous resective surgery, with bone grafting of the deeper bone defects, was performed for the mandibular quadrants, and the patient seen every 3 to 4 months for periodontal maintenance. This surgical treatment reduced pocketing to low levels, and they were maintained at that level 2 years after the surgery by periodic periodontal maintenance.

Pocket depths 2 years after surgery are as follows:

Facial		1	2	3	4	5	6	7	8	9	10	11	12	13	14	15	16
	PD				223	323	323	323	323			223	323	323			
	BOP				1												
Lingual	PD				323	323	332	323	323			334	433	423			
	BOP				111	111	111	1 1									
Lingual		32	31	30	29	28	27	26	25	24	23	22	21	20	19	18	17
	PD	545	434	424	323	323	322	222	222	422	232	323	323	333	434	444	
	BOP	1	1	1	1		1	1	1 1						1		
Facial	PD			1	1		1	1	1							111	
	BOP	324	334	424	423	323	323	323	323	323	323	323	323	323	423	433	

What can be learned from this case?

This case illustrates that successful pocket reduction may require both nonsurgical and surgical treatments. The case benefited from a patient who is reasonably healthy and is committed to improving his health as shown by his effective, although abrasive oral hygiene technique, apparent compliance with medical treatment, and his apparent ability to reduce his blood pressure with lifestyle changes. Unlike Chapter 5 case, this patient has more bony irregularities and these likely explain the need for surgery in this case. The bony defects probably harbor deep subgingival plaque and calculus accretions on the root surfaces adjacent to these defects, and the shape of the bone defect with surrounding tissue made it impossible to remove all deposits. When these were exposed and removed surgically, this allowed proper healing and reduced pocket depths. Patients with low probing depths can be predictably maintained, and this is the reason for the observed periodontal stability.

6.3 Recognize Indications for Pocket-reduction Surgery

Generally, the indications for pocket-reduction surgery are residual deep pockets after high-quality nonsurgical periodontal treatment in a compliant patient.

6.3.1 Risks Associated with Residual Deep Pocketing

Residual deep pocketing poses the following risks:
- Increased risk of further attachment loss and eventual tooth loss.
- Continues active disease and possible systemic risks of periodontal disease.
- Deep pocketing and gingival bleeding may cause inaccurate impressions, resulting in poor restorations and premature treatment failure.
- Increased risk of periodontal abscesses and associated pain.
- Increased risk of peri-implant disease.
- Less predictable orthodontic tooth movement and risk of tooth loss during therapy.
- Longer and more difficult periodontal maintenance, which also may not be effective.

Consequently, deep pocketing needs to be eliminated prior to orthodontics and complex restorative procedures such as implant therapy, crown fabrication, and fixed and removable partial denture therapy.

6.3.2 Causes of Residual Deep Pocketing

Residual deep pocketing is usually caused by residual subgingival plaque or calculus left after nonsurgical therapy. Besides operator error or lack of experience, the following factors may prevent complete calculus removal:

- *Deep pockets*: In pockets deeper than 5 mm, complete calculus removal is unlikely.
- *Pocket anatomy*: Some pockets have curved anatomy, and pocket gingiva prevents visualization of calculus and instrumentation access.
- *Bone defects*: Narrow entrances to bone defects covered with pocket tissue prevent access.
- *Furcation entrances*: For molars, this is the typical cause of residual pockets.
- Root surface abnormalities such as developmental grooves, enamel projections, ridges, root concavities, and enamel pearls are associated with residual pockets. Failing to remove these abnormalities is a common reason for residual pockets after periodontal surgery. Common sites are as follows:
  - Mid-lingual at **palatogingival grooves** at maxillary lateral incisors.
  - Deep mesial root concavities on maxillary 1st premolars.
  - **Cervical enamel projections** at furcation entrances.
  - **Enamel pearls** near furcation entrances of 2nd and 3rd maxillary molars.

Residual pocketing may also be caused by persistent inflammation caused by caries, defective restorations, **biologic width invasion**, occlusal trauma, and endodontic infections.

6.3.3 General Indications for Pocket-reduction Surgery

Typically, the need for periodontal surgery is determined at the periodontal reevaluation appointment about 1 to 2 months after the last round of SRP and before orthodontics and complex restorative treatment, such as crown and bridge, partial dentures, and implant therapy are initiated. If SRP have been completed, but the removal of teeth, caries control, and management of occlusion, endodontic infections, and oral pathology are still in progress, the dentition should be maintained with frequent periodontal maintenance and oral hygiene instruction until initial therapy is complete.

Pocket-reduction surgery is indicated if:
- The patient is interested and able to maintain his or her teeth as evidenced by low plaque levels.
- Initial therapy is complete.
- Residual pocketing equals or exceeds 5 mm (The cutoff or "critical probing depth" may vary between dentists depending on treatment philosophy).

6.3.4 Pocket-reduction and Correction of Biologic Width Issues

A special case of pocketing happens when a restoration invades biologic width, which then produces persistent inflammation, which leads to persistent pocketing around the offensive restoration. If this is not corrected, it leads to attachment and bone loss, which then eventually restores the biologic width, but at the cost of uncontrolled recession and potential transition to locally enhanced chronic periodontitis.

Correction of biologic width invasion can be achieved with crown-lengthening techniques that are very similar to surgery techniques used for pocket-reduction surgery. Consequently,

the end of this chapter will describe indications and the procedure for clinical crown lengthening.

6.3.5 Medical Contraindications

Periodontal surgery is never indicated in patients with unresolved life-threatening medical conditions such as recent (less than 6 months ago) myocardial infarct or stroke, and any condition that requires urgent medical treatment.

Periodontal surgery can be performed on most patients with chronic medical conditions including cancer history, HIV, epilepsy, diabetes, liver cirrhosis, kidney disease, bleeding disorders, asthma, and stable cardiovascular conditions. In those cases, the patient's physician needs to be consulted to check on the current state of the medical condition, and a pre- and postoperative medical management plan should be developed in collaboration with the physician. For consent purposes, a detailed discussion of surgical risks and management steps needs to take place prior to the surgery and documented in the chart.

Neurologic and psychologic conditions that impair the ability to give consent, such as dementia, schizophrenia, and bipolar disorders, require special care. Beyond having appropriate discussions with the patient, risks, benefits, postoperative care, need for sedation and alternatives should be discussed with the patient's caregiver or legal guardian. The patient should be involved in the decision process as much as feasible, and the informed consent process should be carefully documented. The same process should also be used for the rare circumstance when periodontal surgery is considered for a minor.

For patients with a history of bisphosphonate use or radiation therapy in the head and neck region, the low risk of osteonecrosis of the jaw needs to be discussed prior to surgery. Currently, the risk for periodontal surgery is unknown, but is likely similar to the risk from extractions (about 1 to 90 per 100,000 patient-years) for patients on oral bisphosphonates. For informed consent purposes, the discussion needs to describe signs and symptoms of osteonecrosis, and how it is treated.

6.3.6 Dental Contraindications

Periodontal surgery is never indicated for teeth with severe mobility caused by near complete loss of bone as surgical exposure would cause immediate tooth loss.

Generally, pocket-reduction surgery is not performed for 3rd molars because of poor access, and usually the treatment of choice is removal either prior to surgery or during periodontal surgery. Similarly, extraction is the treatment of choice for teeth that will not have an opposing tooth or prosthesis.

6.3.7 Consent Issues

Informed consent must be obtained prior to periodontal surgery, and if a patient is unable to give consent it precludes surgery. Informed consent requires discussion of the benefits, surgical risks, surgical procedure, what to expect after surgery, alternatives, and materials used during the surgery. Chart notes should indicate that this discussion took place, and a form signed by the patient can provide evidence of this discussion.

Typically, benefits of pocket-reduction surgery include increased long-term survival of teeth and restorations including implants, along with better oral health.

Risks of periodontal surgery include typical surgery risks such as postoperative bleeding, pain, infection, and delayed healing. Generally, pocket-reduction surgery exchanges deep pocketing for increased recession, which causes longer-appearing teeth, loss of gum tissue between teeth, and tooth sensitivity that may take several months to resolve. Pocket-reduction surgery may also cause temporary tooth mobility while the tissue heals, especially for teeth with poor crown-to-root ratios.

Alternatives to periodontal surgery always should be discussed during treatment planning. Generally, the alternatives are either periodontal maintenance, which may not eliminate periodontal disease, or extractions of diseased teeth, which require expensive tooth replacement such as implants or dentures.

6.3.8 When to Refer

Generally, the decision to refer to or treat depends on many factors such as practice policies, comfort level and skill with surgical procedures, availability of surgical equipment, economic feasibility, chair time considerations, patient preference and access to a periodontist, and also the extent and type of surgery that is needed. While there are published recommendations on what patient may benefit from treatment by a periodontist, the following characteristics suggest a case suitable for general practice:
- Good overall health.
- Tolerant of long appointment.
- Low esthetic demand (surgery outside of anterior maxilla).
- Easy access and normal mouth opening.
- Isolated pocketing (1 to 2 teeth per quadrant).
- Moderately deep residual pockets (4 to 6 mm).
- Mild bone loss with at most minor bone defects.
- Provider is capable of elevating a mucoperiosteal flap, root planing, and suturing for the simplest type of pocket reduction surgery. For more complex surgeries, the dentist needs to be able to:
  - Create normal physiologic bone contours with surgical instruments.
  - Manipulate bone graft materials.
  - Apply membrane materials over bony defects.
  - Perform more complex sutures for best clinical results.

6.4 Develop a Surgical Treatment Plan for Reducing Periodontal Pockets

Surgical treatment planning has benefits from a generalist and specialist perspective. As generalist it is useful to predict procedures a specialist may use since it allows explaining likely treatments to patients which then improves later treatment acceptance and compliance. If planning to perform the surgery, proper treatment planning improves the likelihood of insurance reimbursement and enables preparation for the surgery including having the proper materials and instruments ready for surgery.

6.4.1 Pocket Types—Suprabony and Infrabony

When planning pocket-reduction surgery, the first decision that needs to be made is whether bone removal is required. This is mostly determined by assessing if the residual pockets are **suprabony** or **infrabony** through comparing radiographic appearance with clinical measurements:
- *Suprabony pockets*: Base of pocket is coronal the alveolar crest. Clinically, there will be a moderately deep pocket (4 to 5 mm usually[1]), but radiographic distinct crestal bone will be parallel to the cementoenamel junction (CEJ) without local defects. Clinical attachment level will be smaller than the distance between the CEJ and the coronal-most tip of crestal bone.
  - **Pseudopockets** are a subtype of suprabony pockets characterized by no attachment loss (CAL = 0). Radiographically, a thick dark gray soft tissue shadow may be present, and clinically, the adjacent gingiva will appear thick. Typically, these are associated with conditions causing gingival overgrowth, the retromolar pad, and maxillary tuberosity.
- *Infrabony pockets*: Base of pocket is apical to the alveolar crest. Deep probing depths will be associated with radiographic changes at the alveolar crest ranging from a fading crestal bone to funnel-shaped bone defects or appearance several distinct bone levels. In areas of narrow interproximal bone, there also may be an isolated sudden drop in bone level.

6.4.2 Treatment of Suprabony Pockets

Suprabony pockets are most likely associated with residual subgingival calculus but may also be associated with excess gingival tissue, and pocket reduction usually does not require bone removal. The choice of one pocket-reduction surgery technique over another depends on what other abnormal tissue characteristics need to be corrected (► Table 6.1).

Gingivectomy

If the goal is to simply remove excess gingiva, gingivectomy is a suitable surgery. This requires:

Table 6.1 Treatment planning for suprabony pockets

Surgical problem				Treatment
Suprabony pocket	Lack of keratinized gingiva	Excess distal/mesial tissue next to edentulous site	Excess gingival thickness	
✓	P	P	P	Gingival flap
✓	✓	P	P	Apical positioned flap
✓	N/A	✓	✓	Distal wedge
✓	✗	P	✓	Gingivectomy

Abbreviations: ✓ addresses problem; ✗, procedure should not be used if this problem is present; N/A, procedure is not affected by this problem; P, procedure possibly solves this problem if creatively applied.

- Gingiva that appears excessively thick, fibrous, and enlarged as around pseudopockets.
- The tooth surface within the pocket feels clean with a fine calculus explorer.

Gingival Flap Surgery/Surgical Debridement

If the goal is to remove residual calculus in a suprabony pocket, the procedure of choice is usually some variation of gingival flap surgery. For best clinical results, this requires:
- Suprabony pockets—the procedure by itself does not address bone defects.
- Calculus can be detected as "rough" tooth surface within the pocket.

Gingival flap surgery can be used as alternative to:
- Gingivectomy if the tissue is excessively bulky.
- Osseous surgery for less gingival recession at the expense of less pocket reduction.

Gingival flap surgery can serve as initial procedure for regenerative surgery. For treatment planning and billing, gingival flap surgery is typically charged by quadrant and the size of the flap. For example, the appropriate ADA CDT code for a single pocket is D4241, and for multiple pockets in a quadrant, D4240.

While the gingival flap procedure is suitable for most suprabony pockets, specialized procedures exist.

Distal Wedge Procedure

For the treatment of a single suprabony pocket at a tooth surface facing an edentulous space, the distal wedge procedure can be used. Typically, this is the distal surface of a 2nd molar facing an extraction scar from the removal of 3rd molars, or excessively thick soft tissue on the retromolar pad or maxillary tuberosity.

Apically Positioned Flap

If an area with suprabony pockets also displays minimal keratinized gingiva, the apical positioned flap is a variant of a gingival flap that conserves keratinized tissue. A variant of the apical positioned flap can be used to increase keratinized tissue (see Chapter 8).

6.4.3 Treatment of Infrabony Pockets

Even though gingival flap surgery can produce pocket depth reduction in infrabony pockets, resective surgery or regenerative techniques are usually more effective. Whether to use resective or regenerative techniques depends on the depth of bone defects present at the affected sites. The type and location of bone defects along with the surgeon's preference determines which regenerative procedure should be chosen for a particular site.

6.4.4 Bone Defect Types

Depth and type of bone defect can be assessed by viewing digital radiographs of the same area (i.e., bitewing and molar/premolar periapical radiographs) with varying brightness and contrast settings (see Chapter 2, for radiographic evaluation). The depth of bone defects can be classified as:
- *Shallow*: About 1 to 2 mm in apical extent; not suitable for regeneration as regeneration is unlikely.

- *Deep*: Greater than 2 mm in apical extent; a regenerative approach may be beneficial.
- *Wide*: Greater than 1 mm in mesial/distal extent; suitable for bone grafting.
- *Narrow*: Less than 1 mm in mesial/distal extent; may need surgical widening for access.

Bone defect types can be classified as follows:
- *3-wall bone defects*: Well-defined pyramid shaped bone defects usually found at 2nd mandibular molars. With increasing brightness on radiographs, the mesial/distal wall appears first, followed by the faint coronal border of the facial and lingual walls.
- *2-wall bone defects*: These are the most common types of defect.
  - Interproximal craters have a facial and lingual wall and are most commonly found between molars. Increasing brightness reveals first the apical floor of the defect, followed by the faint lines of buccal and lingual walls on all radiographs.
  - Compound 2 to 3 wall defects are funnel-shaped defects surrounding an interproximal furcation entrance with a high buccal wall, an intermediate interproximal wall and a very low (if existing) palatal wall. Radiographically, these appear as diffuse defects.
- *1-wall bone defects*: Typically, a well-defined sloping mesial/distal wall between teeth with narrow bucco-lingual interproximal bone such as premolars and anterior teeth.
  - Ramp-like defects are 1-wall defects found at teeth tipped toward an edentulous space.
- *0-wall bone defects*: An area of enhanced bone loss, found usually at mandibular incisors and premolars. Radiographically, these defects are clearly identifiable as distinct localized drop of the alveolar crest, and a distinct cutoff at the border of the alveolar crest.
- *Dehiscence*: An area of facial/lingual bone loss exposing part of the cervical 1/2 of a root, and often associated with malposition of the tooth outside of the arch. Radiographically, these are difficult to detect, and may be suspected in areas localized recession or thin tissue.
- *Fenestration*: A rare type of window-like bone defect exposing part of tooth root, usually near the apex of canines or first premolars. Radiographically, these are practically undetectable on conventional radiographs, and usually discovered during surgery.
- Wide, flat interproximal bone can appear as a 2-wall defect, radiographically. Typically, the bitewing will show a very dense, bright interproximal cortex while the periapical radiograph will show two distinct lines mimicking a 2-wall defect. Clinically, there usually is no pocketing.
- *Pointed interproximal bone*: Mimics compound 2 to 3 wall defects as faded crestal bone, but lacks associated pocketing. Typically, this is seen interproximally between maxillary incisors.

6.4.5 Shallow Infrabony Pockets—Osseous Surgery

Even though regenerative techniques can be used for shallow bone defects, osseous surgery, which removes these defects, leads to more predictable pocket reduction. It also produces the greatest amount of recession of all pocket-reduction surgeries

and therefore should not be used for the anterior maxilla. Osseous surgery is most suitable for bone defects that have the following characteristics:
- Shallow.
- Have few walls:
  o 1-wall and 0-wall defects, including ramp-like defects.
  o Irregular bone level caused by bony ledges and spikes.

For treatment planning and billing, osseous surgery is typically charged by quadrant and the size of the flap. For example, the ADA CDT code for a single infrabony pocket is "D4261 Osseous surgery, 1 to 3 teeth" for the quadrant, and "D4260" for multiple pockets in a quadrant.

6.4.6 Deep Infrabony Pockets—Regenerative Techniques

If the bone defects are more than 2-mm deep, regenerative techniques may be useful since osseous surgery would require excessive bone removal.[1] All regenerative techniques require for treatment planning an access surgery, either a gingival flap surgery or osseous surgery, for the quadrant, and the regenerative technique(s) chosen for each site.

Any Type of Defect—Biologics

Biologics are any materials that aid the regeneration of lost tissues. The most commonly used material is enamel matrix derivative (Emdogain), which is a protein mixture derived of porcine tooth buds and said to stimulate regeneration through simulating the process of root development. It can be easily applied to any site, but the decision to use it hinges on the preference of the surgeon and if the predictable, but relatively small gain in clinical improvement is worth the added expense.

Other materials are recombinant platelet derived growth factor (rhPDGF-BB, commercially available as GEM21), Fibroblast growth factor-2 (FGF-2, in development, may be eventually distributed by Sunstar),[2,3] and autogenous platelet concentrates obtained by a blood draw from a patient's own peripheral blood.[4] Regardless of material, it is typically planned and charged for each site (i.e., using CDT code D4265) in addition to the access surgery and other regenerative techniques.

Wide 2- or 3-wall Defects—Bone Grafting

Bone grafts are solid or semisolid materials applied into bone defects that stimulate regrowth of lost hard tissue. Many bone grafting materials are available and supported by scientific evidence, and grafting generally reduces defects to a half or a third of the original size. Freeze-dried bone allograft (FDBA) is the preferred material when available. Xenograft or alloplast can be used alternatively, if FDBA use is not feasible or if the patient has a documented allergy against gentamycin or bacitracin, which is a preservative in most FDBA grafts. FDBA has the following advantages:
- Resorbs at a slower rate than demineralized bone graft for more predictable regeneration.
- Replaced by soft and hard tissue unlike xenograft (i.e., bone derived from cows or other nonhuman animals) or some alloplasts (i.e., synthetic materials such as solid hydroxyapatite).

- Does not require a second bone harvesting surgery unlike autograft (i.e., bone from patient or genetically identical twin).

Bone grafting is most predictable for bone defects with the following characteristics:
- Wide enough to accept bone particles (>1 mm).
- Has sufficient walls to retain the graft material such as:
  o 3-wall defects.
  o Interproximal craters.
  o 2- and 3-wall defects associated with interproximal furcation defects.

Since deep bone defects are typically associated also with irregular bone contours and bone ledges, osseous surgery should be planned in addition to bone grafting. Bone grafting is typically charged per site, and there is an ADA CDT code for the first site (D4263) and for any additional sites (D4264).

Narrow Defects with Good Surgical Access—Guided Tissue Regeneration

In guided tissue regeneration, a membrane is draped over a bone defect to allow preferential growth of bone and periodontal ligament cells into the defect while keeping epithelial cells out. Guided tissue regeneration can reduce deep defects by about 3 mm in depth on average. In order for this to work, the defect has to be well-defined and well accessible surgically so that a membrane can be adapted tightly around a tooth. Typically, guided tissue regeneration by itself is most predictable for:
- Narrow defects (as long as the exposed root surface is completely decontaminated).
- *Well-defined bone defects with good surgical access.*
  o 3-wall defects not associated with interproximal furcation entrances.
  o Interproximal craters in the mandible.
  o Bone defects associated with buccal furcation entrances.

Even though nonresorbable membranes can be used for guided tissue regeneration, resorbable membranes designed for periodontal regenerative surgery are the material of choice since they do not require a 2nd re-entry surgery and have fewer complications. Typically, guided tissue regeneration is planned and charged for each tooth (i.e., CDT code D4266) in addition to an access surgery such as a gingival flap or osseous surgery for the quadrant.

Other Defects—Combination of Regenerative Techniques

There is no clear-cut evidence proving clinical superiority of one regenerative technique over others, and combining various regenerative techniques may not be superior to a single technique. However, periodontal surgeons will often combine bone grafting and guided tissue regeneration along with possible biologics for the regeneration of bony defects that are difficult to regenerate such as:
- Very large bone defects (i.e., residual defects associated with 3rd molar extraction sites).
- Deep 1-wall and 0-wall defects, although regeneration is highly unpredictable.
- Dehiscences and fenestrations.
- Deep and wide bone defects associated with furcation entrances.

For these circumstances, an access surgery is chosen (osseous surgery or gingival flap) along with a combination of bone grafting, guided tissue regeneration, or biologics for each site.

A summary of surgical treatment planning for residual pocket is given in ▶ Table 6.2.

6.4.7 Specific Consent Issues

Part of the treatment planning process is discussion of the risks and limitations of the planned surgery along with an easily understood description of the surgery, benefits, and alternative treatments. While the generic discussion can be done prior to treatment planning to gauge patient interest in surgical periodontal therapy, there are some specific discussions that need to take place depending on the planned surgery:
* *Materials used for bone grafts, membranes, and biologics*: Patients need to know where any regenerative materials come from, and should be given a chance to voice concerns and discuss alternatives if a material is objectionable to a patient (i.e., bovine bone; Emdogain and some membranes derived from porcine tissue; allograft materials from organ donors).
* Chance for incomplete pocket resolution or no pocket reduction with regenerative techniques.
* Issues that may arise with regenerative materials, i.e., painful exposure of nonresorbable membrane; emergence of bone graft particles; delayed healing; more than usual postoperative swelling; higher postoperative infection risk.

6.4.8 Postoperative Care

Postoperative care begins by providing preventive medications and setting reasonable expectations for wound healing prior to surgery.

In order to reduce postoperative pain, patients should take an analgesic 1 hour before the surgery:
* For most patients, 400-mg Ibuprofen 1 hour prior to surgery and taken every 4 hours as needed for up to 5 days after the surgery is effective along with intermittent ice application. Ibuprofen can also be taken in 600 mg doses every 6 hours, or 800 mg every 8 hours depending on patient preference.
* If Ibuprofen is not feasible, alternatives are 325-mg Aspirin or 325-mg Acetaminophen 1 hour prior to surgery and taken every 4 hours as need along with intermittent ice application.

Even though there is no consistent evidence that it prevents postoperative instructions, there may be a benefit in having a patient take antibiotics starting 1 hour prior to surgery whenever bone graft or membrane materials are used.

Patient postoperative instructions should include the following (see ▶ Video 1.1):
* Leave the surgery area alone for 24 hours by not brushing, rinsing, spitting, or using a straw.
* In case of bleeding, apply pressure with wet gauze or wet black tea bags for 10 to 15 minutes on any bleeding area.
* Some pain is normal, and usually worst the night after the surgery. It should diminish quickly after that and typically is gone by the end of the week. Increasing pain usually indicates a postoperative infection, which needs treatment with an antibiotic (i.e., 300-mg Clindamycin every 6 hours). Longer-lasting pain is caused by delayed healing, and will slowly resolve.
* Teeth may be sensitive or feel slightly loose for the first few months, and this will gradually resolve on its own. Persistent tooth sensitivity can be treated with the application of potassium oxalate gels (i.e., Thermatrol) or other desensitizing agents (i.e., Gluma).
* Healthy tissue appearance usually is achieved few weeks after the surgery, and dental treatments can usually be done after 6 weeks. Pocket reduction can be checked after 3 months and the definite effect on pocket reduction may take up to 2 years to develop.
* Normal oral hygiene should not be delayed for more than 1 week, and it is important to continue periodontal maintenance starting 6 weeks after surgery and continuing every 3 months for best long-term success.

Table 6.2 A treatment planning guide for surgical pocket reduction

Site	Pocket type	Defect depth	Defect width	Defect type	Surgery
Anterior maxilla	Pseudopocket				Gingivectomy
	Suprabony				Gingival flap*
	Infrabony	Shallow			Gingival flap*
		Deep			Gingival flap* + biologic or bone graft
Other sites	Suprabony				Gingival flap
	Infrabony	Shallow			Osseous surgery
		Deep	Narrow	3-wall	Osseous surgery + GTR†
				Craters (mandible)	
				Buccal/lingual furcation	
			Wide	3-wall	Osseous surgery + bone graft†
				2- and 3-wall	
				Craters	
				All other types (0, 1-wall; very large defects >3 mm; dehiscence; fenestration)	Osseous surgery + GTR and bone graft†

* Minimally invasive or uses papilla preservation technique; † and optional application of biologics.
To use this table, read from left to right. GTR, bone graft and biologics are typically planned by site, whereas osseous surgery and gingival flap are treatments planned by quadrant.

6.5 Describe Surgical Pocket-reduction Techniques

6.5.1 Instrumentation

Pocket-reduction surgery can be done with a typical infection control setup for dental procedures and a basic periodontal surgery setup that includes:
- Local anesthesia instruments and supplies.
- Mirror and periodontal probe.
- Scalpel and blade (i.e., no. 15c blade for most incisions, 12 and 12d blades for wedge and some split thickness incisions).
- Periodontal knives for removal of tissue tags (i.e., ½ Orban knife for interproximal tissue; 15/16 Kirkland knife for wedge incisions and gingivectomies).
- Periosteal elevators (i.e., Molt-9 and Prichard).
- SRP instruments (i.e., 1/2, 7/8, 11/12, 13/14, sickle scaler, ultrasonic tips, and ultrasonic unit).
- A surgical handpiece.
- Supplies for sterile irrigation (i.e., Monojet syringes filled with sterile saline, steel bowl filled with sterile saline for refills, steel bowl filled with sterile saline for storing bloodied burs).
- Surgical burs for hard tissue removal (i.e., round diamonds nos. 4 to 8, end-cutting diamond for most bone removal; carbide burs (nos. 4 to 8) for removal of exostoses, cylindrical or tapered diamond burs if needed for tooth preparation).
- Tissue forceps.
- Hemostat.
- Suturing supplies (i.e., "4-0" for posterior areas and "5-0" sutures for anterior areas and vertical releases; reverse cutting, half-circle, or 3/8 circle needle), needle holder (i.e., Castroviejo), and suture scissors.
- Sterile 2 × 2 gauze.
- Surgical suction tip.
- *Good to have, but not required*: Bone graft syringe; Rhodes back action chisel (minor bone harvesting); and Hirschfeld files (smoothening of bone).

As with most periodontal surgery, this technique can be accomplished using conventional local anesthesia using 2% lidocaine and 1:100,000 epinephrine. Local infiltration about 5 mm from the anticipated flap edge, with 2% lidocaine and 1:50,000 epinephrine, is useful to produce a drier surgical field. Local infiltration, with 0.5% bupivacaine and 1:100,000 epinephrine (i.e., Marcaine), at the end of surgery may help reduce postoperative pain along with preoperative analgesics.

6.5.2 Flap Design

Typically, all pocket-reduction surgeries create a full thickness or mucoperiosteal flap that folds back the entire gingiva including epithelium, loose connective tissue, and periosteum to expose alveolar bone.

Terminology

For designing the flap, some terminology is useful to describe incision and flap types ▶ Fig. 6.3):
- *Full thickness flap or mucoperiosteal flap*: An effort is made to push the scalpel blade all the way to the hard alveolar bone and kept in contact with it at all times. The gingiva and mucosa can then be pushed off the bone with a blunt instrument.

- *Split thickness flap*: The gingiva is sharply dissected with a scalpel, leaving a layer of connective tissue and periosteum attached to the underlying bone.
- *Envelope flap*: Only incises the gingiva next to the teeth from distal to mesial, and when opened, reveals the teeth and surrounding bone in a pouch or envelope-like tissue opening.
- *Straight incision*: The scalpel blade cuts perpendicular through the gingiva.
- *Externally beveled incision*: An oblique cut that removes mostly epithelium.
- *Internally beveled incision*: An oblique cut that undermines the epithelium.
- *Linear incision*: A cut that follows a straight line from one point to another.
- *Scalloped incision*: A cut that follows the buccal/lingual contours of adjacent teeth.
- *Intrasulcular incision*: The incision is made as close as possible to involved teeth.
- *Step-back incision*: The incision is made parallel to buccal/lingual tooth surfaces at some distance.
- *Vertical releases*: Straight, linear, full thickness incisions from the flap edges toward the vestibule. This should be done with a slight slant away from the body of the flap, and the length of the release needs to be less than half of the flap height from the base of the flap.
- *Triangular flap*: An envelope flap with an added vertical release at either mesial or distal end.
- *Rectangular flap*: An envelope flap with vertical releases at both mesial and distal ends.

Envelope Flap Design Principles

Generally, the flap design for pocket reduction can be done as follows:
- Posterior teeth and anterior mandible:
  - *Single pocket*: Envelope flap for sextant in which pocket occurs.
  - *Multiple pockets*: Triangular flap with vertical release at distobuccal line angle of canine.
  - The envelope incision part is step-back wherever there is a pocket, otherwise the incision is intrasulcular.
- Anterior maxilla:
  - *Single pocket*: Small envelope flap with papilla preservation incision (see below).
  - *Multiple pockets*: Rectangular flap with vertical releases at distobuccal line angle of both canines and papilla preservation incisions.

The flap design is modified under the following conditions:
- *Edentulous area*: The incision is made on the center of the ridge.
- *Lack of keratinized gingiva*: No step-back incision even if there is pocketing.
- *Excessively thick gingiva*: Increase step-back distance from tooth to remove more tissue.
- *Excessive distal/mesial tissue adjacent to edentulous site*: Distal wedge incision design.

Conventional Incision and Flap Elevation

After good local anesthesia has been obtained, typical incision and flap elevation are done as follows (▶ Video 6.1):
- Plan the incision:

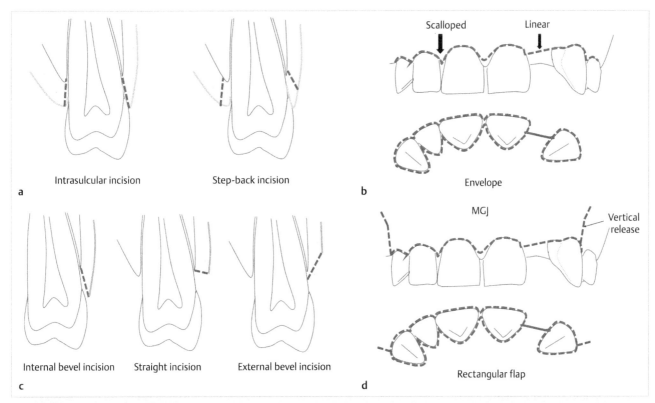

Fig. 6.3 Incision types and basic flap designs. (**a**) Intrasulcular incision inside the sulcus as close as possible to the tooth versus step-back incision aiming for the alveolar crest at some distance from the tooth as determined by pocket depth. (**b**) Envelope flap with scalloped incisions and linear incision for edentulous area. (**c**) Internal bevel incisions undermine the flap edge, straight incisions leave a blunt tissue edge, and external bevel incisions remove epithelium and excess connective tissue. (**d**) A rectangular flap is an envelope flap (**b**) with added vertical releasing full thickness incisions at the ends of the envelope. Note that the height of the flap is less than half of the height of the vertical releases, and that the base of the flap is wider than the tip of the flap.

○ Visualize and remember vital structures in the area (i.e., mental foramen).

○ In areas lacking keratinized tissue, there is no step-back.

○ Determine the number and position of vertical releases as described before. Vertical releases should never be made over the mental foramen or lingual surfaces.

○ Check pocket depths and measure palatal tissue thickness by pushing a periodontal probe through the tissue until bone is encountered. Determine step-back incision as follows (▶Table 6.3).

○ If there is pocketing on a distal/mesial surface facing and edentulous area, plan for a wedge incision.

• *Perform the envelope portion of the flap from distal to mesial*: Aim the blade parallel to the tooth at the predetermined step-back distance, and begin the incision by pushing the blade (i.e., no. 15c) all the way through the tissue contacting bone.

• Move the blade in a smooth motion and firmly in contact with bone mesially, either intrasulcularly or with step-back in areas of pocketing and keratinized gingiva.

• Perform wedge incisions where needed (see below).

• If needed, make any vertical releases as determined before by making a straight, vertical incision to the bone from the gingival margin to the mucogingival junction at the distobuccal of the canine(s). Once the incision reaches the mucogingival junction, slightly slant the incision to broaden the flap base and extend it about halfway to the floor of the vestibule.

• Elevate the flap edges by first using a twisting motion with the scalpel blade full inserted into the incision line at the flap edges and papilla tips, and then elevate the entire flap

off the bone with progressively larger-sized periosteal elevators (see ▶Fig. 6.4, for elevation steps). This should yield a clean, lightly yellow bone surface with few if any red tissue tags attached. Elevate the tissue just past the mucogingival junction where it exists, or about halfway toward the floor of the palate. Be mindful of vital structures such as the mental foramen.

• Remove the interproximal papilla remnant by detaching it from the tooth and alveolar crest with a scalpel or Orban knives inserted on the mesial, distal, and apical side of the soft tissue remnant. Dislodge and remove each interproximal tissue remnant with a sharp scaler or curette.

Basic periodontal flap surgery, also known as surgical debridement, consists of elevating a full thickness flap, cleaning the root surfaces, and suturing the tissues back together closely adapted to the underlying bone. This is usually effective for areas with residual 4 to 6 mm supragingival pockets after nonsurgical SRP.

Variations

There are several useful variations on flap design.

Modified Widman Flap

This technique is useful for minimally deep pocketing (4 to 5 mm) around anterior teeth where minimal recession is sought. Compared to a conventional flap, step-back is minimal (0.5 to 1 mm) and there is just enough reflection of the flap to allow visualization of the root surface.

Table 6.3 Size of step-back

Probing depths (margin to sulcus)	Tissue thickness (margin to bone)	Blade/mark position away from tooth
0–3 mm	0–5 mm	Next to tooth (intrasulcular)
4–5 mm	6–7 mm	1–2 mm*
6–7 mm	7–8 mm	3–4 mm*
7+ mm	9+ mm	5 mm*

* Make sure to keep more than 4-mm keratinized gingiva. If there is less than 5-mm keratinized gingiva, stay closer to the tooth to preserve keratinized gingiva. In this case, try to suture the tissue apically and use periodontal dressing to keep tissue more apically.

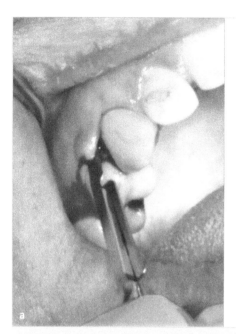 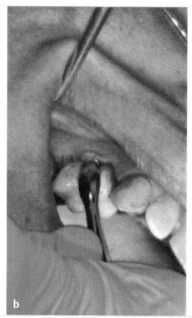 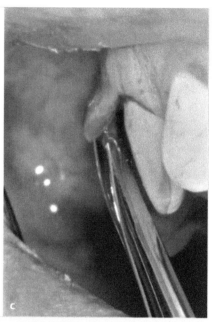

Fig. 6.4 Key initial steps for flap elevation. (**a**) Perform all incisions and begin flap elevation by fully inserting the scalpel into the interproximal incision and twisting the blade to begin reflecting the papilla tip. (**b, c**) Use the tip of a Molt-9 to continue flap elevation by firmly resting against the bone and pushing against the base of the flap. Once the entire papilla is elevated to the mid-buccal/mid-lingual, use the broad base of the Molt-9 to continue elevating the tissue.

Apically Displaced Flap

For pocket depth reduction, this a variant of the gingival flap where the flap edges are sutured at the level of the alveolar crest using inverting mattress sutures, sling sutures, and tacking sutures. This procedure allows the preservation of keratinized gingiva by moving it apically, and produces the greatest amount of recession compared to conventional gingival flap and modified Widman flap procedures. This procedure does not work well with regenerative surgeries that require complete wound closure. A variant of the apical displaced flap using split thickness incisions can be used to generate additional keratinized gingiva (see Chapter 8).

Wedge Incisions

Wedge incisions are made whenever there is excessive soft tissue thickness next to a mesial or distal root surface facing an edentulous space. For maximum pocket reduction, the wedge incision is done as follows (see ▶ Fig. 6.5):

- Determine the endpoint of the wedge incision by pushing a periodontal probe through the tissue toward the distal (or mesial depending on location of the tissue) of the area of thickened tissue. Continue probing the tissue until encountering either tissue of normal thickness (3 to 4 mm), the end of the edentulous space (i.e., end of tuberosity, intersection of occlusal plane with retromolar pad, next tooth), or 1-cm distance from the tooth.
- From this endpoint, make a straight linear incision across the area of thick tissue toward the tooth. A 12d blade is useful for this step.
- If the endpoint of the wedge incision is closer than 1 cm to the tooth, make a small full thickness vertical release that runs from the lingual edge of the ridge to the buccal edge of the ridge.
- Connect the end point(s) of the wedge incision with a full thickness, linear, internally beveled (aim the blade edge toward the alveolar bone edge) incision toward the buccal line angle of the tooth. A 12d blade is useful for this and the next step.
- Connect the end point(s) of the wedge incision with a full thickness, linear, internally beveled (aim the blade edge toward the alveolar bone edge) incision toward the lingual line angle of the tooth.

- With a periosteal elevator, elevate the flap edges, revealing the underlying alveolar bone.
- With a periosteal elevator, a Kirkland knife, and a round surgical diamond bur, remove the piece of gingiva sitting on the alveolar bone between the flap edges. Make sure not to damage either flap edge or root surfaces.
- Continue with the remaining surgery.
- Use an inverting vertical mattress suture to minimize tissue thickness.

Papilla Preservation Incisions

If pocket reduction is needed in the anterior maxilla, papilla-preservation techniques can limit unsightly loss of interdental papilla tissue after pocket-reduction surgery.

Papilla preservation can be done as follows (▶ Fig. 6.6, Video 6.2):
- Create full thickness intrasulcular incisions around each tooth surrounding the defect(s), making sure not to cut the papilla.

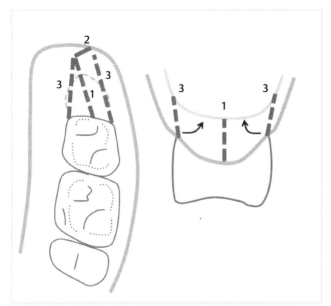

Fig. 6.5 Wedge incision. For suprabony pockets, a resective technique removing the entire area of excessive tissue is needed.

- Create the papilla preservation incision:
  o If the interproximal area is wider than 2 mm, make a linear, slightly internally beveled, full thickness incision from the mid-facial of the teeth adjacent to the bone defect(s) aiming the blade so that the blade tip touches the bone slightly apical to the buccal edge of the bone defect.
  o If the interproximal area is narrow, make a linear, slightly internally beveled, full thickness incision from the adjacent line angles of the teeth next to the bone defect, aiming the blade just apical to the buccal edge of the bone defect.
- Insert a scalpel into the incision, aim at the crest of the bone defect toward the lingual and sweep horizontally across the defect to dissect the papilla tissue from the granulation tissue within the defect.
- Using small periosteal elevators or Orban knives, gently lift the entire papilla toward the contact point to the point that it becomes freely movable.
- Push the papilla tissue under the contact point with a blunt instrument toward the lingual side.
- Elevate the facial tissue past the mucogingival junction apical to the papilla.
- Perform SRP and bone grafting.
- Suture the flap closed using vertical everting mattress sutures connecting the base of both flap edges using 6 to 0 sutures.

Gingivectomy

The gingivectomy technique is used to excise excessively thick gingiva, and uses external bevel incisions.

The steps for this procedure are as follows:
- Infiltrate tissue to be cut with additional 2% lidocaine/ 1:50,000 epinephrine.
- Measure probing depths interproximally and facially. Mark the location of the pocket base on the external surface of the gingiva by piercing the gingiva with a sharp instrument at the level of the pocket base all the way through to the tooth. At this time, check if the probe passes through soft tissue, or if it is stopped prematurely by hard tissue. Adjust the gingivectomy outline coronally until no bone is encountered.

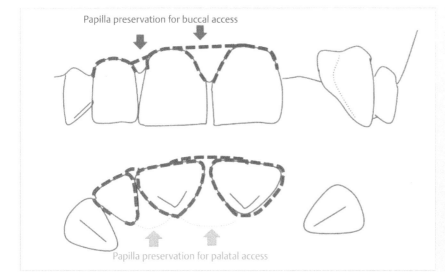

Fig. 6.6 Incision design for papilla preservation depends on if pocketing is more centered facially or lingual.

- Based on the pocket depth markings, picture a normal appearing gingiva with pointed papilla, flat tissue profile against teeth (at most 3-mm thick) and normal probing depth (at most, 3 mm).
- *Cut outlined soft tissue with a sharp scalpel*: The scalpel is pointed from the vestibule toward the pocket base, and moved along the pocket depth margins.
- Remove detached gingiva with Kirkland knife.
- Firmly apply wet gauze to stop bleeding for 10 minutes. Some minor bleeding will occur over the next day.
- Prescribe alcohol-free antiseptic mouthrinse for the patient. Instruct the patient to begin using it 24 hours after the surgery.

6.5.3 Surgical Debridement and Odontoplasty

The key to successful elimination of pockets is elimination of all plaque and calculus deposits on the root surface. Follow the following steps:

- Remove tissue tags and granulation tissue from bony defects with ultrasonics and curettes.
- Use ultrasonics to remove all visible residual calculus, leaving only off-white root surfaces.
- Check for root defects such as dentin ridges, pointed furcation roofs, enamel projections.
- Remove any root defects with surgical diamond burs.
- Remove smear layer with Gracey curettes producing a glassy smooth root surface.

6.5.4 Osseous Resective Technique

If there are infrabony pockets, correct shallow defects with osseous surgery and modify deep defects with the following steps (▶ Fig. 6.7, Video 6.3):
- *Remove ledges, minor tori, and exostoses*: Fully expose these, and place large periosteal elevator apical to it. With large surgical round carbide and copious irrigation, shave bone until it is flat.

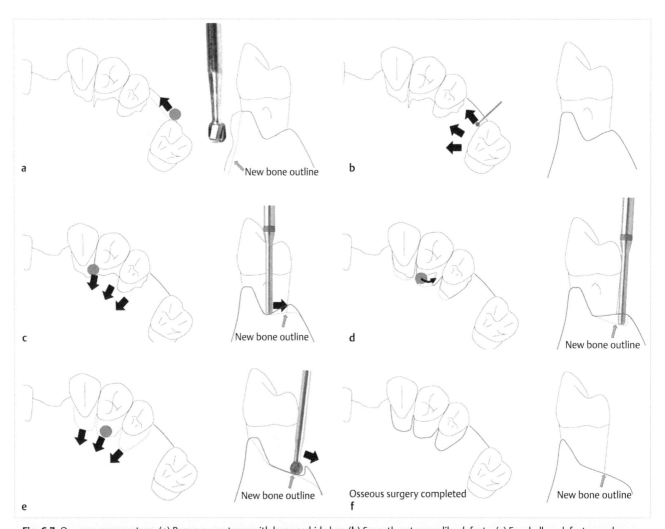

Fig. 6.7 Osseous surgery steps. (**a**) Remove exostoses with large carbide bur. (**b**) Smooth out ramp-like defects. (**c**) For shallow defects, mark depth of defect toward lingual. For deep defects, reduce and smooth defect walls so that they become well-defined 3-wall defects prior to regenerative techniques. (**d**) Recreate parabolic architecture by removing bone next to the root surfaces using the depth created in step 3 as a guide. (**e**) Use diamond burs to smooth bone and tooth surfaces. Note the preserved buccal bone height as little bone is removed toward the buccal. This prevents excessive interproximal recession. (**f**) Check to ensure that the bone preparation is smooth and follow normal physiologic contours.

- Remove ramp-like defects by removing crestal bone with a round bur so that it forms saddle-shaped ridge toward the adjacent tooth.
- For shallow interproximal defects (less than 2-mm deep), take an end-cutting surgical bur, place the tip on the defect floor, and get a feel for the depth of the location. Activate the bur, and move the bur toward the lingual aspect of the ridge to mark the most apical extent of the defect on the lingual side.
- For shallow bone defects associated with buccal/lingual furcations, mark the extent of the defect on the buccal/lingual wall using an end-cutting bur. See Chapter 7 for details on dealing with furcation involvement, and consider biologic shaping techniques as described in Chapter 7.
- For moderate and deep defects, visualize the defect and see if the defect can be converted into a more well-defined 3-wall defect by removing some bone around it. If it appears doable, use an end-cutting bur to round the edges of the defect, focusing mostly on the lingual side for any bone removal.
- With an end-cutting bur, remove bone next to the root surfaces and smoothly connect the marks made previously. Make sure that the lingual bone on the mid-lingual root surface is lower than the interproximal and furcation bone. For the buccal bone, maintain interproximal bone as high as possible, and create a scalloped bone architecture where mid-facial root surface bone is slightly lower than interproximal and furcal bone.
- Use a round surgical diamond bur to eliminate any troughs and ledges on the alveolar bone. The bone-tooth interface should always follow a smooth scalloped pattern.
- Scale and root plane any areas that were not accessible before.
- Continue with the remaining surgery.

6.5.5 Biologics Application

Generally, follow the manufacturer's instructions. For enamel matrix derivative, it is a two-step process:
- Apply root conditioning by depositing the clear gel containing EDTA root conditioner on a root surface.
- After 10 to 20 seconds, rinse it off, and deposit the milky enamel matrix derivative gel on the root.

For growth factors, reconstitute the protein with the provided sterile solution, mix it (or drip it) on the provided carrier (i.e., sponges or particles) and apply this into the defect.

6.5.6 Bone Grafting Technique

While bone grafting using bone graft putty may be as simple as using composite materials, it may not always be available, and particulate bone graft does not contain inert gel material. However, it is more difficult to use. Using commercially available particulate graft materials, the process is as follows (unless specified differently by the graft manufacturer) (▶ Video 6.4):
- Make sure the bone defect is completely clear of tissue tags, blood clot, and debris.
- Have an assistant carefully slide the sterile graft container from the outer packaging onto a sterile work surface. Carefully open the bone graft container. Static electricity may cause some bone graft particles to escape. Save bone graft labels for record keeping.

- Gently drip a sterile solution (i.e., sterile saline; if available, platelet poor plasma) into the container until there is a sizeable puddle of solution in the container.
- Gently stir the particles with a sterile instrument to thoroughly wet the particles and break up air bubbles.
- Let the bone graft stand and absorb the liquid for a few minutes.
- Draw off excess liquid with the tip of a saline-moistened sterile 2 × 2 gauze. The graft material should have consistency and stickiness of wet sand (▶ Fig. 6.8). This step is key, and the proper consistency or "wetness" allows relatively simple handling.
- Repeat second to fifth points, if instructed by graft material instructions.
- Quickly rinse out the bone defect with sterile saline. If there is no bleeding in the bone defect, quickly scrape the bone defect walls to induce some bleeding.
- For typical small bone defects encountered during periodontal surgery, use the flat side of a sterile periosteal elevator to carry the material to the patient's defect without dropping it, and gently pat particles into place. For very large defects (such as residual extraction sockets), load a bone graft syringe with bone graft in a manner similar to filling an amalgam condenser, and gently insert bone graft with syringe into defect.
- Lightly pack the bone graft material into the bone defect. Do not overfill.
- After the surgery, complete any required bone graft records and mail back the bone graft survey if required by tissue bank regulations.

6.5.7 Membrane Application

The steps for membrane application are as follows (▶ Video 6.5):
- Make sure that area of membrane application is free of soft tissue debris, the flap is elevated at least 2 cm away from the defect margins, and it can cover the defect with 1 to 2 mm overlap.
- Have an assistant carefully slide the sterile envelope containing the membrane from the outer packaging onto a

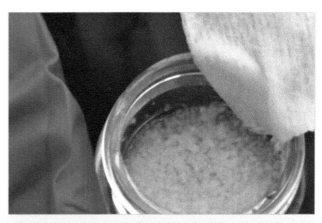

Fig. 6.8 A key step to make handling of allograft particulate bone easier is to hydrate it with sterile saline, and draw off excess liquid with sterile gauze. This makes the allograft particles acquire a consistency similar to wet sand, and allows placement and adaptation of the bone graft.

sterile workspace. Carefully open this envelope, separating the actual membrane from sterile wrapping.

- Using small iris scissors, make a template from the sterile inner envelope until it fits neatly over the defect and over-laps it by about 3 mm.
- Clean and dry template with gauze, and cut actual membrane to the same shape.
- Thread small resorbable suture (i.e., gut 5 to 0) through a corner of the membrane facing root (▶ Fig. 6.9).
- Hydrate membrane if required by manufacturer. Drape over defect. For interproximal use, roll up half of membrane into an L-shape, insert roll into interproximal space and unfold over defect.
- Feed the suture around the tooth, insert it from the under-side up through the membrane corner, wrap it back around the tooth, and tie a suture knot that anchors membrane at tooth (▶ Fig. 6.9).
- Advance the flap over the membrane and suture with a vertical everting mattress suture.

6.5.8 Suturing

Suturing is critical to the success of periodontal surgery. In general, the tissue will heal in the position where it is sutured, and the success of regenerative techniques depends on the flap edges not moving and exposing the underlying membrane or graft material.

General Suturing Principles

When suturing, keep the following principles in mind:
- The 2–1–1 knot is a secure knot for most common suture materials other than nylon and polytetrafluoroethylene (PTFE). This surgical knot is created by two clockwise suture throws around the needle holder, followed by a single counterclockwise and another single clockwise throw.
- When tying surgical knots, tighten by pulling on the suture end containing the needle (needle end).
- Keep the free end of the suture no longer than 1 inch.
- *Rule of 3s*: The point where the suture enters the flap should be at least 3-mm away from the flap edge, and 3 mm from adjacent suture points. The free ends of the suturing knot should be 3-mm long. This applies especially to continuous sutures.

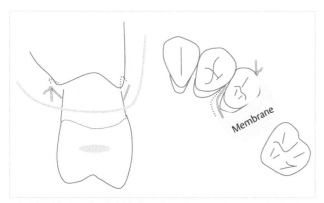

Fig. 6.9 An internal sling suture is used to secure the membrane tightly against a tooth and drape it over the adjacent bone defect.

- Keep tissue pink.
- Suture from distal to mesial, vestibule to crest, buccal to lingual, and mobile flap to attached tissue.
- Suture the tissue where it needs to be.
- For pocket reduction, avoid empty space under flaps.
- Make sure that suture knot rests on tissue, as otherwise the knot may interfere with healing.
- Wherever possible, place suture knots interproximally or on buccal side for patient comfort.
- Thin tissue requires small suture sizes and suture points further away from the incision line.

Mattress Sutures (Vertical versus Horizontal, Everting versus Inverting)

Mattress sutures should be the first suture placed in pocket reduction and regenerative surgery as they are placed deeply in the flap base and require access to the mucoperiosteal side of the flap. These sutures can reposition tissue apically, advance flap edges coronally, and secure membranes. Generally, for:
- Maximum pocket depth reduction use inverting mattress sutures.
- Regenerative techniques use everting mattress sutures.

Typically, vertical (everting/inverting) mattress sutures are used between teeth, and horizontal (everting/inverting) mattress sutures for edentulous areas.

The **inverting vertical mattress** suture is created with the following steps (▶ Fig. 6.10a, ▶ Video 6.6):
- Insert needle into buccal flap base. For apical traction, engage un-elevated tissue near floor of vestibule with the needle. For coronal traction, engage tissue near mucogingival junction.
- Feed suture underneath contact point to lingual.
- Insert needle at mid-section of lingual flap, and emerge 3 mm more apically.
- Feed suture back to buccal underneath contact point.
- Gently tighten suture until flap edges are adapted to underlying bone, and tie 2–1–1 knot.

An **everting vertical mattress suture** is created with the following steps (▶ Fig. 6.10c, ▶ Video 6.7):
- *Release periosteum*: Visualize underside of mucoperiosteal flap, which is periosteum. Incise this layer with sharp scalpel by 1 mm in distomesial direction for the entire length of flap at the base of the flap. Bleeding can be controlled with epinephrine, suctioning, and gauze pressure.
- Insert needle at base of buccal flap from epithelial side. Do not engage membrane/graft.
- Pass through and run over membrane/graft underneath contact point to lingual.
- Insert needle at base of lingual flap from the periosteum side and pass through.
- Insert needle at some distance coronal to base of lingual flap back into the tissue.
- Pass through and run over membrane/graft underneath contact point to buccal.
- Insert needle coronal to the base of buccal flap in periosteal side and pass through.
- Gently tighten suture until flap edges can be brought into contact, and tie 2–1–1 knot.

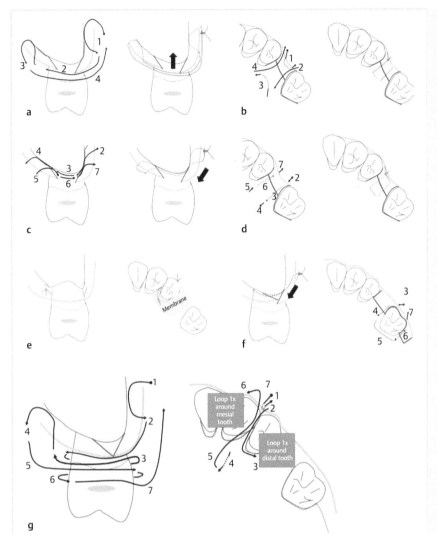

Fig. 6.10 Complex suturing to position flaps. (a) Vertical inverting mattress suture for pocket reduction between teeth. (b) Horizontal inverting mattress suture for close adaptation of tissue to edentulous ridges. (c) Vertical everting mattress suture for advancing tissue over graft materials and creating tissue thickness. (d) Horizontal everting mattress suture for covering grafts on edentulous ridges. (e) Internal sling suture for adapting a membrane to a tooth. (f) External sling suture for advancing or laterally positioning of a flap. (g) Combination sling-mattress suture for firm adaptation to teeth and underlying bone, and particularly useful for osseous surgery.

An **inverting horizontal mattress suture** is created with the following steps (▶ Fig. 6.10b, ▶ Video 6.8):
- Insert needle into buccal flap base. For apical traction, engage un-elevated tissue near floor of vestibule with the needle. For coronal traction, engage tissue near mucogingival junction.
- Insert needle at base of lingual flap (but not the floor of the mouth or near the greater palatine blood vessels), and have it reemerge mesially (or distally, but this is harder).
- Run suture back to buccal over tissue.
- Gently tighten suture until flap edges are adapted to underlying bone, and tie 2–1–1 knot.

An **everting horizontal mattress suture** is created with the following steps (▶ Fig. 6.10d, ▶ Video 6.9:
- Release periosteum as for the vertical everting mattress suture.
- Insert needle into buccal flap at some apical distance from the flap edge.
- Run suture over the alveolar crest and graft/membrane to the lingual.
- Insert needle into lingual flap from periosteal side at some distance to vestibule.
- Insert needle into lingual flap at some point mesial to the emergence point of third point.

- Run suture over the alveolar crest and graft/membrane to the buccal.
- Insert needle into buccal flap from periosteal side at some mesial to insertion of first point.
- Gently tighten suture until flap edges can be brought into contact, and tie 2–1–1 knot.

Sling Sutures (Internal versus External)

Sling sutures are used to secure membranes and advance flaps coronally or laterally. An internal sling suture is used to secure membranes against a tooth, and needs to be resorbable as it is completely buried under the tissue (▶ Fig. 6.10e, ▶ Video 6.10). An external sling suture anchors a flap against a tooth, and is at least partially exposed to the oral cavity. Sling sutures need to be placed prior to other sutures that close flap edges (i.e., simple interrupted and continuous sutures).

To tie an external sling suture for tissue repositioning, follow the following steps (▶ Fig. 6.10f, ▶ Video 6.11):
- Select the flap that needs advancement.
- Release the flap (as for everting mattress sutures).
- Insert the needle 2-mm mesial to the center of the flap to be moved.
- Grab the needle from the underside of the flap.

- Select a suitable anchor tooth in line with the desired movement.
- Feed suture through the mesial contact point of the selected anchor tooth, wrap it around, and feed it back through the distal contact point.
- Insert needle through periosteal side of flap 2-mm distal to the center of the flap.
- Tighten suture gradually, and until tissue is in desired position.
- Once satisfied with the flap position, tie a 2–1–1 knot.
- Finish suturing to achieve flap closure.

Sling-mattress Combination Sutures

Sling-mattress combination sutures firmly secure tissues against the underlying teeth and produce great flap stability. The following vertical inverting mattress-sling suture combination can be used as a workhorse suture for pocket-reduction surgeries and crown-lengthening procedures (▶Fig. 6.10g, ▶Video 6.12).
- Insert needle at base of buccal flap near the vestibule and apical to the interproximal contact. Aim the needle so that it reemerges coronally slightly below the alveolar crest.
- Feed the needle over the flap edge underneath the contact point toward the lingual.
- If there is no distal tooth, skip this step. Otherwise, wrap it around the distal tooth; feed it back to the buccal underneath the next distal contact point. Wrap it around the tooth, and feed it back again through the original interproximal contact toward the lingual.
- Insert the needle into lingual flap slightly apical to the ridge crest and have the needle reemerge about 3 to 4 mm apical to the insertion point.
- Feed the needle over the flap edge underneath the contact point toward the buccal.
- If there is no mesial tooth, skip this step. Otherwise, wrap it around the mesial tooth; feed it back to the lingual underneath the next mesial contact point. Wrap it around the tooth, and feed it back again through the original interproximal contact toward the buccal.
- Tighten the suture and watch the tissue both retract apically and constrict against the teeth. Once the tissue looks securely tightened, but still pink, tie the 2–1–1 knot.
- If needed, connect flap edges with simple interrupted sutures near incision line.

Simple Interrupted

After the initial mattress suture(s), the flap edges need to be brought together and connected with adjacent tissues at any vertical release. This can be accomplished with simple interrupted sutures that:
- Line up the corners of a flap with surrounding tissue (For a rectangular flap, tie the first corner sutures slightly loose).
- Close vertical releases.
- Connect flap edges at palatal papilla preservation incisions.
- Connect papilla tips between teeth after the placement of everting mattress sutures.

Suturing follows the following simple steps (▶Video 6.13):
- Insert needle apical to buccal flap edge.
- Pass under contact point to lingual.
- Feed needle through underside of lingual flap/non elevated flap.

- Pass back under contact point to buccal.
- Tie 2–1–1 knot.

Tacking Suture

As final suture(s) for apical flaps, a tacking suture is a simple interrupted suture within the flap for:
- Securing apical positioned flaps to underlying periosteum (use 6 to 0 sutures).
- Pulling apical positioned flaps toward the vestibule (use 3 to 0 sutures).

The steps for creating a tacking suture are as follows:
- Hold tissue to new position.
- For split-thickness flaps, insert needle through both flap and periosteum in coronal to apical direction. For vestibular pull, engage deep vestibular tissue.
- Rotate the needle through the tissue so that it emerges near the vestibular floor.
- Tie 2–1–1 knot, but only tight enough to maintain the knot and creating some tissue bunching.

Continuous (Locking and Nonlocking)

Continuous sutures are a more efficient alternative to simple interrupted sutures for long vertical releases and edentulous areas. Continuous non-locking sutures are a fast method to close a long straight flap edge (▶Video 6.14). Locking continuous sutures (▶Video 6.15) provide more tissue control than non-locking sutures.

For continuous sutures, follow the following steps:
- Insert needle in loose flap toward incision line.
- Feed needle through underside of the other flap edge.
- Tie 2–1–1 knot, but only trim length of free end to 3 mm.
- Go back to the loose flap edge, insert needle again toward incision line 3 mm from last suture point on same side of flap.
- Feed needle through underside of the other flap edge.
  - For a locking suture:
    - Instead of pulling suture tight, leave a 2 inch-long loop of suture (free loop) hanging.
    - Take the free loop, twist it once, and feed the needle through the loop.
- Repeat fourth and fifth points until flap is closed. Make sure to pull suture for each loop uniformly firm.
- For the last loop, leave loop hanging. Grab the apex of this loop and treat it as "free end" for suture knot tying.
- Tie 2–1–1 knot and trim off both needle end "free end."

6.6 Identify Suitable Cases for Crown-lengthening Procedures

Crown-lengthening procedures can rescue some teeth from being unrestorable by exposing additional sound tooth structure at the expense of supporting bone in the area. They also can aid better esthetic appearance in some cases where maxillary anterior teeth appear short or display excessively gingiva.

6.6.1 Indications

Crown-lengthening procedures should be considered for the following restorative problems:
- Subgingival caries.
- Cusp fracture extending below gingival margin.

- *Invasion of supracrestal attached tissues:* Usually, a patient will complain of persistently "sore gums" that started after placement of a restoration, and does not resolve with periodontal treatment. Clinically, there will be no sign of open margins or caries, and the apical margin cannot be felt within the sulcus. Radiographically, the restoration appears close to bone, and closer than the normal CEJ-bone distance on adjacent teeth.
- Short teeth that prevent creation of enough preparation length for crown retention.
- Short crowns.
- *Altered passive eruption*: Facial gingival margin is more than 2-mm coronal of the CEJ, or facial radiographic bone level is closer than 2 mm to the CEJ.

Crown-lengthening procedures use the same technique as resective pocket-reduction techniques and are very predictable surgeries that carry low surgical risks.

6.6.2 Determining if Crown Lengthening is Possible

Medical and dental contraindications are the same as for pocket-reduction surgery. In addition, it needs to be determined if crown lengthening is helpful in a given case. The following points need to be considered (▶ Fig. 6.11, ▶ Video 6.16):
- Should tooth be saved?
  - Tooth is too tilted or malpositioned to be useful and orthodontics is not feasible.
  - Tooth lacks value to patient—3rd molars and teeth that will remain unopposed.
  - Patient cannot maintain or does not want to save tooth.

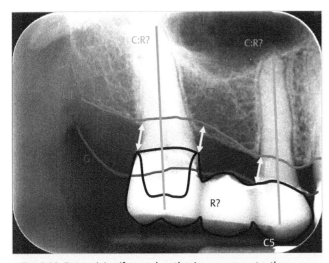

Fig. 6.11 Determining if crown lengthening can save a tooth: 1. Picture the final restoration on the radiograph, and determine if the tooth is restorable ("R?"). There must be enough tooth structure to allow a long enough preparation form (>4 mm), enough occlusal clearance (>1.5 mm), enough dentin at the margin (>1 mm), and root canal therapy possible, if needed. 2. Determine soft tissue thickness as estimate for biologic width (B) by the outline of the gingival shadow (G) or the distance of CEJ or healthy restorative margin to existing bone away from the surgical site. 3. Project biologic width (B) from the planned restoration margin to determine the new bone level (NBL) that parallels the new restorative margin. 4. Check if this new bone level still allows for appropriate crown-to-root ratio ("C:R?") and does not expose furcation entrances ("F?"). If it does, crown lengthening is likely to succeed.

- Is tooth restorable? If this cannot be determined from experience:
  - Remove all caries. Remove tooth if not enough tooth structure remains for restoration.
  - Attempt root canal treatment (RCT) if needed. Remove tooth if RCT cannot be finished.
  - Restore tooth with core-buildup material and prepare tooth to final margin disregarding gingiva or bone. Provisionalize as best as possible. Remove tooth if this cannot be done.
  - Examine tooth. Consider alternatives if preparation lacks proper height and clearance.
- Can crown lengthening reestablish biologic width without compromising teeth in area?
  - On radiographs, picture a new bone level 3-mm below the final margin.
  - With new bone level, does crown-to-root ratio remain 1:1 or better?
  - With new bone level, will furcations be exposed in the area?
  - If the answer is yes to either questions, consider alternatives such as biologic shaping.
- If tooth is visible, is crown lengthening for esthetics possible on contralateral tooth as well?

If the answer is "yes" to all four questions, crown lengthening may aid the restoration and saving of a tooth.

6.6.3 Determining the Coslet Type of a "Gummy Smile"

There are many reasons why a patient may complain about having a "gummy smile" ranging from altered passive eruption to excessive muscle activity and skeletal malformation. The cause of the "gummy smile" should first be assessed through an orthodontic exam after initial disease control. If other causes of a "gummy smile" are ruled out, determining the Coslet type aids treatment planning. This can be done with the following steps using a periapical radiograph and bone sounding of locally anesthetized gingiva:
- Determine the radiographic distance between CEJ and alveolar crest:
  - If the crest is at least 1-mm apical to CEJ, bone relationship is normal: Coslet type A.
  - If the crest is closer than 1 mm, there is excess bone: Coslet type B.
- Determine total tissue thickness at line angles and midfacial by pushing periodontal probe through sulcus and tissue until hard bone is felt. The distance from the probe tip to gingival margin is the total tissue thickness.
- Measure the width of keratinized gingiva.
  - If total thickness > 4 mm and less than keratinized gingiva, it is Coslet type 1.
  - If total thickness > 4 mm and more than keratinized gingiva, it is Coslet type 2.
  - If total thickness is up to 4 mm, it is normal and thus "Coslet type 0."
- Combine the "Coslet types" for treatment planning, i.e., "type 1 + B," "type 0 + A."
- Treatment plan the appropriate procedure (see below).

6.6.4 Treatment Planning

Treatment planning of crown-lengthening procedures depends on whether it is done for restorative purposes or treatment of passive eruption.

Crown Lengthening for Restorative Purposes

For treatment planning, the following information needs to be gathered: if a restoration is needed, if there is periodontitis present, and if there is excessive gingival thickness. With these factors in mind, treatment planning follows the pattern shown in ▶Table 6.4.

Crown Exposure for Passive Eruption Treatment

Crown-exposure techniques for the treatment of altered passive eruption follows the Coslet types as determined previously (▶Table 6.5).

6.6.5 Specific Consent Issues for Crown-lengthening Procedures

As with any periodontal surgery, informed consent must be obtained. Beyond the typical surgical risks associated with periodontal surgery, the patient must be aware that teeth in the area of crown lengthening will appear longer. In addition, there is the risk that a tooth may not be restorable despite crown lengthening, especially if the tooth breaks prior to restoration. Repeat crown-lengthening surgery may be needed if insufficient tissue was removed at the first time.

Beyond the usual alternatives to periodontal surgery, such as extraction and keeping the tooth "as is," there are alternatives to crown lengthening that may be helpful in some cases:
- Orthodontic extrusion on teeth with long remaining roots.
- Biologic shaping (see Chapter 7).
- Conversion to overdenture abutment.

6.6.6 Crown-lengthening Surgery Technique

Crown lengthening is similar to osseous surgery,[5] and includes the following steps (▶Fig. 6.12):
- After local anesthesia, gently rock provisional bucco-lingually with mosquito forceps and remove.
- Create a full thickness envelope flap in sextant containing tooth, and step-back by 1 to 2 mm in area of crown lengthening if there is more than 4 mm of keratinized gingiva.
- Clean off tissue tags and scale and root plane the exposed teeth.
- Note flap thickness "T" on adjacent healthy teeth, which is usually about 2 to 3 mm.
- With end-cutting bur remove bone along tooth until bone is "T" mm apical to preparation margin. This creates a trough-like bone defect around tooth.
- Treat trough-like defect as periodontal defect in osseous surgery, and reestablish smooth, parabolic, and positive architecture by removing adjacent bone with a surgical round bur. Facial/lingual bone should be lower than interproximal bone.
- Flatten any prominence such as exostoses and shelfs from the facial and lingual bone.
- Test for sufficient bone removal by replacing flap and checking if flap rests just below margin.
- Suture the tissue in place with vertical mattress sutures (i.e., 4 to 0 or 5 to 0).
- Recement provisional with small amount of temporary cement, and remove excess cement.
- Wait 8 weeks before the restoration of posterior teeth. Wait at least 3 months for anterior teeth.

6.7 Key Takeaways

- Surgical intervention is indicated when residual deep pockets remain after nonsurgical therapy has been completed. Residual pockets are usually due to hidden subgingival plaque and calculus, irregular bony defects, or root surface abnormalities. Persistent inflammation due to the invasion of biologic width by a restoration is another indication for surgical correction.
- Pockets can be classified as suprabony or infrabony. A pseudopocket has no attachment loss and is a subset of the suprabony pocket.
- Gingival flap surgery addresses the soft tissue. Osseous surgery in the form of a resective or regenerative technique addresses the bony defects. Resective techniques are best for shallow defects whereas regenerative techniques are preferable for deeper defects.
- Grafting bony defects have a better prognosis with an increasing number of remaining walls, i.e., a narrow, 3-wall defect has the best chance for regeneration versus a deep, 0-wall defect which is worst. Grafts with biologics

Table 6.4 Crown-lengthening treatment planning

Periodontal status	Needs bone removal	Needs restoration	Treatment plan
No periodontitis	Yes	Yes	"Clinical crown lengthening" per tooth
		No	"Crown exposure" per tooth
	No—excess tissue		"Gingivectomy" per quadrant
Periodontitis	Yes		"Osseous surgery" per quadrant
	No—excess tissue		"Gingival flap" per quadrant

Table 6.5 Crown-exposure techniques by passive eruption type

Coslet type	0—normal gingiva width	1—excessive keratinized gingiva	2—lack of keratinized gingiva
A—normal CEJ-bone relationship	Normal No treatment needed	"Gingivectomy," per quadrant	"Apical positioned flap"
B—too much bone	"Crown exposure" per tooth	"Crown exposure" per tooth	"Apical positioned flap," per quadrant (also involves bone removal)

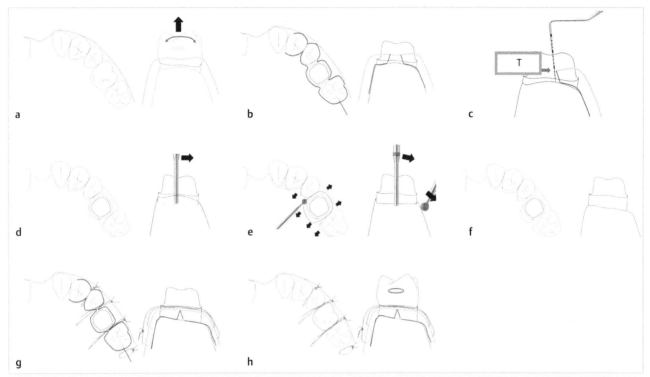

Fig. 6.12 Steps of conventional crown-lengthening surgery. (**a**) Remove provisional. (**b**) If the site has sufficient keratinized gingiva, create envelope flap with appropriate step-back at the tooth receiving crown lengthening. (**c**) Determine thickness (T) of the flap edge, which approximates biologic width. (**d**) With end-cutting bur, remove bone around the tooth forming a trough. Stop when the base of the trough is "T" millimeters away from the restoration. (**e**) Mark the base of trough by moving end-cutting bur facially/lingually and smoothen bone to the level of trough with round burs. Make sure to create smooth, scalloped bone architecture that has facial/lingual bone more apical than interproximal and furcation bone. (**f**) Inspect the area for sufficient bone removal. (**g**) Use vertical inverting mattresses or sling-mattress combination sutures to adapt the flap tightly to underlying bone and teeth. (**h**) Replace provisional with small amount of temporary cement. Make sure to remove any excess cement, and check occlusion for minimal centric contact and no interference contacts.

and membranes have specific uses; the operator must be familiar with their indications.

- *Techniques include crown lengthening*: Flap design base is always wider than the top. Vertical release incisions are no more than ½ the height of the flap and on either side of the papilla. Flap edges always rest on sound bone, so flap size extends 1 to 2 teeth away from the defective area.
- Suturing ensures the tissue stays in the desired position. Mattress sutures can be vertical or horizontal, everting, or inverting. Simple, continuous, and sling suturing techniques properly position the flap to heal in place.
- Crown lengthening can be indicated for restorative or developmental issues and like all osseous surgery, thoughtful treatment planning is a must.

6.8 Review Questions

A 67-year-old African American female presents to you because of pain she is experiencing in the lower right side of her mouth. She did not see a dentist for 2 years, but is now experiencing intermittent pain when she drinks something cold. She is healthy, with no known medical conditions, but years ago developed hives and difficulty breathing when she was given penicillin for tooth pain.

Extraoral exam findings revealed no abnormal findings for the facial skin, lymph nodes, thyroid gland, cranial nerves, salivary glands, masticatory muscles, and temporomandibular joint other than a slight popping sound when she opens her mouth on the left side. Intraorally, no mucosal pathology was apparent other than periodontal disease with signs of gingival inflammation. The grooves of nos. 18 and 17 were stained, and the center portion of no. 18 felt sticky with a sharp explorer.

Blood pressure is 130/70 mm Hg and pulse is 68/min.

Initial presentation is as follows (see ▶ Fig. 6.13 for clinical appearance and ▶ Fig. 6.14 for radiographs).

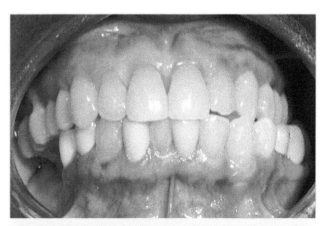

Fig. 6.13 Facial view at initial exam.

Initial periodontal findings are as follows:

Maxilla facial

	1	2	3	4	5	6	7	8	9	10	11	12	13	14	15	16
PD	336	523	522	433	323	333	333	323	333	332	233	323	423	423	333	4410
BOP		1				1			1							
CAL	6	6	2													10
GR	1	1														
MGJ	667	655	532	345	333	333	445	454	444	544	444	544	455	444	434	444
Furc																
PLQ	2	2	2	2	2	2	2	2	2	2	2	2	2	2	2	2

Maxilla lingual

	1	2	3	4	5	6	7	8	9	10	11	12	13	14	15	16
PD	326	844	533	334	334	433	433	434	333	323	424	332	322	334	435	555
BOP	11	1														
CAL	6	8	3													1	1
GR																
Furc																
Mobil							1	2	2	2						
PLQ	2	2	2	2	2	2	2	2	2	2	2	2	2	2	2	2

Mandible lingual

	32	31	30	29	28	27	26	25	24	23	22	21	20	19	18	17
PD				433	334	323	323	323	333	322	332	222	333	333	533	454
BOP																
CAL								1							1	1
GR																
MGJ				777	666	555	555	555	555	555	555	666	778	999	999	999
Furc																
PLQ				3	3	2	2	2	2	2	2	3	3	3	3	3

Mandible facial

	32	31	30	29	28	27	26	25	24	23	22	21	20	19	18	17
PD				534	433	323	322	333	322	333	323	432	434	335	423	333
BOP					1									1		
CAL				2	1									1		
GR																
MGJ				644	657	334	333	333	333	333	333	322	433	343	554	555
Furc																
Mobil							2	2	2	2	1					
PLQ				3	3	2	2	2	2	2	3	3	3	3	3	3

Abbreviations: BOP, bleeding on probing (1), suppuration (2); CAL, clinical attachment level; Furc, furcation involvement (Glickman class); GR, gingival recession; MGJ, position of mucogingival junction from margin; Mobil, tooth mobility (Miller grade); PD, probing depths; PLQ, plaque level (0 none to 5 heavy).

Pocket depths after SRP are as follows:

Facial

	1	2	3	4	5	6	7	8	9	10	11	12	13	14	15	16
PD	333	324	423	323	323	323	324	323	433	323	324	323	323	325	623	
BOP																

Lingual

	1	2	3	4	5	6	7	8	9	10	11	12	13	14	15	16
PD	336	633	422	424	424	333	233	324	423	323	323	323	424	324	445	
BOP	1	1											1			

Lingual

	32	31	30	29	28	27	26	25	24	23	22	21	20	19	18	17
PD				323	423	323	333	323	323	323	323	223	424	433	333	455
BOP																

Facial

	32	31	30	29	28	27	26	25	24	23	22	21	20	19	18	17
PD				1												
BOP				334	323	323	323	323	323	323	323	333	325	633	323	333

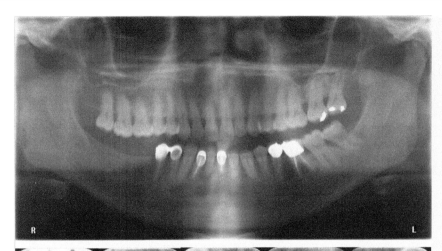

Fig. 6.14 Radiographs for review case.

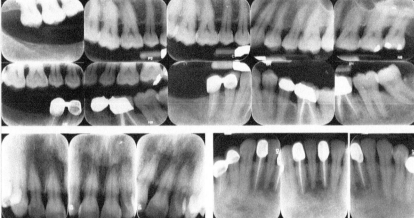

Learning Objective: Recognize indications for pocket reduction surgery.

1. In this case, tooth no. 16 has a deep pocket on the distal side as determined during the initial exam. As you can see, it was no longer present at reevaluation. What might have been the reason for removing it?
   A. Too much bone loss
   B. Low strategic value
   C. Noncompliant patient
   D. No opposing tooth

2. What is the likely reason for the persisting pocket between nos. 14 and 15?
   A. Furcation entrance retaining plaque
   B. Incomplete SRP
   C. Poor interproximal contact
   D. Root canal infection of no. 15

3. If you removed nos. 14 and 15 because of the persisting pocket, which is the LEAST concern with tooth replacement?
   A. Limited ridge height to sinus
   B. Lack of appropriate removable partial denture abutments
   C. Lack of appropriate fixed partial denture abutments
   D. Lack of posterior stops

Learning Objective: Develop a surgical treatment plan for reducing pockets.

4. Your restorative plan includes fabricating a removable partial denture replacing the mandibular molars on the right side. Which treatment plan would allow you to reduce pockets and offer the best chance of regaining attachment?
   A. Gingival flap, 1 to 3 teeth
   B. Osseous surgery, 1 to 3 teeth
   C. Osseous surgery, 1 to 3 teeth + guided tissue regeneration no. 2
   D. Gingival flap, 1 to 3 teeth + bone grafting no. 2

5. For the residual pockets between nos. 14 and 15, which treatment plan offers the best chance of pocket reduction?
   A. Gingival flap, 1 to 3 teeth
   B. Osseous surgery, 1 to 3 teeth
   C. Osseous surgery, 1 to 3 teeth + guided tissue regeneration no. 15
   D. Gingival flap, 1 to 3 teeth + bone grafting no. 15

6. For the residual pocket between nos. 19 and 20, which treatment plan offers the best chance of pocket reduction?
   A. Gingival flap, 1 to 3 teeth
   B. Osseous surgery, 1 to 3 teeth
   C. Gingival flap, 1 to 3 teeth + bone grafting no. 20
   D. None of the above

Learning Objective: Describe surgical pocket-reduction techniques.

7. If you used osseous surgery for reducing the pockets between nos. 2 and 3, which flap and suture design is most appropriate?
   A. Full thickness envelope flap, vertical inverting mattress sutures
   B. Modified Widman flap, vertical inverting mattress sutures
   C. Full thickness envelope flap, simple interrupted sutures
   D. Modified Widman flap, simple interrupted sutures

8. If you used regenerative therapy for the pocket between nos. 2 and 3, which flap and suture design is most appropriate?
   A. Apical displaced flap, tacking suture, and vertical inverting mattress sutures
   B. Apical displaced flap, external sling suture, and everting mattress suture
   C. Triangular flap, external sling suture, and everting mattress suture
   D. Triangular flap, tacking suture, and vertical inverting mattress suture

9. The patient says she does not want any products derived from pigs. Which regenerative procedure is most likely affected by this statement?
   A. Allograft
   B. Xenograft
   C. Guided tissue regeneration with resorbable membranes
   D. Enamel matrix derivative application

Learning Objective: Identify suitable cases for crown-lengthening procedures.

10. You remove the crown at tooth no. 29 since it is bulky and has persistent inflammation. You discover significant caries that removes the top half of the crown. Therefore, you remove the caries, redo the RCT, and rebuild the tooth with core material and a provisional. You are attempting to take the impression, but have a difficult time capturing the subgingival margin as your retraction cord will not stay. What should your treatment plan be?
    A. Extraction
    B. Crown exposure
    C. Crown lengthening
    D. Nothing

11. What limits the amount of crown lengthening you can perform for this tooth no. 29?
    A. Root length
    B. Furcation entrance
    C. Length of no. 28
    D. Amount of coronal tooth structure

6.9 Answers

1. **B.** As seen on the case photographs, the patient has low plaque levels and noncompliance seems unlikely given the presence of multiple restorations and general well-kept appearance of the dentition. Although no. 16 is a 3rd molar and of low importance to the patient, it does seem to occlude with an opposing no. 17 and there is good bone support remaining around the tooth, which may make extraction more challenging.

2. **A.** At least one radiograph shows the mesial furcation entrance of no. 15 coronal to the existing bone level. While incomplete SRP in theory is always a possible reason for residual pockets, it is more likely that the furcation entrance cannot be accessed without surgery. The proximal contact appears normal, which likely rules it out as contributing factor. While on the panoramic radiograph, it appears that there is a periapical radiolucency at no. 15, closer inspection on periapicals reveals it as uneven sinus floor anatomy with normal periapical periodontal ligament space.

3. **C.** If nos. 14, 15, and 16 were missing, the premolars, canines, and contralateral molars could still serve as removable partial denture abutment. Obviously, lacking a distal abutment prevents you from placing a fixed partial denture, and the uneven sinus floor anatomy coupled with some bone loss after extraction may prevent you from placing implants without sinus augmentation. Lack of posterior stops is a restorative concern as without the left maxillary molars, you have no molar occlusion. This would cause a collapse in vertical dimension, which you then have to determine with occlusal rims.

4. **D.** The problem here is that no. 2 has a moderate well-defined 2-wall defect with a mesial slope and most likely a buccal wall as it surrounds a furcation that opens toward the lingual. Since the goal includes regeneration, a regenerative procedure is needed for best regeneration. Gingival flap surgery can stimulate limited regeneration, but numerous clinical trials show that most regenerative therapy is always superior in stimulating bone growth compared to a gingival flap. Osseous surgery usually results in some attachment loss, and not gain. Since this is a maxillary molar with a narrow interproximal area, it is probably more difficult to place a membrane than a bone graft, which makes the bone graft a preferred option here.

5. **B.** The goal here is maximum pocket reduction, which is achieved by osseous surgery. In addition, the defect here is smaller than on the right side, which makes either regeneration procedure less predictable. Gingival flap surgery produces some pocket reduction in the presence of bone defects, but osseous surgery is more effective.

6. **D.** The problem here is the large recurrent caries on the distal of no. 20, which none of the proposed periodontal surgeries will address. This really is a crown lengthening case as there is no periodontitis-induced bone loss in the area, but an issue of biologic width violation by the caries as seen on the bitewing radiograph.

7. **A.** Modified Widman flaps do not provide enough access for osseous surgery, but a fully reflected envelope flap does. Simple interrupted sutures bring the flap edges together, but do not control tissue thickness and likely are not as efficient in reducing pockets. Vertical inverting mattress sutures apply pressure on the incision area and can retract tissue toward the vestibule. Both properties favor pocket reduction, which makes these sutures preferred to simple interrupted sutures in this case.

8. **C.** For regeneration, you need to make sure to advance the tissue over the membrane and graft, which is done with sling sutures and everting mattress sutures. Tacking sutures cannot be used over grafted sites since there is no anchorage in grafted sites. An apical displaced flap does not work for regeneration, as it will expose the graft material, likely resulting in less regenerative potential. A full thickness triangular flap works well for regeneration as it provides access to the bone and has some potential for advancement.

9. **D.** Enamel matrix derivative is made from tooth buds of pig embryos, and would very likely discomfort this patient. Xenograft may be an issue if you happen to use pig-derived bone. However, xenograft typically is derived from cows and so not an issue. Allografts are from organ donors and the patient's statement does not apply. Non-resorbable guided tissue regeneration membranes are synthetic, whereas nonresorbable membranes often are derived from cows. You have to be careful though, as it may be possible that a resorbable membrane derived of pig material exists.

10. **C.** You need to restore no. 29, which eliminates crown exposure as this procedure is only used to expose a tooth that does not need a restoration. Doing nothing is not an option, as you need to get an accurate impression. You could try electrosurgery or soft tissue laser ablation to artificially increase the sulcus before impression taking, but because you seem to be close the sulcus based on the information presented here, you will run the risk of biologic width violation. Extraction is always an option, but in this case should be avoided, as it seems that the tooth can be crown lengthened and therefore made restorable.

11. **A.** No. 29 has the shortest tooth root in the area, which limits the amount of crown lengthening you can do as you still need to maintain a good crown-to-root ratio better than 1:1. There is no furcation nearby, and there is no radiographic evidence of furcations for the premolars.

6.10 Evidence-based Activities

- Find studies that evaluate other methods in reducing pockets (i.e., lasers, growth factors, tissue-engineered materials, and flowable membranes), and debate their merit.
- Obtain a clinical case from your instructor/institution or the internet and discuss what surgical treatment may be most suitable for it. Have your instructor (or mentor) provide insights on his or her experience with these treatments.
- Critically evaluate the surgical cases presented in this chapter and debate how the surgical technique can be improved. Have your instructor (or mentor) describe how he or she performs pocket-reduction surgeries and compare it with the methods presented here.
- Go to the University of Texas Health Science Center School of Dentistry at San Antonio's library of critically appraised topics (CAT) at https://cats.uthscsa.edu/ and search for a review on regeneration. Read any CAT you can find, and debate if the conclusion is still correct based on current literature.
- Create a CAT on treating Class III furcation involvement (or any other topic for which a CAT is not available) following the outline provided by Sauve S, et al. in "The critically appraised topic: a practical approach to learning critical appraisal" (Ann R Coll Physicians Surg Can. 1995; 28:396–398).

References

[1] Carnevale G, Kaldahl WB. Osseous resective surgery. Periodontol 2000 2000;22:59–87

[2] Cochran DL, Oh TJ, Mills MP, et al. A Randomized Clinical Trial Evaluating rh-FGF-2/β-TCP in Periodontal Defects. J Dent Res 2016;95(5):523–530

[3] Kitamura M, Nakashima K, Kowashi Y, et al. Periodontal tissue regeneration using fibroblast growth factor-2: randomized controlled phase II clinical trial. PLoS One 2008;3(7):e2611

[4] Dohan DM, Choukroun J, Diss A, et al. Platelet-rich fibrin (PRF): a second-generation platelet concentrate. Part I: technological concepts and evolution. Oral Surg Oral Med Oral Pathol Oral Radiol Endod 2006;101(3):e37–e44

[5] Rosenberg ES, Cho SC, Garber DA. Crown lengthening revisited. Compend Contin Educ Dent 1999;20(6):527–532, 534, 536–538 passim, quiz 542

7 Treating Teeth with Furcation Involvement

Abstract

Furcation involvement presents a special challenge to nonsurgical and surgical periodontal techniques, and the management of furcation involvement has to be approached from both periodontal and restorative perspectives. This chapter reviews the challenge posed by furcation involvement, and presents multiple approaches for treatment.

Keywords: furcation treatment, biologic shaping, root resection

7.1 Learning Objectives

- Recognize the effect of furcation involvement on tooth prognosis.
- Develop strategies for managing furcation involvement.
- Describe surgical methods for Class I and Class II furcation involvement.
- Describe surgical methods for deep Class II and Class III furcation involvement.

7.2 Case

A 44-year-old East Asian female was referred from a local dental hygiene school clinic for periodontal evaluation. She was concerned about the bone loss she had and that the supervising dentist at the hygiene clinic told her that she will lose all her teeth. She had no known medical conditions or allergies, and saw a physician for a check-up 3 or 4 years ago. She described that she had four uneventful pregnancies and that since the last one 5 years ago, her gums bled more frequently. For dental care, she did not see a dentist for about 20 years until she felt she needed a tooth cleaning and sought care at a dental hygienic clinic because of the low cost. Lately, she felt some discomfort when chewing and felt that some teeth (nos. 15, 23 to 25) had become loose. She explained that she brushes her teeth with a soft brush after every meal, and flosses once daily. When questioned, she explained that her husband noticed that she grinds her teeth at night.

Other than periodontal disease the extra and intraoral exams revealed no signs of disease. This was especially pronounced in the upper right quadrant, where tooth no. 3 had deep pocketing and a furcation involvement that appeared to be through-and-through from the mesial entrance to the distal entrance, and a deep buccal furcation entrance (▶ Fig. 7.1).

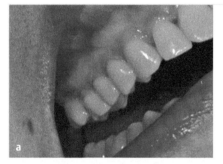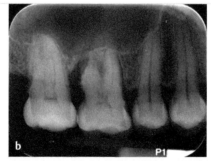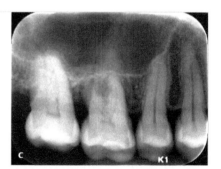

Fig. 7.1 (a) Initial presentation of upper right quadrant. (b) Initial periapical radiograph showing deep bone defect and furcation involvement at tooth no. 3. (c) A radiograph taken 4 months after surgical treatment shows partial radiographic fill of the furcation area.

Initial periodontal findings for the upper right quadrant are as follows:

Maxilla facial		1	2	3	4	5	6	7	8
	PD		526	643	323	424	323	333	322
	BOP		1	1 1		1			1
	CAL		6	7	2	1	1	1	1
	GR		1	22	1	1			
	MGJ		646	647	747	757	767	757	858
	Furc			2					
	PLQ								
Maxilla lingual	PD		735	646	324	323	233	233	332
	BOP		1						
	CAL		3	8					
	GR		11	22					
	Furc			3 3					
	Mobil							1	1
	PLQ								

Abbreviations: BOP, bleeding on probing (1), suppuration (2); CAL, clinical attachment level; Furc, furcation involvement (Glickman class); GR, gingival recession; MGJ, position of mucogingival junction from margin; Mobil, tooth mobility (Miller grade); PD, probing depths; PLQ, plaque level (0 = none, 5 = heavy).

The patient was taught how to use interproximal brushes in the molar area, and scaling and root planning (SRP) was performed, which improved bleeding on probing, but did not otherwise improve the condition and allowed easier detection of furcation entrances:

Maxilla facial		1	2	3	4	5	6	7	8
	PD		324	622	314	313	223	322	212
	BOP								
	CAL		3	8	3	1	1	1	1
	Furc		1	2					
	PLQ			1					
Maxilla lingual	PD		523	423	223	323	323	322	213
	BOP		1			1			
	CAL			8					
	Furc			2					
	Mobil							1	1
	PLQ		1						

Abbreviations: BOP, bleeding on probing (1), suppuration (2); CAL, clinical attachment level; Furc, furcation involvement (Glickman class); GR, gingival recession; MGJ, position of mucogingival junction from margin; Mobil, tooth mobility (Miller grade); PD, probing depths; PLQ, plaque level (0 = none, 5 = heavy).

Periodontal surgery was then performed, which cleaned and reshaped the furcation entrance to remove root concavities, and placed bone graft material. This reduced pocketing more and made the furcation involvement shallower, while also improving radiographic presentation (▶ Fig. 7.1c).

Maxilla facial		1	2	3	4	5	6	7	8
	PD		322	422	212	212	212	213	222
	BOP		1	1					
	CAL		3	5	3	1	1	1	1
	Furc			1					
	PLQ								
Maxilla lingual	PD		322	225	213	213	322	213	312
	BOP			11		1			
	CAL								
	Furc			2					
	Mobil							1	1
	PLQ								

Abbreviations: PD, probing depths; CAL, clinical attachment level; BOP, bleeding on probing (1), suppuration (2); GR, gingival recession; MGJ, position of mucogingival junction; Furc, furcation involvement (Glickman class); Mobil, tooth mobility (Miller grade); PLQ, plaque level (0 = none, 5 = heavy).

What can be learned from this case?

This case stresses the importance of comprehensive periodontal treatment in patients with furcation involvement as a combination of nonsurgical and surgical therapy usually is needed to manage furcation involvement. The goal in furcation management is not necessarily to eliminate a furcation involvement, but to be able to create a local environment with low probing depths that can easily be kept clean. While a regenerative approach was successful in reducing pockets and improving radiographic appearance, this case could benefit from further restorative and surgical treatment that improves the shape of the tooth. However, the patient declined additional treatment, and the furcation involvement presents a long-term risk for continued disease.

7.3 Recognize the Effect of Furcation Involvement on Tooth Prognosis

As seen in this case, furcation involvement makes it more likely that pocketing persists after nonsurgical periodontal therapy. Furcation involvement also presents a long-term risk of recurrent periodontal disease activity.

7.3.1 Describing Furcation Involvement

While many furcation classification systems exist, the Glickmann classification is the most commonly used system. For surgical treatment planning, the following characteristics of a periodontally involved furcation are important.
- Location of furcation:
  - *Mandibular molars vs. maxillary molars*: Guided tissue regeneration is more predictable on mandibular molars.
  - *Buccal/lingual vs. interproximal*: Guided tissue regeneration is unlikely to be effective on closing interproximal furcation entrances.
- *Association with a bone defect*: Bone defects can benefit from regenerative procedures.
  - *Depth of the defect*: Regeneration is more predictable for deep defects (>2 mm deep).
  - *Bony walls*: For furcation involvement, the presence of bony walls may aid the retention of regenerative material and improve the likelihood of regeneration. Typically, bone defects at a buccal or lingual furcation have a single wall fronting the furcation entrance.
- Shape of furcation:
  - *Peaked, inverted "V"-shape*: Needed to be rounded out to improve regenerative success.
  - *Round, inverted "U" shape*: More accessible to SRP than inverted V-shape.
- Width of furcation entrance: Narrow (<1 mm) vs. wide:
  - Narrow furcation entrances need to be widened surgically. If this is not possible, the chance of treatment success diminishes and extraction should be considered.
  - Wide furcation entrances are more conducive to regeneration and SRP. A wide mandibular molar furcation may also allow tunneling of a furcation for oral hygiene access.

- Horizontal depth of furcation:
  - *Glickmann Class I, "shallow" Glickman Class II furcation*: Bone loss in the furcation entrance does not protrude under the pulp chamber (about 1/3 tooth width from buccal/lingual side, or more with increasing age). Tooth shaping (odontoplasty, and biologic shaping) will likely not require root canal treatment.
  - *"Deep" Glickman Class II furcation*: Bone loss in furcation extends under pulp chamber. Odontoplasty will likely require previous root canal therapy. More aggressive forms of tooth shaping such as root amputation or hemisection should be considered.
  - *Glickman Class III furcation*: Chance of regeneration is much reduced.
- Presence of root surface abnormalities such as cervical enamel projection, pearls, ridges:
  - If these are not removable, they diminish the likelihood of treatment success.

7.3.2 Challenges Associated with Furcation Involvement

The increased risk of periodontal disease progression of furcation-involved teeth is related to the anatomy of multi-rooted teeth.

Furcation Anatomy

Any multirooted tooth is at risk for furcation involvement, along with teeth prone to having root deep root concavities:
- *Maxillary 1st and 2nd molars*: Mid-buccal, distolingual, and mesiolingual furcation entrances.
- *Mandibular 1st and 2nd molars*: Mid-buccal and mid-lingual furcation entrances.
- Maxillary premolars (especially the 1st) have mesial and distal root concavities.
- Mandibular incisors have mesial and distal root concavities.

The risk for periodontal disease involvement depends on the length of the root trunk, which is the segment of the tooth between the cemento-enamel junction (CEJ) and the furcation entrance. Short root trunks create a risk for early furcation involvement as it takes little attachment or bone loss to expose the furcation to the oral cavity (▶Fig. 7.2a).

The buccal furcation entrance is closest to the CEJ on all molars, making it the easiest to detect. On average, furcation entrances are about 3 mm apical to the CEJ in mandibular molars and almost 5 mm apical to the CEJ in maxillary molars.

The size of the furcation varies considerably between individual teeth. The width of a furcation entrance typically ranges from 0.5 mm near the roof of the furcation to 3 mm at the widest aspect, and the angle created by the tooth roots usually is about 15 to 30 degrees. The depth of the furcation area is about 7–8 mm for molars (from one side to another furcation entrance) and about 3 ½ mm for premolars. For comparison, the blade of a typical new standard-size Gracey curette is 0.9 mm wide and 4 mm long. This makes it difficult to fully clean some furcation entrances with curettes (▶Fig. 7.2b) as the blade cannot reach the roof of the furcation, and surrounding tissue usually blocks full entry of the blade into the furcation.

In addition to the limited size of the furcation, root surface abnormalities can make it difficult to access furcation entrances

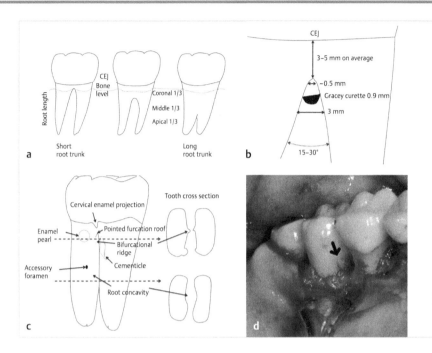

Fig. 7.2 Furcation characteristics that are associated with furcation involvement. **(a)** Root trunk configurations can range from short to long, and teeth where the furcation entrances is located in the coronal third of the root are likely to have furcation involvement even with minor attachment/bone loss. **(b)** Average dimensions of furcation entrances impede use of curettes and often preclude successful nonsurgical treatment of teeth with furcation involvement. **(c)** Various tooth root surface abnormalities may prevent additional obstacles to SRP furcation entrances. **(d)** Root surface defects are commonly associated with persistent deep pocketing at furcation entrances. An example is this small enamel pearl near furcation entrance of no. 15 observed during surgery.

(▶Fig. 7.2c) and often are the main contributing factor that leads to local furcation involvement. Root surface abnormalities associated with furcation involvement can include any of the following:

- *Cervical enamel projections*: Small wedge-shaped tongues of enamel pointed at the furcation entrance, and found on about 80% of all molars with furcation involvement. Most commonly found at mandibular 1st molars, followed by maxillary 1st molars and 2nd molars. Cervical enamel projections are difficult to detect clinically or radiographically, and usually found at surgery.
- Enamel pearls are round, smooth enamel islands on the root surface and can contain dentin and even pulp. Enamel pearls are found in up to 10% of molars and are most common on maxillary first and second molars. Since enamel pearls do not support periodontal attachment, exposure of an enamel pearl by a periodontal pocket results in sudden attachment loss by several millimeters, and they are often associated with severe localized periodontal breakdown.[1]
- Cementicles are usually found as clusters of small sharp projections on a root surface, and sometimes are associated with molar furcation entrances.
- Bifurcation ridges are dentinal ridges that run across the roof of a furcation entrance and create niches where plaque can hide. There are commonly found on teeth which also have cervical enamel projections.
- *Furcation and root concavities*: Almost all mandibular molars have root concavities on the mesial and distal root, and these concavities are about 0.4–0.9 mm deep. On maxillary molars, the mesiobuccal root usually contains a root concavity that may be up to 0.7 mm deep, whereas the palatal root is usually convex and the distobuccal root has a flat profile toward the furcation entrance. Given the restricted space of a furcation entrance, root concavities are very difficult to clean completely.
- Accessory root canals opening into the furcation area of molars are found in about half of molars, and may be

involved in furcation involvement of teeth with pulpal necrosis.
- Restorations near the furcation entrances can provide an additional locus of plaque collection, and interproximal restorations are associated with an increased risk of furcation involvement.

The effect of these anatomic factors poses several risks to dental treatment, and ultimately tooth survival at the following levels.

Oral Hygiene

At a very basic level, furcation involvement produces concavities and corners on a root surface that may not be accessible to tooth brush bristles, and floss will skip over these concavities as demonstrated in Chapter 5. While interproximal brushes may be able to reach into shallow root concavities, deep, wedge-shaped furcation involvement is beyond the reach of an interproximal brush. While rubber-tipped interproximal stimulators and toothpicks may reach into facial furcation involvement, they also cannot completely clean a furcation entrance, especially if it contains dentin ridges and grooves. Therefore, furcation entrances tend to retain plaque, which leads to a greater likelihood of gingival inflammation, which in turn favors localized attachment and bone loss.

Scaling and Soot Planning

Furcation anatomy is a major impediment to scaling and root planing, as the furcation in about 50–60% of molars is smaller than the blade of a curette. Since the roof of a furcation is almost invariably pointed and narrower than a curette, it is nearly impossible to completely scale and root plane a Class II or Class III furcation involvement with a curette. Ultrasonics tend to do better since the ultrasonic tip is smaller than a curette blade. However, since even the round tip of an ultrasonic insert may not completely fit into a furcation groove, the only solution to make a furcation cleansable is to reshape the roof into a wider round structure with diamond burs.

Abscess Risk

Exposed furcation entrances can become the nidus for a periodontal abscess as they present a small space that can be easily enclosed by soft tissue, and a study found that almost 90% of periodontal abscesses on multirooted teeth were associated with furcation involvement.

Surgical Access

Furcation involvement also poses a surgical challenge since successful periodontal surgery depends on the ability to thoroughly scale and root plane a root surface, which is difficult to accomplish in furcation involvement as already described. In addition, the interproximal location of most furcation entrances makes it challenging to scale and root plane these entrances, place bone graft or place a barrier membrane that can seal these furcation entrances. Consequently, regenerative approaches work less predictably on interproximal furcation involvement of maxillary molars compared to buccal and lingual furcation involvement.

Restoration

Placing a restorative margin on the convex, inward sloping dentin/cementum surface of a furcation entrance is more difficult that placing it in sound enamel coronal to the CEJ. It is also difficult for a laboratory technician to create good marginal fit of metal castings into these areas. Porcelain tends to slump onto margins placed into furcation entrances leading to overhanging restorations unless corrected by the lab technician or dentist prior to crown placement. Moreover, furcation involvement poses a risk for tooth preparation as it is easy to perforate the gingival floor of a cavity preparation overlying a furcation entrance. This then makes it extremely difficult to apply and seal off the cavity preparation with a matrix band, which then produces amalgam or resin overhangs into the furcation entrance.

Effect on Prognosis

While furcation involvement definitely increases the risk of periodontal disease and worsens prognosis, periodontal therapy can maintain teeth with furcation involvement for years. Survival ranges from 77–93% over 10 years after the surgical treatment of the furcation.[2] For comparison, the 10-year survival rate of teeth after root canal treatment ranges between 74 and 97%.

Even hopeless teeth with "through-and-through" furcation involvement can occasionally be successfully treated and retained with regenerative therapy.[3] It is also possible to maintain these teeth and hold off tooth loss for about 5 to 10 years on average[4] with either tunneling procedures that provide oral hygiene access for diligent patients, or with resective procedures that eliminate a diseased root and maintain the function of the tooth. Therefore, teeth with furcation involvement should not be extracted without considering the cost of tooth replacement versus maintaining the tooth with periodontal therapy.

7.4 Develop Strategies for Managing Furcation Involvement

Generally, the following strategies exist for treating teeth with furcation involvement:
- Maintain "as is."
- Extract.
- Reduce pocketing and reshape tooth (▶ Fig. 7.3).

7.4.1 Maintenance "as is"

Maintenance "as is" is the least invasive treatment. Indications are as follows:
- Patient finished SRP, but other initial therapy is still in progress.
- Patient refuses other treatment and understands risk of new disease, tooth loss.
- No other treatment is feasible and patient wants to keep tooth "as is," understands the compromised nature of tooth and accepts the risk of eventual tooth loss.
- *Tooth with furcation involvement is maintainable*:
  ○ Low probing depths (no more than 4–5 mm) with no bleeding on probing.
  ○ Furcation entrance is easily accessible for oral hygiene and professional cleaning:
    – Convex shape of the furcation area.
    – Wide entrance to the furcation (>1 mm).
    – Shallow horizontal furcation depth.

If any of these indications apply, routine periodontal maintenance every 3–4 months should be performed. If the tooth with furcation involvement is maintainable, tooth loss is unlikely.

The advantage of this treatment is that it is the least invasive option, and allows further treatment when necessary along with staving off extraction and tooth replacement.

The disadvantage of this treatment is that it only provides definite "treatment" if there is no disease associated with the furcation. In most clinical situations with active disease, periodontal maintenance is just a stop-gap procedure until more definite treatment can be performed.

7.4.2 Extraction

A definite treatment for furcation involvement is extraction. Although hopeless teeth are usually extracted, specific indications for extraction of teeth with furcation involvement include the following:
- Patient is not interested in saving the tooth.
- Tooth has no strategic value for treatment or patient.
- Periodontal therapy is unlikely to improve prognosis of tooth and chance of success is too low for patient and dentist. This usually applies to teeth with:
  ○ Miller II or III tooth mobility.
  ○ Severe generalized bone loss >60%.
  ○ Concurrent endodontic infection.
  ○ *Poor root anatomy*: Narrow furcation entrance, root proximity, enamel pearls, and etc.

The advantage of this approach is that it will eliminate teeth at risk for future periodontal disease at a low initial cost, and

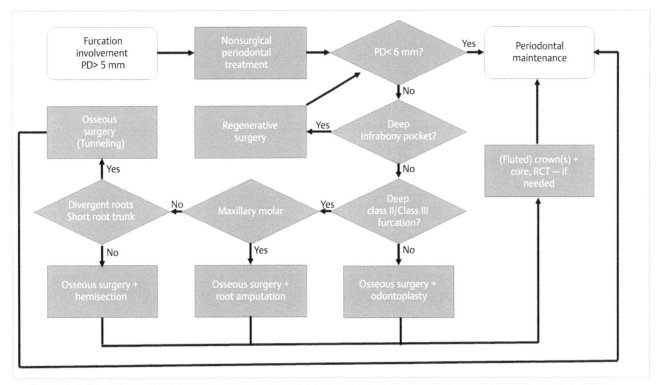

Fig. 7.3 Treatment planning for furcation involvement other than maintenance "as is" or extraction. If a tooth presents with furcation involvement, deep pocketing and it is desired to keep tooth and improve it with treatment, the next step is nonsurgical periodontal treatment including oral hygiene instruction and SRP. If this fails to resolve pocketing, regenerative surgery should be attempted first for deep infrabony pockets suitable for regeneration as it may improve the condition. If regeneration is not indicated, or did not resolve pocketing, osseous surgery combined with odontoplasty should reshape tooth and surrounding bone of teeth with shallow Class II or I defects. If the furcation has a deep horizontal depth on a maxillary molar, root amputation may eliminate the furcation involvement. For mandibular molars, tunneling can provide oral hygiene access on teeth with shallow root trunks and divergent roots. Otherwise, hemisection can remove the furcation roof in mandibular molars by either removing a root or transforming each half of the tooth into a premolar-like tooth. Hemisection, root amputation, and odontoplasty require a new full coverage restoration for each retained tooth. Root canal therapy and core build-up typically are required after hemisection and root amputation, and may be needed after odontoplasty.

it is a useful approach for simplifying periodontal treatment in arches containing second and third molars with furcation involvement.

The major disadvantage with this approach is the loss of occlusal function and bone that comes with tooth extraction. Tooth replacement is most likely necessary for any teeth other than 2nd or 3rd molars. Tooth replacement is costly with implant therapy the most expensive dental treatment. Moreover, restorations replacing missing teeth most likely need periodic replacement, and pose a risk for recurrent disease. Therefore, for most patients, the goal of dental therapy should be to maintain natural teeth as long as possible.

7.4.3 Combined Pocket Reduction and Tooth Shaping Approach

The goal should be to preserve most teeth with furcation involvement with periodontal and restorative therapy. Indications for the tooth in question are as follows:
- Tooth is of importance to the patient and overall treatment (especially first molars).
- Tooth lacks mobility.
- Restoration is possible.

- Patient is willing to undergo procedures and willing to maintain teeth long term.

The advantage of this method is that it preserves teeth and function at a relatively low cost and facilitates long-term periodontal maintenance. There is no real disadvantage to this approach.

7.4.4 Pocket-reduction Strategy

Initially, pocket reduction should be attempted with nonsurgical therapy including oral hygiene and SRP, even though this will likely not resolve the furcation involvement. It will, however, simplify the remaining treatment through better gingival health.

For oral hygiene, the following may be effective:
- End-tufted tooth brush for very wide, exposed buccal, and distalmost furcation entrances.
- Small interproximal brushes for insertion into wide, exposed furcation entrances.
- Rubber-tipped stimulators (i.e., GUM Stimudent) for narrow furcation entrances.
- Oral irrigators (with subgingival tip, if available) for any furcation involvement.

For SRP, the following instrumentation may be useful:
• Ultrasonic tips including fine periodontal tips.
• DeMarco furcation curettes.
• Diamond-coated Nabor probes for narrow furcation entrances.

Commonly, nonsurgical techniques will not reduce pocketing associated with a furcation entrance. Regenerative techniques should be attempted next, especially if the furcation entrance is associated with a large bone defect. In most cases, this will create a smaller, shallower furcation involvement that is easier to manage for definite treatment, and regenerative treatment is unlikely to worsen furcation involvement. For this reason, regenerative surgery should even be attempted at nonmobile teeth with accessible Class III furcation involvement as long as the patient is willing to undergo this procedure.

7.4.5 Osseous Surgery Alone is not Sufficient for Furcation Treatment

Osseous surgery by itself should not be used for the sole purpose of furcation treatment, as it does not resolve the furcation involvement. After osseous surgery, pockets likely will be reduced around the furcation and furcation may now be accessible for professional cleaning, but is still difficult to near impossible for patients to clean. Consequently, the tooth is still at risk for new disease.

7.4.6 Reshaping of Tooth

While pocket reduction should be done for most furcation-involved teeth with pocketing, it does not eliminate the furcation involvement unless a regenerative procedure by chance filled the furcation completely. Most likely, the furcation

remains and continues to present an oral hygiene and maintenance problem, which may lead to new disease at the site.

The only treatment that can directly eliminate furcation involvement is reshaping the tooth with a biologic shaping technique.

Reshaping the tooth usually requires full coverage, fluted restoration (▶ Fig. 7.4), which provides easy oral hygiene and scaling access to the former furcation area. Key to this restoration is that the restoration does not form an overhang over the furcation area, but features a smooth metallic groove in this area that extends to the occlusal surface.

Root reshaping is treatment planned in different ways depending on the depth and location of the furcation:
• Depth of furcation extends less than 1/3 third of tooth from both directions—Odontoplasty:
  ○ This can be done as part of pocket-reduction surgery (i.e., osseous surgery).
  ○ Core-build up may be needed, depending on the amount of tooth structure remaining after removal of old restorative material and caries.
  ○ Root canal therapy may be needed, if the pulp is exposed.
  ○ A new full coverage restoration (i.e., porcelain fused to metal [PFM] crown) is needed unless no dentin is exposed.
• Depth of furcation extends a 1/3 of the tooth from both directions:
  ○ *If maxilla*: Consider root amputation if palatal root and one of the buccal roots are sound and have no periodontal involvement.
  ○ *If mandible*: Consider hemisection and removal of a root or transforming roots into two premolar-type teeth.
  ○ Either scenario requires root canal treatment, core build-up, and full coverage restoration (or two restorations for each root of a hemisected tooth).

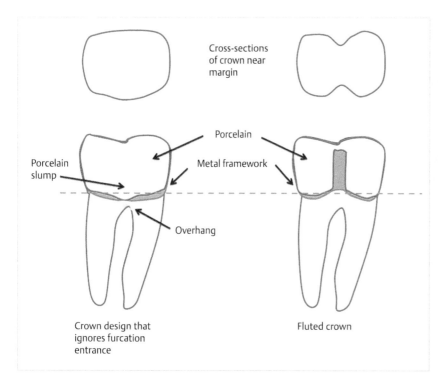

Cross-sections of crown near margin

Porcelain

Metal framework

Porcelain slump

Overhang

Crown design that ignores furcation entrance

Fluted crown

Fig. 7.4 In areas of furcation involvement, the crown margin must follow the furcation contour and the lab technician making the crown must be aware of the furcation in this area. Since the master cast die for the crown fabrication will not indicate the furcation area, the lab technician will create the typical convex crown over the furcation entrance, and applied porcelain tends to slump, especially on the mid-facial or mid-lingual aspect. If this is not corrected prior to crown placement, the metal margin will traverse the furcation entrance and form together with the slumped porcelain an overhang. In order to avoid this overhang, alert the lab technician that this area should be "fluted" and be kept as polished metal.

○ If the root trunk is short, roots long and the furcation is wide (>1 mm) on a mandibular molar, tunneling is an option. Tunneling is treatment planned as part of "osseous surgery," and tunneled teeth do not require restoration.

7.5 Surgical Methods for Class I and Class II Furcation Treatment

The focus of furcation treatment is to create a tooth that is maintainable. The goals of surgical therapy of furcation involvement are: elimination of contributing factors such as subgingival calculus and root surface abnormalities; creation of tooth surfaces that are less likely to retain plaque, and recreation of normal local anatomy that favors wound healing and periodontal health. There are three different surgical techniques to treat furcations: resection, regeneration, and biologic shaping.

7.5.1 General Consent Issues and Patient Preparation

Regardless of the technique chosen, the benefits, risks, and alternatives need to be discussed with the patient prior to surgery, and this discussion properly documented in the patient's chart. In general, the benefit of surgical furcation treatment is the increased likelihood of tooth survival. The risks are the typical surgical risks such as injury, bleeding, swelling, pain, local bruising, and infection along with the typical periodontal risks of periodontal surgery such as increased tooth length, gum recession, root sensitivity, increased tooth mobility, and potential for the therapy not to produce desired results. In addition to these risks, the patient needs to be aware that restorative treatment including root canal therapy may be needed in some cases, and that long-term success depends on good home care and frequent professional tooth cleaning. As with general pocket-reduction surgery, the alternative to surgical treatment of furcation is either no treatment at all, continued nonsurgical treatment or tooth removal. All alternatives may carry a higher risk of tooth loss, and patients need to understand this risk if they chose not to undergo periodontal surgery.

The preoperative preparation is similar to general pocket-reduction surgery techniques. Patients should be premedicated in the hours preceding surgery with analgesics such as Ibuprofen (i.e., 400 mg every 4 hours) and have enough tablets (either as over-the-counter medicines like Motrin or generic Ibuprofen 200 mg; or as prescription for 400 mg tablets) for 4 to 7 days depending on the size and depth of the surgery. If bone graft materials or membranes are used for the surgery, or if a patient has compromised immunity (i.e., poorly controlled diabetes mellitus), patients need to be premedicated with antibiotics such as Amoxicillin as well. Typically, a simple course of Amoxicillin 500 mg every 8 hours, for a week starting 1 hour prior to surgery is appropriate for most regenerative surgeries and patients.

7.5.2 Regenerative Technique

Regenerative treatment of furcation-involved teeth can improve the longevity of teeth and create a more manageable furcation involvement if it works.

Indications

Prior to definite resective treatment of furcation involvement, regeneration should be attempted whenever there is a chance of improvement and the patient is willing to undergo this procedure as part of periodontal treatment for a tooth with furcation involvement.

Generally, regenerative techniques should be attempted for furcation involvements associated with:
- Deep bone defects.
- Buccal or lingual Glickman Class II furcation involvement with a deep horizontal component.
  ○ Guided tissue regeneration works best on mandibular molars, but not on interproximal furcation defects of maxillary molars.

Even though much less predictable, regenerative techniques may be attempted for the following:
- Interproximal Glickman class II furcation involvement using bone grafts.
- Mandibular molar Glickman class III furcation involvement using guided tissue regeneration.
- Shallow bone defects.

Even though in these cases guided tissue regeneration is not predictable, it still may improve the clinical outlook of a tooth, especially if done by an experienced surgeon.

Risks

The surgical risks for regenerative therapy are generally the same as for periodontal surgery. The main risk of regenerative surgery is that it does not work, and fails to improve the outlook of a given tooth. If it does not resolve the furcation, a second resective surgery is needed for definite treatment of the furcation involvement. The addition of graft materials and membranes may pose an increased risk of postoperative infections, delayed healing, premature membrane or graft exposure, swelling, and pain compared to resective treatment.

Benefits

Regenerative treatment can resolve furcation involvement or simplify subsequent definite treatment without excessive risk.

Technique

The technique is similar to regenerative procedures aimed at pocket reduction.

Instrumentation and Anesthesia

The following instruments are needed:
- Local anesthesia syringe and short/extra short needle.
- Mirror and periodontal probe.
- Scalpel and blade (i.e., no. 15c blade).
- Periosteal elevators.
- SRP instruments.
- Surgical handpiece, supplies for sterile irrigation (i.e., Monojet syringes filled with sterile saline).
- Regenerative materials (i.e., bone graft, membranes, and biologics).
- Surgical burs for hard tissue removal.

- Suturing supplies (i.e., 5–0 sutures; P3 needle is useful for delicate tissue suturing, FS-2 useful for suturing between molars).
- Needle holder (i.e., Castroviejo) and suture scissors.
- Bone grafting syringe, tissue forceps for handling the membrane.
- Orban knifes for interproximal tissue removal.

As with most periodontal surgery, this technique can be accomplished using local infiltration anesthesia with 2% lidocaine and 1:100,000 epinephrine. Local infiltration with 2% lidocaine and 1:50,000 epinephrine is useful to produce a drier surgical field.

Flap Design

The flap design for the regenerative approach needs to preserve the gingival tissue as much as possible so that it can fully cover membranes and bone graft materials. For full access to the bone and root surfaces, a full thickness flap is used. The steps for the incision are as follows:

- Inspect the gingiva and determine where areas of inflammation and puffiness are. These areas tend to tear during the flap elevation process, resulting in possible areas where the flap may expose the graft or membrane. Handle these areas with extra care when manipulating the tissue. Note areas of thin gingiva as regeneration is less likely to succeed there.
- Create envelope flap for affected sextant:
  - *Determine distal-most point of flap*: If regeneration involves distal-most tooth, begin at distal end of maxillary tuberosity or intersection of occlusal plane with retromolar pad. If regeneration does not involve distal-most tooth, begin at distal surface of distal-most tooth.
  - Begin the incision on the distal-most aspect as determined before, pushing the blade (i.e., no. 15c) all the way through the tissue contacting bone, and in a smooth motion and firmly in contact with bone, move the scalpel straight along the ridge crest to the distal surface of the last tooth. From there, for both buccal and lingual side of the tooth, continue to move the scalpel mesially, following the sulcus of each tooth as much as possible and maintaining contact with the alveolar crest at all times until the distobuccal and distolingual of the canine is reached.
- Create vertical release at distobuccal line angle of canine in the same sextant to a point near the floor of the buccal vestibule.
- Elevate the flap edges by first using a twisting motion with the scalpel blade full inserted into the incision line at the flap edges and papilla tips, and then elevate the entire flap off the bone with progressively larger-sized periosteal elevators. This should yield a clean, lightly yellow bone surface with few if any red tissue tags attached. Elevate the tissue just past the mucogingival junction where it exists, or about half-way toward the floor of the palate.
- On the buccal side, pull back the flap with tissue forceps, exposing the periosteum underside of the flap. Just about at the level of the mucogingival junction, gently incise the periosteum by 1 mm along the entire flap and feel the flap edge gaining a small amount of elasticity. This will help advancing the flap over membranes or graft material.

- Remove the interproximal papilla remnant by detaching it from the tooth and alveolar crest with a scalpel or Orban knives inserted on the mesial, distal, and apical side of the soft tissue remnant. Dislodge and remove each interproximal tissue remnant with a sharp scaler or curette.

Bone Removal

Inspect the exposed defect. If the bone defect is too narrow to allow root planing of the furcation surfaces, widened the moth of the bone defect slightly with a round carbide surgical bur. Remove any ledges or small tori adjacent to the furcation entrance to make membrane application easier.

Root Surface Preparation

Perform scaling and root planing as described previously, achieving a smooth root surface finish devoid of any calculus or plaque. Use rotary diamond instrumentation to remove enamel pearls, enamel projections, grooves, root concavities, and other root surface abnormalities known to interfere with regeneration. Widen the furcation entrance to at least 3 mm in diameter, and make sure that the entrance has an inverted "U" shape. Be careful not to accidentally expose pulp tissue. Rescale and root plane furcation entrances to a smooth finish after rotary instrumentation. If instructed by a biologics manufacturer, apply root conditioning agent (i.e., EDTA gel from Emdogain kit) followed by actual biologic according to instructions.

Bone Graft Application

Have an assistant carefully drop sterile graft package from outer package shell onto sterile work surface, and have the assistant safe keep any required bone graft documentation including tissue bank mailing card.

Hydrate particulate bone graft material according to instructions supplied with the graft container. Usually, this involves dripping a sterile wetting solution (i.e., sterile saline or the content of an unused local anesthetic cartridge) into the bone graft container, gently tapping the container to release trapped air bubbles in the graft material and letting the graft soak in the liquid for a few minutes. Excess moisture can be drawn out with a damp sterile 2 × 2 sponge pad, leaving a graft material with the consistency and stickiness of wet sand. If using autogenous bone chips, harvest these with a harvesting device from an area of excess bone according to the device instructions, taking care not to damage roots and vital structures.

Scoop bone graft particles with a clean periosteal elevator into any bone defect. Gently pad bone graft into the defect, taking care not to pack the graft tightly or overfilling the defect.

Membrane Application

Carefully have an assistant drop the sterile envelope containing membrane from outer packaging onto sterile work surface.

Separate envelope from actual membrane and set aside membrane. Cut a piece off the envelope using suture scissors or take the template material provided with the membrane. Apply this material to the bone defect and use suture scissors to trim it until it passively drapes over the bone defect or graft material. The template should fit over the defect and tooth similar to an apron and extend at least several millimeters past the defect edge onto the bone. The template also needs to be able to rest against the tooth at the CEJ. Once it fits, take this template, blot it dry, overlay it on the actual membrane and trim the membrane to match the template. Make sure to keep track of the actual membrane and discard the template. Unless the membrane comes with an attached suture, take a small resorbable suture (i.e., chromic gut 4–0) and carefully thread it half-way through one corner of the membrane. The side of the membrane with the suture needle will be facing toward the tooth.

For some membranes, it is easiest to place the membrane in a dry state since blood-soaked membranes are too sticky and friable to be handled easily. For interproximal application, it may help to roll up the membrane into a stick form, stick it through the interproximal space and then unroll the buccal and lingual sides of the membrane. Place the membrane over the defect or graft material, feed the suture through the nearest interproximal space around the opposite site of the tooth to the far interproximal space. Pass the suture from the underside of the membrane to the surface, and tie a surgical knot. This should secure the membrane tightly against the root surface, and make the membrane drape over the defect or graft material.

Suturing

The goal of suturing for regenerative procedures is to ensure coverage of the graft or membrane by soft tissue and minimize flap movement. Inverting vertical mattress sling combination sutures can accomplish these requirements by firmly holding flap edges to teeth and anchor the flap firmly against the underlying graft or membrane while minimizing tissue thickness. For this suturing technique, a suitable suture material (i.e., chromic gut 5–0 with a reverse cutting 3/8 circle FS-2 needle) and a small needle holder (i.e., Castroviejo) are useful.

- If vertical releases were used, align each mesial and distal flap edge to the surrounding tissues with a simple interrupted suture, making sure not to exert any pull on the tissue.
- Connect the interproximal flap edges with vertical inverting mattress sling combination sutures.
  - For each interproximal space, insert the needle into the tissue at the base of the flap in unelevated tissue apical to the interproximal space and have the needle return to the flap surface just coronal to the mucogingival junction.
  - Feed the needle and suture under the contact point and outside of the flap tissue to the lingual side.
  - If there is a tooth distal to the interproximal contact, wrap the suture around the tooth distal to this interproximal contact by passing the suture back to the buccal on the distal side of the tooth and back again to the lingual side through the original interproximal contact. If there is no distal tooth, wrap the suture around the mesial tooth. Pull the suture snug against the tooth.
  - Insert the needle into the lingual flap about 5-mm apical to the flap edge and interproximal space, and let it resurface over the still unelevated base of the flap.
  - Feed the needle and suture under the contact point and just outside of the flap tissue back to the buccal.
  - As long as there is a mesial tooth to the interproximal space, wrap the suture around the tooth by passing the suture back to the lingual on the mesial side of the tooth and back again to the buccal through the original interproximal contact. If there is no mesial tooth, wrap the

suture around the distal tooth again. Pull the suture snug against the tooth.
  - Tie the suture and watch the tissue being pushed against the tooth and underlying bone.
  - Repeat for every interproximal contact and the distal and mesialmost tooth surface.
- With simple interrupted sutures, connect the flap and surrounding tissues at the vertical releases.
- Apply pressure with wet gauze until bleeding stops. The tissue usually stops bleeding after the suturing is applied.

7.5.3 Biologic Shaping

Biologic shaping is a very predictable technique that aims to *shape tooth surfaces* for improved maintenance. It was developed by Dr Melker[5–7] and uses specific burs to address the entire root surface (▶Fig. 7.5 and ▶Fig. 7.6).

Indications

This method can directly eliminate furcation involvement. This method can be used for the treatment of the following:
- Glickman Class I and shallow Glickman Class II furcation involvement.
- Glickman Class III and deep Glickman Class II furcation involvement if combined with hemisection or root amputation techniques.

In addition to furcation treatment, biologic shaping also allows definite treatment of root surface defects such as developmental grooves, enamel projections, dentin ridges, and abnormal root surfaces such as ledges, gouges, and restorative flash.

It also is an alternative to conventional crown lengthening procedures (▶Fig. 7.7), where it requires less bone removal than conventional crown lengthening.

Regardless of indication, biologic shaping usually requires fabrication of (a) new crown(s), and may require core build-up and root canal treatment if the furcation is deep or the tooth has been compromised by recurrent caries.

Risks

From a patient perspective, there are no risks other than the typical surgical risks of minimal bleeding during the procedure, limited postoperative pain, and minimal risk of postoperative infection. Patients need to understand that this technique requires restoration of teeth and that these teeth will be shaped slightly different than the original tooth.

While there is a possibility of tooth sensitivity from exposed dentin during the healing time, root surface medications applied after treatment effectively prevent tooth sensitivity. For teeth with shallow Classes I and II furcation involvement, the chance of accidental root exposure is very low. For the practitioner, the technique requires the ability to raise a split thickness flap and good restorative skills.

Benefits

This technique is more predictable than the regenerative approach. From a patient perspective, this approach preserves existing teeth, gum tissue and bone, avoids reentry and revision procedures needed after some types of

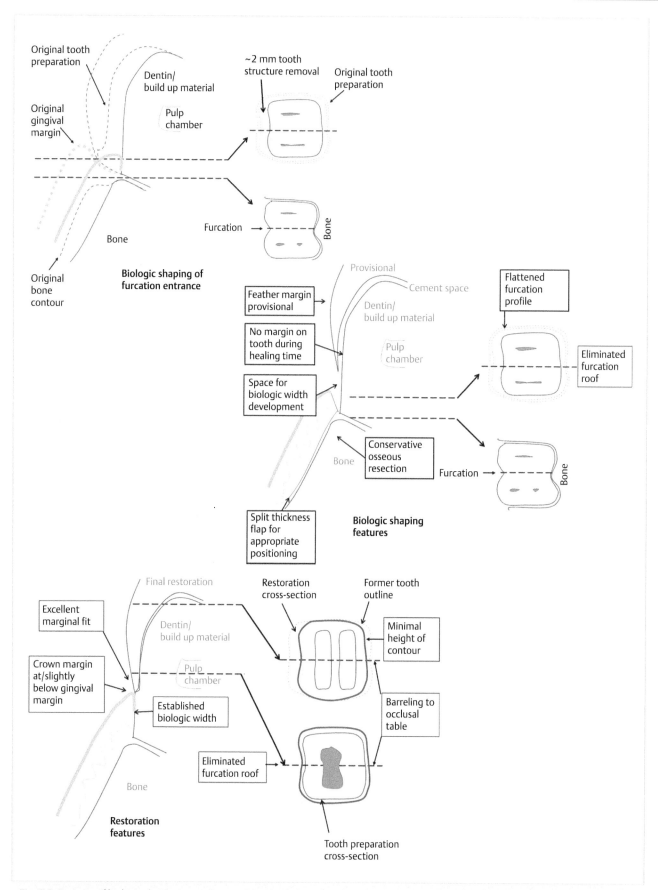

Fig. 7.5 Features of biologic shaping.

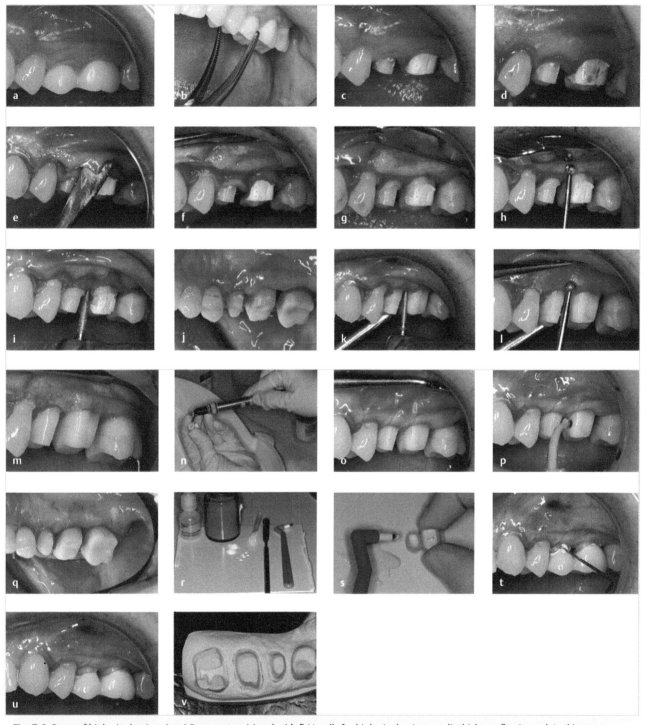

Fig. 7.6 Steps of biologic shaping. (**a–c**) Remove provisionals. (**d–f**) Usually for biologic shaping, a split thickness flap is used. In this case, because of the exostosis, a full thickness flap was raised to uncover the exostosis and the tissue was split after the blade passed the exostosis. The initial step back removed hyperplastic tissue in this case. (**g–i**) Remove bone shelfs and old margins. (**j–k**) Remove furcation roofs, root concavities, and other root defects. (**l–m**) Create parabolic and smooth bony architecture. (**n**). Air blow provisional to remove oils. (**o**) Suture flaps together. (**p–q**) Apply desensitizing solution and let it seal dentinal tubules. (**r–u**) Recement provisionals that have feather margins and supply room for the gingiva to reattach and redevelop biologic width. (**v**) Get impressions with the final margins once tissue is stable. (These images are provided courtesy of Dr. Melker.)

regenerative surgery, and carries little surgical risk. From a dentist's perspective, this technique can preserve teeth that have a poor prognosis and would otherwise be replaced with implant-supported restorations. This technique can also be used to restore teeth with furcation involvement that are poor candidates for conventional crown lengthening technique.

Compared to conventional crown lengthening, it has several benefits: it removes the old margin entirely thus allowing for minimal removal of bone. By preserving bone, the integrity of the furcation area is preserved and does not worsen the existing crown-to-root ratio; creates a smooth root surface that is predictable to restore and maintain.

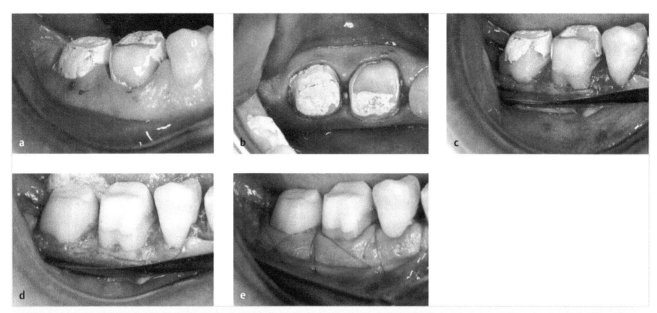

Fig. 7.7 Biologic shaping as a bone-sparing alternative to conventional crown lengthening surgery. (**a–b**). After removal of provisionals existing tooth surface can be seen. (**c**) A split thickness flap reveals proximity of the furcations on nos. 30 and 31. A significant problem is the location of the previous margin location approximating the bone on the mesial aspect of no. 30. With conventional crown lengthening, 3–5 mm of bone on the mesial to create a space for the Biologic width. Unfortunately to create a proper biologic osseous contour, several mm of bone will need to be removed on both the buccal and lingual to create a parabolic architecture. This would significantly weaken the tooth as it is removing supporting bone as well as the adjacent tooth where the same amount of bone would need removal. Biologic shaping instead removes any existing furcation issues, existing margins and requires only minimal bone removal to create a parabolic architecture. Biologic shaping allows a new biologic width to establish many times coronal to the original location of the old margins thus preventing needless removal of bone and preserving the stability of the teeth. (**d**) Completed biologic shaping. Note conservative bone removal and furcation elimination. (**e**) Suturing adapts the tissue tightly to underlying bone and teeth for uneventful healing. (These images are provided courtesy of Dr. Melker.)

The key to the success of biologic shaping is the creation of a tooth surface that is amenable to the hygienists' curettes and patient home care.

Technique

The technique requires important presurgical and postsurgical preparation, and the steps are as follows (▶ Fig. 7.6).

Instruments and Local Anesthesia

The instruments are the same as for pocket-reduction surgery:
- Local anesthesia syringe and supplies.
- Mirror and periodontal probe.
- Mosquito forceps.
- Round scalpel handle and blades (i.e., nos. 15c, 12d blade).
- Periosteal elevators.
- Goldman-Fox periodontal knife (or other suitable periodontal knives).
- SRP instruments.
- A surgical handpiece and supplies for sterile irrigation (i.e., Monojet syringes filled with sterile saline).
- Surgical burs for hard tissue removal (F-82 coarse and superfine diamond burs for teeth, no. 6 round carbide, and no. 8 round diamond).
- Restorative burs and materials for the adjustment of provisional restorations.
- Tissue forceps.
- Suturing supplies (i.e., chromic gut 5–0 for superficial sutures, Ethicon FS-2 needle is useful for interproximal suturing between molars, P-3 for thin tissue).

- Needle holder (i.e., Castroviejo) and suture scissors. Bone chisels, files, and periodontal knives can be useful but are not required.
- Potassium oxalate gel (i.e., Thermatrol).
- Polycarboxylate cement (i.e., Duralon, Tylok).

As with most periodontal surgery, this technique can be accomplished using local infiltration anesthesia from buccal and lingual sides. Local infiltration, with 2% lidocaine and 1:50,000 epinephrine, is useful to produce a drier urgical field.

Presurgical Preparation

- Assess the gingival tissue surrounding the tooth. Treatment plan a connective tissue graft in addition to the osseous surgery and odontoplasty if the gingiva appears thin and translucent.
- Remove all caries, existing restorative materials. Perform endodontic treatment if pulp exposure occurs.
- Build-up tooth with resin-based core material (if needed).
- Prepare tooth with a feather edge margin on sound tooth structure. The feather edge margin at this step preserves tooth structure.
- Provisionalize tooth with acrylic provisional and cement with polycarboxylate cement (i.e., Durelon, Tylok).

Surgical Appointment

- Provide local anesthesia.
- Engage provisional crown with a mosquito forceps at the incisal third and remove with a gentle rocking motion to avoid fracture of the provisional.

- Assess the surgical area and determine mesio-distal extent of flap, usually 1–2 teeth mesial and distal to the tooth needing biologic shaping. Make a smooth incision that follows the sulcus and steps back from tooth whenever needed to remove hyperplastic/diseased tissue as described previously. If exostoses or tori are present, elevate a full thickness flap to fully expose these bony protuberances. Otherwise, create a split thickness flap by carefully dissecting the flap edge so that there is a layer of connective tissue remaining on alveolar bone. A 15C blade is useful in splitting the interdental papilla and beginning the split thickness flap there. A no. 4 Goldman fox blade is useful in removing tissue tags adhering to the tooth.
- Remove bone with surgical diamond burs (i.e., no. 6) to reestablish biologic width, create physiologic contours, and remove exostoses with a carbide round bur (i.e., no. 8). Accidental nicks in the root surface will be corrected at the next step.
- Perform biologic shaping using diamond burs such as the F-82 coarse and superfine burs:
  - Remove any enamel remnants and the CEJ. Remove any old chamfer/shoulder margins.
  - Remove cervical enamel projections.
  - Remove furcation roofs.
  - Flatten roots/eliminate concavities.
  - Use an ultra-fine diamond bur (F-82) for the final root surface finish.
- Smooth bone with round diamond to eliminate bone shelves. Make sure that positive architecture has been achieved.
- If needed to correct thin gingival tissue, harvest connective tissue (as described in Chapter 8) and place connective tissue graft if needed.
- Suture tissue firmly against the alveolar crest with 5–0 gut (see photographs as a guide).
- Apply potassium oxylate (i.e., Thermatrol) on exposed root surfaces for 45–60 seconds and air dry lightly repeat. Repeat 2–3 times.
- Clean provisional.
- Adjust and recement provisional with polycarboxylate cement (i.e., Durelon). When cementing the provisional following suturing, it must be 1-mm shy of the sutured tissue to allow for continued biologic width growth in a coronal direction. Therefore, the provisional will need adjustment at the apical area (margin) to avoid contact with the tissue.
- *Provide postoperative and specific oral hygiene instruction*: Rinse with chlorhexidine prescription mouthrinse (i.e., PerioGuard 0.12% Chlorhexidine, 16 oz., rinse with ½ oz., for 30 seconds after brushing and flossing at least twice daily) starting in evening after the surgery; use prescription fluoride toothpaste (i.e., Prevident 1.1% sodium fluoride) at bedtime starting on the surgery day; water/Listerine rinse after meals.

Postsurgical Treatment

- Four weeks after surgery, remake/reline provisional with margin 1-mm coronal to tissue margin to allow tissue regrowth; recement.
- Fourteen weeks after surgery, re-prepare tooth with chamfer margins just coronal to the gingival collar. If endodontic treatment was done and the remaining tooth structure is dark, the margin can be extended slightly into sulcus to avoid cosmetic issue.

- Restore tooth. In furcation areas, the furcation must be barreled in to the occlusal surface.
- Provide continued oral hygiene instruction when needed and ensure adequate maintenance. Consider continued fluoride therapy (i.e., daily stannous fluoride rinse) to prevent recurrent decay.

Treating Postoperative Sensitivity after Biologic Shaping

While uncommon, some patients may experience more significant tooth sensitivity after biologic shaping. For patients needing more extensive biologic shaping, the following treatment addresses this issue.

Desensitizers

- Prednisilone acetate ophthalmic suspension USP 1%.
- Phoenix Dental, Inc. Super Seal dental desensitizer liner.
- Colgate Prevident gel (1.1% sodium fluoride).
- Colgate Prevident Varnish (Vanish) 5% fluoride.
- Colgate Sensitive Pro-relief desensitizing paste.
- 3M Espe CavityShield 5% sodium fluoride.
- Sultan Topex in-office fluoride rinse.

Desensitizing Treatments

Surgery

Super seal is used after suturing. Teeth must be dry and one drop is placed on each tooth and lightly air blow dry after 30–40 seconds—repeat 3 to 4 times. If the teeth have been severely barreled into the furcation, a drop of Prednisolone 1% is also placed on the teeth.

Patient is given Prevident Gel 1.1% sodium fluoride to rinse with at home twice daily.

Week 1

Patient is scaled with a universal implant scaler (double end) because it is made with plastic and more comfortable for the patient.

Patient is polished with Colgate Sensitive Pro-Relief desensitizing paste—the wooden end of a cotton-tipped applicator is used to spread paste inter-proximally.

If patient cannot brush, a drop of prednisolone is placed on the teeth. Patient rinses with Sultan Topex in-office fluoride rinse for 1 minute. Patient is to keep rinsing 2 × a day with Prevident Gel. Prevident Gel is to be expectorated after use and they cannot eat, drink or rinse for 30 minutes after use.

If the patient is able to start brushing, a drop of Prednisolone is placed on the teeth. Prevident Varnish or 3M Cavity Shield is placed on the teeth. Patient is instructed to brush off in 4 hours with regular toothpaste. Patient is to start brushing with Prevident Gel 2 × a day for 1 minute after they have brushed with regular toothpaste. Prevident Gel is to be expectorated after brushing and they cannot eat, drink or rinse for 30 minutes after use.

Following Weeks

All treatments are based on whether a patient is allowed to brush or not.

If the patient cannot brush, a drop of Prednisolone is placed on the teeth. Patient is to keep rinsing 2× a day with Prevident

Gel. Patient rinses with Sultan Topex in-office fluoride rinse for 1 minute.

If the patient is able to start brushing, a drop of Prednisolone is placed on the teeth. Prevident Varnish or 3M Cavity Shield is placed on the teeth. Patient is instructed to brush off in 4 hours with regular toothpaste. Patient is to start brushing with Prevident Gel 2 × a day for 1 minute after they have brushed with regular toothpaste.

Treatments are continued until patient is comfortable.

General Postoperative Care

Surgical treatment of furcation involvement produces the same healing as pocket-reduction surgery as the surgical approach is largely the same. In general, bleeding from periodontal surgery is usually capillary-based and usually stops with proper suturing technique. If there is postoperative bleeding after periodontal surgery, it can be predictably stopped with pressing wet gauze or wet black tea bags for 10–15 minutes on any bleeding area. Postoperative pain is best prevented by setting the expectation for minor discomfort after the surgery, good surgical technique, a preoperative single dose of non-steroidal anti-inflammatory drugs such as Aspirin, Ibuprofen or Acetaminophen, and the postoperative intermittent application of ice packs. In our experience, discomfort is worst immediately after the anesthesia wears off, and it quickly tapers off within a day of the surgery. Dentinal hypersensitivity can predictably be treated with dentinal tube sealing agents such as potassium oxalate gels. If using a resective or regenerative approach, the most important instruction to give to patients receiving this surgery is to leave the surgery area alone for 24 hours by not rinsing, spitting, or drinking from a straw to allow proper blood coagulation and the start of wound healing. Occasionally, a patient may develop a postoperative infection, which manifests itself in a sudden increase in pain during the healing time. The infection usually can be aborted by prescribing a broad-spectrum, bone-accumulating antibiotic such as clindamycin (i.e., 300 mg every 6 hours).

7.6 Describe Surgical Methods for Deep Class II and Class III Furcation Treatment

Deep Class II and Class III furcations generally bode poorly for tooth survival and often these teeth are removed early on during initial treatment. However, deep furcation involvement can be treated successfully and such teeth maintained for many years given proper case selection. As noted before, regeneration can be used to reduce or eliminate deep furcation involvement, although unpredictable. More predictably and long term, biologic shaping techniques can also be used reliably to eliminate deep furcations as well, although they will require the restoration of the tooth. Similarly, the traditional root resection and hemisection techniques require restoration of the tooth, along with root canal treatment, as they aim to eliminate the furcation by either removing the roof of the furcation or removing one side of the furcation by removing a tooth root. Conversely, the tunneling technique makes a Class III furcation involvement a virtue by enlarging it and providing oral hygiene access for patients.

7.6.1 Root Resection and Hemisection

Root resection and hemisection extend the principles of odontoplasty and eliminate the furcation by removing a tooth root and reshaping the tooth so that there is no longer a furcation roof. Since these procedures will expose the pulp chamber, root canal treatment, core build-up, and a crown are required treatment for these teeth.

Indications

In general, teeth were root resection or hemisection is considered need to have the following criteria besides a deep furcation involvement:

- *Good surgical access to the furcation*: This is best for teeth with short root trunks and wide furcation entrances. Root resection is difficult for teeth that have closely spaced tooth roots. Teeth with long root trunks are difficult to resect and likely will not have enough bone support to make this technique worthwhile.
- *Good crown-to-root ratio*: Root resection removes bony support and these teeth need strong remaining roots to support continued occlusion.
- *Strong remaining tooth roots*: Ribbon-shaped, narrow tooth roots are prone to fracture and are not suitable for this technique. Likewise, teeth that either have large root canals or had multiple endodontic retreatment.
- *Root and crown axis coincide*: Since the area of root resection is a mechanical weak point of the resected tooth, occlusal forces need to be directed parallel to the long axis of the remaining roots.
- *Normal bony architecture*: In order to make these teeth maintainable, there cannot be deep pocket depths around these tooth roots. To prevent pocketing, it is important to make ensure that the alveolar bone level still follows smoothly the remaining tooth roots with facial/lingual bone levels lower than interproximal/furcation bone levels.
- *Absence of excessive occlusal forces*: Root-resected teeth are prone to fractures since they are root canal treated and lack root support, and this is particularly true if the root resected tooth is the most distal tooth in the arch. To avoid fracture, the occlusal table of root resected teeth has to be smaller than that of normal molars, and is usually L-shaped to account for the missing tooth root in maxillary molars. For mandibular molars, the crown for each tooth half is usually shaped into a premolar-like tooth. Cantilevers should not be added to root-resected teeth and root resection should not be performed in patients with parafunctional habits.
- *Good oral hygiene*: Root-resected teeth are prone to caries because of their unique contours which tend to retain plaque. Therefore, this technique is reserved for patients who are willing and able to use Superfloss or other oral hygiene aid to keep these teeth clean.
- *Restorative skill of dentist/laboratory technician*: Creating a sound restorative margin on root resected teeth is more challenging than for typical crowns and requires great attention from both lab technician and dentist.

Treatment planning for root resective surgeries including hemisection involves the following steps:
- *Root canal treatment*: This step is easier to perform with the intact tooth as applying a rubber dam for isolation and

clamping the tooth is more difficult with the triangular or bisected shape of an amputated tooth.
- *Core build-up*: This is easier to perform with an intact tooth, and in the case of some build-up materials may strengthen the tooth which makes resection easier to perform. Depending on the remaining root shape, it may be necessary to add a post for retention of the build-up material.
- Root resective procedure—either:
  ○ Root amputation for maxillary molars and other multi-rooted teeth except mandibular molars with a mesial and distal root.
  ○ Hemisection for mandibular molars with a mesial and distal root.
- *Crown (either PFM or cast metal)*: This crown must have an emergence profile that matches the tooth shape after root resection, and needs to be easily cleansable by the patient. Full ceramic crowns and ceramic reconstruction (CEREC) crowns may not be possible their greater demand on tooth structure reduction.

Benefits

Prior to the widespread use of dental implants in replacing teeth with poor prognosis, root resective techniques were commonly used to retain teeth with deep furcation involvement. With good patient cooperation, surgical skill, and high-quality restorations, it is possible to maintain root resected teeth and surrounding gingiva in good healthy condition for many years (▶ Fig. 7.8).

Risks

Prior to surgery, the patient in addition to usual consent issues related to periodontal surgery needs to understand the importance of oral hygiene, and that the tooth will be smaller than the original tooth. The patient also needs to understand that root resected teeth likely will fail after a decade, as tooth survival ranges from 56 to 97% over 10–15 years.

Technique

The surgical procedure is similar to the resective approach already described, and uses odontoplasty techniques, which are as follows:
- Create a split thickness flap for the sextant as described for biologic shaping.
- Starting from the furcation entrance, insert a round carbide or diamond of at least 1-mm diameter into the furcation area and pull the bur toward the occlusal table. This removes the roof of the furcation.

- Follow the furcation anatomy by either bisecting the tooth as in a mandibular molar, or following the L-shaped furcation path of the furcation root in a maxillary molar, repeating the first step.
- When the tooth root is completely separated from the remaining tooth, use a tapered bur to flatten the sides of the channel now separating the tooth roots, taking care to eliminate any undercut.
- If root removal is needed (typically for maxillary molars), gently elevate root with a small apexo elevator and retrieve it with a small forceps or Rongeur.
- With a chamfer or shoulder bur (depending on preference for a restorative margin) create a continuous restorative margin that is about 3-mm coronal to the alveolar bone. The distance may be more for patients who have a thick gingival biotype as evidenced by a flap edge that is more than 3-mm thick. Make sure that the margin is well defined around the entire tooth including the furcation areas, and that there are no undercuts in the tooth preparation.
- Smooth any rough bone or tooth surface with hand instruments or a fine grit diamond bur.
- Complete remaining surgery steps (i.e., grafting) and suture flap edges to achieve minimal soft tissue thickness at the crest.
- Provisionalize crown(s).

7.6.2 Tunneling

While root resection and hemisection approaches can be effective for treating deep furcation involvement, a tooth-conservative approach is the tunneling procedure, which converts a deep furcation involvement into a wider channel that allows oral hygiene access through the entire furcation. Clinically, this leads to teeth with obvious Glickman Class IV furcation involvement which looks dramatic, but actually can maintain teeth with "hopeless" prognosis for a long time as tunneled teeth do not lose additional furcation bone after successful tunneling. The benefit of this procedure is that it does not require root canal therapy or restoration, and it can be a useful procedure for some teeth that have no caries, but deep furcation involvement (▶ Fig. 7.9).

Indications

In general, teeth were tunneling is considered need to have the following criteria besides deep furcation involvement:
- *Good surgical access to the furcation*: This is best for teeth with short root trunks, wide furcation entrances, and divergent roots. Typically, this is the case for mandibular molars

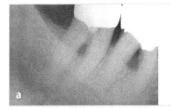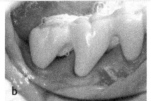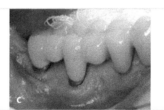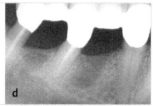

Fig. 7.8 Teeth with deep furcation involvement that have seemingly guarded or hopeless prognosis can be successfully treated long term with root resective approaches and diligent maintenance. This patient was seen 30 years ago and furcation involvement (**a**) was resolved with hemisection and restoration (**c**). 30 years after treatment, maintenance, and replacement of the restoration, bone levels are essentially unchanged (**b**) and the gingiva appears healthy (**d**). (These images are provided courtesy of Dr. Melker.)

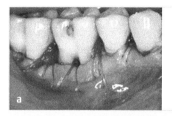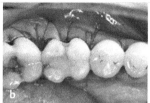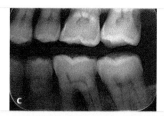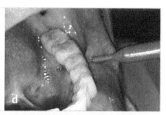

Fig. 7.9 Tunneling procedure. (**a, b**) Surgery completely exposes furcation and a suture is passed through the furcation to maintain the tunnel so that an interproximal brush can be inserted from both sides. (**c**) Radiograph of a tunneled no. 19. (**d**) The patient can maintain the furcation entrance by inserting an interproximal brush into the furcation entrance twice daily. ([**a–c**] These images are provided courtesy of Dr. Melker.)

with Class III furcation involvement. Tunneling without exposing the root canals is nearly impossible with closely spaced roots, and there is too much bone that has to be removed if tunneling is attempted on teeth with long root trunks.

- *Good oral hygiene*: This is absolutely essential for maintenance of these teeth as patients need to clean the furcation tunnel diligently to prevent root caries within the furcation tunnel.
- *Normal bony architecture*: In order to make these teeth maintainable, there cannot be deep pocket depths around these tooth roots. To prevent pocketing, it is important to make ensure that the alveolar bone level still follows smoothly the remaining tooth roots with facial/lingual bone levels lower than interproximal bone levels.
- *Absence of excessive occlusal forces*: The tunneling procedure may weaken the furcation area of a tooth by removing tooth structure, which possibly could invite tooth fracture.

Treatment planning a tunneling procedure is simple as it is a variant of osseous resective surgery, and no restorative procedures are required for tunneling. All that needs to be planned is "osseous surgery" and "odontoplasty."

Benefits

As with root resective techniques, this technique also was used to retain teeth with deep furcation involvement, especially prior to the advent of contemporary implant therapy. In contrast to root resective techniques, this technique rarely requires root canal treatment and restoration of the tooth.

Risks

Prior to surgery, the patient in addition to usual consent issues related to periodontal surgery needs to understand the importance of oral hygiene in preventing caries and tooth failure. In addition, the patient needs to understand that the tooth will look much longer than before, and have a "hole near the gum tissue on both sides of the tooth" where the patient needs to insert an interproximal brush from both sides at least twice daily to maintain the tooth. The patient also needs to understand that tunneled teeth are a method of preserving "hopeless" teeth, and that these teeth most often fail because of "cavities."

From a dentist's perspective, a major disadvantage of this procedure is the removal of furcation bone. When the tunneled tooth fails and is eventually extracted, the alveolar bone height will be substantially reduced. Since this procedure is

done mostly for mandibular molars, the reduced bone height may then preclude implant therapy as there will not be sufficient bone height to the inferior alveolar nerve for implant placement.

Technique

The surgical procedure is similar to the resective approach already described, and resembles the osseous surgery approach, as follows:

- Create a split thickness flap for the sextant as described for biologic shaping.
- Remove facial and lingual bone with an end-cutting bur so that it is apical to the interproximal bone level and clearly exposes the furcation entrance on both facial and lingual side. This requires exposure of about 4 mm of furcation entrance in apico-coronal direction.
- Starting from the furcation entrance, insert a round carbide or diamond of at least 1-mm diameter into the furcation area and carefully remove furcation bone following the furcation. Be careful not to drill into the tooth. Carefully remove bone from both sides of the furcation until there is a clear tunnel under the tooth.
- Lower the floor of the furcation tunnel until the floor is about 4-mm below the furcation roof.
- Gently odontoplasty the furcation entrance to round the furcation roof and eliminate root concavities within the furcation. Be careful not to perforate into the root canal or pulp chamber.
- Test if there is enough bone removal by replacing the flap tissue and inserting an interproximal brush. If the brush does not easily pass through to the other side, more bone removal is needed to lower the floor of the furcation tunnel.
- Smooth any rough bone or tooth surface with hand instruments or a fine grit diamond bur.
- Suture the flap area closed. For the furcation entrance, make sure to use a vertical inverting mattress suture with the suture running through the furcation entrance.

Instruct the patient to begin accessing the furcation channel with an interproximal brush within days of the surgery to keep the channel open and prevent food impaction.

7.7 Key Takeaways

- Furcation involvement is typically caused by local factors such as root concavities, ridges, and enamel projections.
- Furcation involvement by itself is not detrimental to prognosis.

- The goal of furcation treatment is to reduce pocketing around furcation entrances and make furcations more maintainable.
- Treatment of furcation involvement includes nonsurgical treatment and may involve flap surgery, osseous resective surgery, and regeneration for shallow and deep furcation involvement. Deep furcation involvement may involve root amputation, hemisection, or tunneling.
- Teeth with treated furcation defects can survive for about a decade, and usually fail because of caries or root fracture.

7.8 Review Questions

A 58-year-old African American male with a history of hypertension and high blood cholesterol presents for a dental exam after several years without dental treatment. He takes hydrochlorothiazide 12.5 mg, atorvastatin 20 mg, and tamsulosin 0.4 mg once daily. He has no known allergies. He has no dental complaint other than wanting a check-up since his gums bleed when he brushes. He brushes twice a day, but says he has a hard time flossing the back teeth.

Blood pressure is 125/78 mm Hg and he has a pulse of 69/min.

There are no significant extraoral findings, and there intraoral mucosal and salivary tissues appear normal other than signs of gingival inflammation near the molars.

Occlusion is canine-guided, Angle Class I with 2-mm overjet, and no overbite.

Findings in the periodontal chart are as follows (see ▶Fig. 7.10 for clinical appearance and ▶Fig. 7.11 for radiographs):

Maxilla

	1	2	3	4	5	6	7	8	9	10	11	12	13	14	15	16
Maxilla facial																
PD		437	848	725	636	535	323	333	633	343	627	527	638	636	734	
BOP		111	111	111	111	111	111	111	111	111	111	111	111	111	111	
CAL		5	6	6	2	2	2		1	1	2	3				
GR														2	2	
MGJ		888	888	888	888	888	888	888	888	888	888	888	888	856	655	
Furc		1	1											1	1	
PLQ		2	2	2	2	2	2	2	2	2	2	2	2	2	2	
Maxilla lingual																
PD		337	637	634	426	525	524	423	323	323	235	636	637	526	633	
BOP		111	111	111	111	111	111	111	111	111	111	111	111	111	111	
CAL													5	5	6	
GR		2	2													
Furc		1 1	1 1	1 1	1 1							1 1	1 1	1 1	1 1	
Mobil																
PLQ		2	2	2	2	2	2	2	2	2	2	2	2	2	2	

Mandible

	32	31	30	29	28	27	26	25	24	23	22	21	20	19	18	17
Mandible lingual																
PD	647	534		424	533	333	323	323	323	323	323	427	637	648	736	
BOP	111	111		111	111	111	111	111	111	111	111	111	111	111	111	
CAL	5										2	5	5	5	5	
GR																
MGJ	555	555	555	555	555	555	555	555	555	555	555	555	555	555	555	
Furc	2	2												2	2	
PLQ	2	2		2	2	2	2	2	2	2	2	2	2	2	2	
Mandible facial																
PD	527	833		424	423	425	323	323	323	323	323	426	323	335	536	
BOP	111	111		111	111	111	111	111	111	111	111	111	111	111	111	
CAL		4		2	1	1	1									
GR																
MGJ	555	555		555	555	555	555	555	555	555	555	555	555	555	555	
Furc	2	2												2	2	
Mobil																
PLQ	2	2		2	2	2	2	2	2	2	2	2	2	2	2	

Abbreviations: BOP, bleeding on probing (1), suppuration (2); CAL, clinical attachment level; Furc, furcation involvement (Glickman class); GR, gingival recession; MGJ, position of mucogingival junction from margin; Mobil, tooth mobility (Miller grade); PD, probing depths; PLQ, plaque level (0 = none, 5 = heavy).

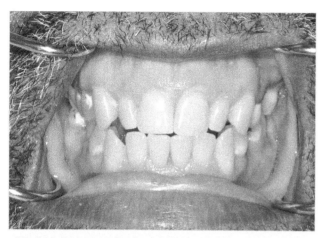

Fig. 7.10 Review case facial view.

Learning Objective: Recognize the effect of furcation involvement on tooth prognosis.

1. For tooth no. 3, besides plaque, what is an obvious factor that has contributed to the furcation involvement seen on the distal side of the tooth?
   A. Enamel pearl
   B. Root fracture
   C. Amalgam overhang
   D. Dentin ridge

2. For tooth no. 14, which of the following factors is UNLIKELY to have contributed to the furcation involvement seen on the mesial side of the tooth?
   A. Caries
   B. Lack of interproximal hygiene
   C. Bulky contour
   D. Enamel pearl

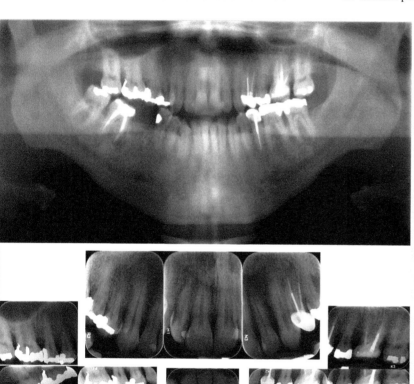

Fig. 7.11 Radiographic series for review case, taken at initial exam.

3. Evaluate the following statements:
   Statement 1: The mesial furcation of tooth no. 15 presents a problem for the restoration of the carious lesion on the mesial side of this tooth.
   Statement 2: Lingual furcation involvement is the most difficult to access surgically.
   A. Both statements are correct
   B. Neither statement is correct
   C. Only the first statement is correct
   D. Only the second statement is correct

Learning Objective: Develop strategies for managing furcation involvement.

4. This patient has deep probing depths and furcation involvement at the initial exam, and wishes to keep as many teeth as possible. Along with oral hygiene instruction, what treatment should you do next?
   A. SRP
   B. Pocket-reduction surgery
   C. Root amputation/Hemisection
   D. Regenerative therapy

5. After nonsurgical therapy including replacement of the amalgam restoration on tooth no. 19, probing depth now is 4 mm and the gingiva is coral-pink with no bleeding on probing. However, tissue recession exposed more of the furcation involvement on no. 19, which is now a deep Class II furcation involvement. What needs to be done?
   A. Osseous resective surgery
   B. Periodontal maintenance
   C. Regenerative therapy
   D. Tunneling procedure

6. Calculus and plaque levels are low, and tooth no. 31 has a deep Class II furcation involvement and unchanged probing depths. Which of the following techniques is most likely able to fill the furcation entrance with bone?
   A. Osseous resective surgery
   B. Regenerative therapy
   C. Surgical debridement
   D. Odontoplasty

Learning Objective: Describe surgical methods for Class I and Class II furcation involvement.

7. Evaluate the following statements:

   Statement 1: Surgical treatment of furcation usually involves raising a full thickness flap.
   Statement 2: Since this allows more possibilities apically position the flap.
   A. Both statement and reasoning are correct
   B. Neither statement nor reasoning is correct
   C. The reasoning is correct, but not the statement
   D. The statement is correct, but not the reasoning

8. From the case, which of the following teeth requires the least amount of preparatory work for odontoplasty?
   A. No. 31
   B. No. 18
   C. No. 3
   D. No. 14

9. Which of the following suture designs would be best suited to hold the flap close to the bone after furcation treatment of nos. 14 and 15?
   A. Vertical inverting mattress suture
   B. Figure 8 suture
   C. Simple interrupted
   D. Deep sling suture

Learning Objective: Describe surgical methods for Class II and Class III involvements.

10. Which of the following teeth is best suited for root amputation?
    A. Tooth no. 14
    B. Tooth no. 2
    C. Tooth no. 18
    D. Tooth no. 31

11. Which of the following teeth is best suited for tunneling?
    A. Tooth no. 14
    B. Tooth no. 2
    C. Tooth no. 18
    D. Tooth no. 31

7.9 Answers

1. **C.** The amalgam overhang is likely a contributing factor to the patient's periodontal disease at this tooth. There is no sign of an enamel pearl on the radiograph, which would appear as round radiodense area on the root surface. Dentin ridges are rarely seen on radiographs as they are too small to be seen on conventional radiographs unless location on the tooth root and film exposure accidentally highlight its position. Root fracture is highly unlikely as there is no radiographic sign for it. Root fractures usually are seen as cracks or separation of tooth pieces, and result in large areas of bone loss.

2. **D.** There is no sign of an enamel pearl. However, contributing factors are the caries on the root surface, the patient's self-professed inability to floss and the bulky mesial contour of the tooth.

3. **C.** There is significant caries on the mesial side of the tooth and just coronal to the furcation entrance, which poses a problem for caries removal. While access to lingual furcation involvement may be complicated by a tongue, it is less difficult than mesial or distal furcation entrances blocked by neighboring teeth.

4. **A.** This patient was seen for initial exam and has untreated periodontal disease. As with any untreated periodontal disease, the first step is nonsurgical treatment such as SRP. Although various surgical interventions can be performed, it is not advised since the tissue will be inflamed and difficult to handle. In addition, surgery time is limited and there may not be enough time to perform SRP during the surgery.

5. **B.** Periodontal maintenance. The key is to remember that furcation involvement only needs to be treated if there is disease. In this case scenario, probing depths are low and there is no inflammation suggesting periodontal healthy even if there is furcation involvement. Osseous surgery is possible, and could be used along odontoplasty to open up the furcation entrance to make it more cleansable. However, since there is no sign of disease—bleeding on

probing—it must be assumed the patient is already able to keep the area clean and maintain the furcation-involved tooth. Likewise, regenerative therapy is possible, but not needed as this already is disease-free. Tunneling can be done since it is a deep furcation involvement, but even if disease is present, you would want to attempt regenerating it first before undergoing such destructive treatment.

6. **B.** Regeneration. While some regrowth of bone occurs with surgical debridement, only regenerative techniques with either bone grafting or membrane application can regrow lost bone. Osseous resective surgery always results in net bone loss. Odontoplasty is a prerequisite for regeneration in most cases, but by itself it does little to regenerate bone.

7. **D.** Furcation treatment requires access to the bone, which means a full thickness flap. However, apical positioning can be achieved with either split or full thickness flap. A split thickness flap is used for soft tissue procedures such as pedicle flaps and soft tissue grafting as with these surgeries a graft devoid of blood supply needs to be embedded in soft tissue so it can get a blood supply.

8. **D.** Tooth no. 14 already is root canal treated and has a core build-up, in addition to shallow furcation involvement (at least clinically). Tooth no. 3 still has vital pulp and likely will need root canal treatment since preparation of the distal furcation will likely expose the pulp horn that reaches over the amalgam overhang. Tooth no. 18 has a Class II furcation involvement and likely needs root canal treatment. Tooth no. 31 is root canal treatment, but has a radiographic furcation arrow, meaning that the furcation involvement is deep and this tooth may be better served by hemisection or tunneling.

9. **A.** Inverting mattress sutures hold the tissue close to the bone as the suture is anchored in tissue deep in the vestibule and applies pressure on the coronal aspect of the flap as it runs across the ridge and over the flap edges. A simple interrupted suture simply pulls two flap edges together, and if anything, it pushes tissue upward at the flap edge. A figure 8 suture pulls tissue toward the center of the "8" and is used mostly for extraction sites. A sling suture usually is anchored around a tooth and pulls the tissue toward the tooth, which may cause the tissue to ride up against the tooth, leading to thicker tissue thickness as it heals.

10. **A.** Tooth no. 14. The tooth is already root canal treated, as divergent roots, and the mesiobuccal root is mostly exposed due to bone loss. No. 3 would need a root canal treatment, and has closely spaced roots that may be difficult to remove. Nos. 18 and 31 are mandibular teeth where hemisection is more appropriate.

11. **D.** Tooth no. 31 has the most divergent roots, and is already root canal treated. Hemisection and tunneling do not work well with maxillary molars as they have three roots and the furcation tunnel. Tooth no. 18 is not root canal treated and hence may be a candidate for tunneling as the roots are divergent and a good amount of bone is already missing in the furcation area. The only downside is that the remaining roots in the bone are not very long.

7.10 Evidence-based Activities

- Find studies that evaluate or report other rare methods in treating furcation involvement (i.e., lasers, furcation sealing) not described in this chapter, and debate their merit.
- Obtain a clinical case of furcation involvement from your institution (or look for cases on the web) and discuss which method presented in this chapter is best suited for your case. Make sure to discuss risks and benefits for each method, and determine which method is most likely to maintain teeth in your case.
- Critically evaluate the surgeries presented in this chapter, consult published case literature or other textbooks, and discuss if and how you would improve each surgery. Even though evidence may be limited, explain what you would differently and why.
- Go to the University of Texas Health Science Center School of Dentistry at San Antonio's library of critically appraised topics (CAT) at https://cats.uthscsa.edu/ and search for a review on regenerative furcation treatment. Read any CAT you can find, and debate if the conclusion is still correct based on current literature.
- Create a CAT on treating Class III furcation involvement (or any other topic for which a CAT is not available) following the outline provided by Sauve S, et al. in "The critically appraised topic: a practical approach to learning critical appraisal" (Ann R Coll Physicians Surg Can. 1995; 28:396–398).

References

[1] Romeo U, Palaia G, Botti R, et al. Enamel pearls as a predisposing factor to localized periodontitis. Quintessence Int 2011;42(1):69–71

[2] De Beule F, Alsaadi G, Perić M, Brecx M. Periodontal treatment and maintenance of molars affected with severe periodontitis (DPSI = 4): An up to 27-year retrospective study in a private practice. Quintessence Int 2017;48(5):391–405

[3] Rosen PS, Froum SJ, Cohen DW. Consecutive case series using a composite allograft containing mesenchymal cells with an amnion-chorion barrier to treat mandibular class III/IV furcations. Int J Periodontics Restorative Dent 2015;35(4):453–460

[4] Needleman I. How long do multirooted teeth with furcation involvement survive with treatment? Evid Based Dent 2010;11(2):38–39

[5] Melker DJ, Richardson CR. Root reshaping: an integral component of periodontal surgery. Int J Periodontics Restorative Dent 2001;21(3):296–304

[6] Strupp WC Jr, Melker DJ. Maximizing aesthetics using a combined periodontal-restorative protocol. Dent Today 2003;22(5):60–62, 64–69

[7] Tucker LM, Melker DJ, Chasolen HM. Combining perio-restorative protocols to maximize function. Gen Dent 2012;60(4):280–287, quiz 288–289

8 Correcting Gingival Recession and Mucogingival Defects

Abstract

While the discovery of deep pocketing seems to be the most common cause of alarm during periodontal exams, soft tissue deficiencies are often overlooked during routine exams. This is problematic as soft tissue deficiencies may worsen without obvious signs of disease, cause restorative difficulty, and may contribute to tooth loss. Treatment of soft tissue deficiencies also becomes progressively more difficult and unpredictable with increasing size of defect and with time, it may become untreatable.

Keywords: recession, mucogingival defect, corrective surgery

8.1 Learning Objectives

- Recall the importance of proper soft tissue dimensions of periodontal health.
- Create treatment plans that prevent, manage, or correct mucogingival problems.
- Describe surgical strategies that augment gingival tissues.
- Describe surgical strategies that reposition gingiva and vestibular mucosa.

8.2 Case

A 57-year old Caucasian female with a history of total joint replacement, gastroesophageal reflux disease, and sulfa drug allergy takes 10 mg pantoprazole once daily and is interested in improving the uneven appearance of her front teeth with the left-side canine appearing longer than any teeth on the right side. She has received regular periodic dental treatment in the past including restorative treatment, endodontic treatment, and orthodontic treatment. Restorative treatment was originally done to treat caries she had as a young adult, and these restorations have been replaced several times since. She also received restorations to fill in erosion lesions on the facial surfaces of teeth that appeared over time. Root canal therapy for tooth no. 3 was done decades ago. Orthodontic treatment was done to relieve severe crowding when she was a teenager, and involved removal of tooth no. 6 and no. 24. She wears a fixed wire retainer on the lingual side of the mandibular incisors. She reported that she clenches her teeth at times during the day, and is interested in an occlusal guard. For oral hygiene, she brushes her teeth twice a day with an Oral-B brush in a sweeping motion running from the gingiva to the facial surfaces, and flosses 2 to 3 times a week.

The extraoral exam does not produce any significant findings with no enlarged lymph nodes, normal muscle palpation, and normal opening range. Intraoral tissues appear all normal except with marginal gingival inflammation at some teeth. Salivary flow is normal and glands palpate normally. Teeth are generally clean and in good repair, although there is attrition on all occlusal surfaces and staining of restorative margins. The patient's occlusion fits the Angle Class I pattern, and teeth display group function during excursive movements.

Blood pressure is 120/90 mm Hg and the pulse is 59/min.

The area of concern are shown in (▶ Fig. 8.1).

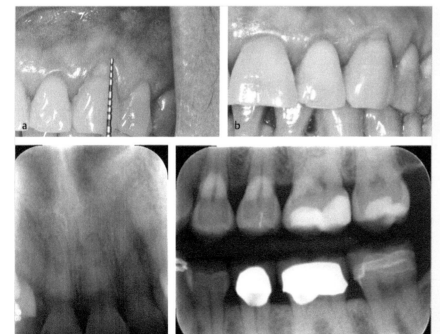

Fig. 8.1 (a–d) Initial presentation of this case (radiographs), and after connective tissue grafting. Note position of gingival margin on tooth no. 11 relative to tooth no. 10, or the line of tooth discoloration on the facial surface of no. 11.

The periodontal findings for the maxillary teeth are as follows:

		1	2	3	4	5	6	7	8	9	10	11	12	13	14	15	16
Maxilla facial																	
	PD		223	322	322	212		212	212	212	212	212	312	212	212	212	
	BOP																
	CAL		1			1					2	5*			2	2	
	GR										1	3*			1	1	
	MGJ		555	767	656	656		656	767	567	767	757	656	656	555	555	
	Furc																
	PLQ											1					
Maxilla lingual	PD		113	314	212	212		112	211	112	212	212	212	212	212	212	
	BOP			1													
	CAL																
	GR																
	Furc																
	Mobil																
	PLQ	1	1	1	1			1	1	1	1	1	1	1	1	1	

Abbreviations: BOP, bleeding on probing (1), suppuration (2); CAL, clinical attachment level; Furc, furcation involvement (Glickman class); GR, gingival recession; MGJ, position of mucogingival junction from margin; Mobil, tooth mobility (Miller grade); PD, probing depths; PLQ, plaque level (0 = none, 5 = heavy).
* Relative to the coronal margin of the facial restoration of this tooth.

Oral hygiene instruction was provided to make sure that the patient could maintain low plaque levels without using an aggressive brushing technique. The old composite restoration at tooth no. 11 was removed as it was stained and had a pitted margin and replaced it with a resin-modified glass ionomer restoration with the same coronal margin position. Prior to surgery, a rigid palatal stent was fabricated to cover and protect the palatal donor site during wound healing. Connective tissue graft surgery was performed, which reduced recession, thickened the gingival margin, and produced improved appearance (compare before and after on ▶Fig. 8.1). Healing was uneventful with no bleeding after surgery, moderate pain only for one day, and no pain within days after the surgery. Within 3 months, tissue appearance matched the surrounding teeth and the teeth in this quadrant had even gingival margins to the satisfaction of the patient. Additional corrective treatment was planned for other quadrants and scheduled as the patient's finances allowed.

What can be learned from this case?

While this patient presented with no severe periodontal disease as evidenced by low probing depths, little or no attachment/bone loss, good oral hygiene, and little bleeding on probing, this patient has multiple mucogingival conditions. As this patient was bothered by the recession at tooth no. 11, treatment was indicated. This patient presented with several factors that may have contributed to the recession such as orthodontic treatment, facial restorations, and parafunctional habits. Aggressive tooth brushing can contribute to facial recession, but in this case, there is limited evidence for it although her oral hygiene regimen could be improved regarding interproximal care.

Resin-modified glass ionomer was used to provide a more hydrophilic surface that promotes tissue adaptation and reduces caries risk as the restoration is now partially submerged in soft tissue. The corrective surgery showed key features of connective tissue graft surgery such as excellent color match, improved root coverage, and tissue thickness with little scarring. Given that the contributing factors for recession in this area occurred in the past, the risk of new recession development in this area seems low.

8.3 Recognize Indications for Mucogingival Surgery

While periodontal treatment usually focuses on reducing inflammation and pocketing, achieving proper soft tissue dimensions and characteristics is also important for periodontal health.

8.3.1 Risks Associated with Gingival Recession

Normal physiologic gingival contours with gentle scalloped facial and lingual margins support good oral hygiene and protect the underlying cementum and dentin from exposure to the oral environment. Gingival recession that exposes root surfaces often presents an esthetic concern. The exposed root surfaces usually are darker than the enamel and are more likely to stain and adhere plaque given the rougher surface of dentin and cementum compared to enamel. These surfaces are also softer and less mineralized than enamel, and prone to root caries, which then necessitate restoration that is different from a natural, healthy tooth surface. Gingival recession also tends to be uneven in severity, resulting in longer and uneven appearing teeth as seen in the case described above.

Besides the esthetic concern, exposed root surfaces also tend to be sensitive, causing short-lived, but intense pain whenever cold material touches the sensitive surface. Sometimes, sensitivity is severe enough that even touching the sensitive surface causes pain.

Ideally, therefore, gingival recession should be avoided and corrected wherever possible. Practically, it is not possible to revert most areas of gingival recession given that it often is the result of irreversible tissue damage caused by periodontal disease. As the ideal situation cannot be attained in most patients with periodontitis, periodontal treatment presents in these patients as a compromise: pocket reduction is traded against increased recession since this allows easier periodontal maintenance and lower risk of tooth loss. The consequent recession then has to be managed with patient education, oral hygiene instruction, fluoride application, and application of desensitizing medications to guard against the consequences of gingival recession.

8.3.2 Causes of Gingival Recession

The following factors are associated with gingival recession, and are often the cause of gingival recession:

- *Gingival inflammation*: Gingival recession often follows attachment and bone loss seen in periodontitis, as the continued destruction of gingival fibers and supporting tissue will cause apical migration of the gingival margin. In many populations, gingival inflammation linked to plaque and calculus deposits is most associated with gingival recession.[1] For similar reasons, older age and male gender are associated with gingival recession, as older and male patients tend to have more severe periodontal disease. For diagnosis, gingival recession caused by persistent inflammation most likely will be interproximally as these sites commonly have the worst plaque level, and there will be signs of significant periodontal disease. For treatment, this means if a site with gingival recession is associated with inflammation, plaque, and calculus build-up, oral hygiene instruction and scaling and root planing need to be performed in order to prevent further tissue damage.
- *Smoking and use of smokeless tobacco*: These factors are often associated with gingival recession as tobacco use will exacerbate periodontal disease leading attachment loss and destruction of gingiva-supporting tissue. Smoking history or exacerbated recession in the area of smokeless tobacco placement will suggest this cause in addition to enhanced periodontal disease. Consequently, periodontal therapy will need to include tobacco-cessation counseling in this case.
- *Aggressive tooth brushing*: Aggressive brushing or using a hard toothbrush has long been associated with gingival injuries, facial gingival recession, and abrasion of tooth surfaces, although this relationship is not seen in all studies.[2] Clinically, this can be evaluated by observing the patient while the patient performs oral hygiene, and noting aggressive brushing techniques. In case of aggressive tooth brushing, recession will be most pronounced at teeth that protrude from the arch such as the canines.
- *Piercing*: Labial or tongue piercing is associated with gingival recession adjacent to the tongue or lip ornament, and patients should be discouraged from wearing intraoral piercings.
- *Occlusal trauma*: This has long been associated with gingival clefting and some studies suggest a general relationship between occlusal interference contacts and localized gingival recession.
- *Chronic trauma*: Chronic trauma from restorative factors (that is ill-fitting RPD clasps) or destructive habits may cause localized recession.

- *Orthodontic therapy*: This is associated with slightly increased gingival recession, but only in few patients this is clinically significant and orthodontic tooth movement can also correct gingival recession in some cases. While labial tooth movement may produce gingival recession, it is more likely that other factors such as aggressive tooth brushing and reduced tissue thickness at the new tooth position may predispose the patient to increased recession. In our experience, this typically becomes a problem in mandibular incisors if there is limited symphysis bone and thin gingiva.
- *Thin gingival tissue thickness*: Thin gingival tissue is more likely associated with gingival recession.
- *Frenum pull*: High frenum attachment is sometimes associated with gingival recession, usually at the facial surfaces of the central incisors, and occasionally near premolars. Frenum pull can be identified by moving the lip and cheek tissues with finger pressure, and observing the mucosa for any tissue bands that pull and blanch the gingiva coronal to these tissue bands.
- *Soft tissue disorders*: Very rare, soft tissue diseases such as mucous membrane pemphigoid are associated with increased gingival recession as the gingiva cannot hold up against normal forces of chewing and brushing.

8.3.3 Risks Associated with Lack of Keratinized Tissue

Another factor that is associated with gingival recession is lack of keratinized gingiva. However, this association is more controversial as various cross-sectional studies show a relationship, whereas several cohort studies failed to find a significant association.

The determining factor, if a site without sufficient keratinized gingiva is prone to develop recession, is inflammation caused by either plaque accumulation or presence of a subgingival restoration that irritates the local tissues. Teeth without sufficient keratinized gingiva are more likely to have higher plaque scores and inflammation, presumably because brushing these teeth is more uncomfortable as toothbrush bristles scrape up against the more delicate mucosa.

While dental implants lack the gingival attachment mechanism of teeth, the question of how much keratinized gingiva is needed to maintain healthy periimplant tissues is similarly controversial. As with teeth, some studies suggest that lack of keratinized gingiva is associated with more inflammation,[3] while other studies fail to show clear evidence for this relationship. Currently, the evidence seems to favor the idea that sufficient amount of keratinized gingiva around implants is better for long-term health and implant survival. The key factor again is oral hygiene, and presence of keratinized gingiva allows for easier hygiene and implant maintenance.

Causes of Insufficient Keratinized Gingiva

The position of the mucogingival junction is likely determined by genetic factors controlling the growth of the jaws and differentiation of oral epithelial cells. Therefore, some individuals are born with low amounts of keratinized gingiva and are more prone to have mucogingival defects. For any individual, lack of keratinized gingiva develops if periodontal disease destroys the marginal gingiva and the gingival margin approaches the fixed mucogingival junction.

How much Keratinized Gingiva Is Needed?

Generally, for implants, it appears that at least 2 mm of keratinized mucosa are needed for improved health. For teeth, this question depends on oral hygiene and if a subgingival restoration is needed as teeth without attached gingiva may never develop recession in the absence of gingival inflammation. For teeth that need restoration, the minimum requirement seems to be at least 2 mm of attached gingiva, and there is one recommendation for 5 mm of keratinized mucosa that includes 3 mm of attached gingiva.

8.3.4 Tissue Thickness, Biotype, and Restorations

Thin gingival tissue poses a greater risk for recession, reduces effectiveness of regenerative procedures, and is easily injured during restorative procedures leading to additional recession.

Thin gingival tissue is associated with a thin biotype, and has the following characteristics:
• Smooth, translucent, delicate gingival tissue.
• Long, thin papillae.
• Able to see the shadow of the periodontal probe through the gingival margin while probing.

If a patient has a thin gingival biotype, consider:
• Prior to placement of subgingival margins in the anterior maxilla, augment gingiva with a connective tissue graft.
• For implant therapy in the anterior maxilla, consider additional connective tissue grafting.
• Careful handling during surgery to avoid flap necrosis and delayed healing.

8.3.5 The Problem of High Frenum Attachments

While frenum attachments are part of normal oral anatomy, a frenum may attach too close to teeth resulting in local lack of keratinized gingiva or a diastema. Such high frenum attachments can be detected by moving the cheek and lips in various directions, and observing how close the frenum inserts to the gingival margin. High frenum attachments should be removed if they cause or are associated with:
• An esthetic concern.
• Speech pathology.
• An obstacle for orthodontic treatment.
• Interference with tooth brushing.
• Interference with denture construction.
• Interference with regenerative periodontal and implant surgery.
• *Gingival recession*: Clinically, activation of the frenum will cause blanching of the gingiva adjacent to the recession defect.

8.3.6 Importance of Sufficient Vestibular Depth

The vestibule is nearly always overlooked during periodontal exams, but vestibular depth may be important for some patients. Typically, the vestibular fold is about 6 to 7 mm apical to the facial gingival margin in the anterior mandible and often this is the area with the shallowest vestibule. While a shallow vestibule by itself usually is not detrimental to periodontal health, teeth in an area of shallow vestibule tend to accumulate plaque and calculus as the shallow vestibule restricts brushing and interproximal cleaning. A shallow vestibule makes retention of dentures more difficult and may also make impression taking more challenging. Shallow vestibular depth also seems to have a negative effect on the health of periimplant tissues.[4]

Surgical procedures, such as the lateral sliding flaps or pedicle flaps, require a sufficiently deep vestibule to allow execution of the surgery procedure. Other surgical procedures such as bone augmentation procedures may shorten the vestibule, which then can cause oral hygiene problems unless this is corrected with another surgery step.

8.3.7 Medical Contraindications

Surgeries that correct soft tissue defects should not be performed in the presence of uncontrolled medical conditions. Typically, such surgery causes more bleeding than pocketreduction surgery and relies more on soft tissue healing. Therefore, patients with bleeding disorders or taking anticoagulants and antiplatelet agents require medical collaboration, and the procedure may not work well in patients with immune and soft tissue disorders.

Dental Contraindications

There are few if any dental contraindications to mucogingival surgery. Mucogingival surgery is easier to perform and likely has better clinical outcomes if the local gingiva is healthy. For this reason, it is usually advisable to correct pocketing and inflammation prior to mucogingival surgery.

Root coverage procedures are more challenging to perform on tooth roots that excessively protrude outside of the dental arch. Orthodontic treatment may help with root coverage procedures if it lines up teeth and reduces root prominence. Consequently, any orthodontic treatment should be completed before mucogingival surgery.

A shallow vestibule makes it difficult to create a pedicle flap or good recipient site for a connective tissue graft. Coronally positioned flaps actually worsen a shallow vestibule by repositioning the gingiva and mucosa even more coronally. In these cases, procedures that increase vestibular depth such as free gingival graft, an apical positioned flap, or vestibuloplasty should be considered.

8.3.8 Consent Issues

As with any surgery, informed consent must be obtained by discussing risks, benefits, and alternatives with the patient.

The specific benefit of mucogingival surgery depends on the specific need it addresses, but in general, mucogingival surgeries promote tooth longevity as they improve oral hygiene, cover sensitive root surfaces, and provide greater resilience during restorative treatment.

The risks of mucogingival surgery are similar to most oral surgery procedures. The most common risk are prolonged bleeding after surgery, moderate pain, and swelling of the treated tissue. For soft tissue grafting, the surgery site may undergo color changes from gray over purple and red to pink during healing. As with any surgery, there is a chance that mucogingival surgery may fail to produce the desired results.

The alternative to mucogingival surgery usually is not to perform the surgery. Often, mucogingival conditions worsen little over long periods of time if the original cause has been removed, and regular periodontal maintenance is a valid alternative to most mucogingival surgery, although the condition may become worse over time.

8.4 Create Treatment Plans that Prevent, Manage, or Correct Mucogingival Problems

Mucogingival conditions such as recession, lack of keratinized tissue, excessively thin tissue, frenum attachments, and shallow vestibule should be treated if any of the following conditions is present.

- Signs of periodontal inflammation: Pocketing, erythema, or edema.
- Evidence that condition is getting worse, i.e., increased recession and attachment loss at subsequent maintenance visits.
- Evidence that condition interferes with oral hygiene, i.e., persistent plaque and calculus accumulation that does not improve despite improved patient effort.
- If the patient has an esthetic concern specific to gingival appearance, and it is correctable with surgery.
- Dentinal hypersensitivity in an area of isolated facial/lingual gingival recession.
- Root caries associated with isolated facial/lingual gingival recession.
- Lack of keratinized tissue or tissue thickness on a tooth that needs a restoration at or below gingival margin.
- Lack of keratinized tissue, thickness, or root coverage, high frenum attachment in an area that will receive orthodontic treatment.
- Lack of keratinized tissue or tissue thickness, high frenum attachments in an edentulous area that will receive periodontal or implant-related surgery.

8.4.1 Prevention of Mucogingival Problems

Since definite correction of mucogingival problems usually requires surgery, it is best to avoid the development of mucogingival problems in the first place. Therefore, risk factors for gingival recession, such as gingival inflammation, tobacco use, intraoral piercings, and aggressive tooth brushing, should be assessed at every dental exam and addressed promptly.

The importance of oral hygiene instruction in preventing mucogingival problems cannot be overstated as in our experience many patients adopt overly aggressive tooth brushing techniques in the hopes of "brushing pockets away." Recently, there is some evidence that teaching patients gentle, but effective plaque-removal techniques can lead to minor improvement of gingival recession over time.[5] For patients with aggressive brushing habits, we recommend using a modified Stillman technique using a toothbrush with extrasoft bristles (i.e., Nimbus Microfine brush) and low abrasive dentifrice (i.e., pure baking soda or Arm & Hammer PeroxiCare toothpaste).

In order to prevent the development of mucogingival problems as a result of dental treatment, soft tissue dimensions need to be assessed prior to restorative treatment or orthodontic treatment. If tissue amounts are deficient, the patient needs to be advised of the possibility of recession development and corrective mucogingival surgery should be planned after orthodontic or restorative treatment.

8.4.2 Management of Mucogingival Problems

Treatment of mucogingival problems involves first identifying the mucogingival problem, correcting contributing factors and planning the corrective procedure(s) for each mucogingival problem.

Identifying the Mucogingival Problem

For any tooth or site with a mucogingival problem, it is important to identify each mucogingival deficiency and determine its importance for the patient and for dental treatment. Mucogingival problems can be categorized as follows:

- Recession/lack of root coverage. If this is a concern, note:
  - Depth of the recession (does it go past the mucogingival junction).
  - Width of the recession (narrow or wide).
  - Location of the recession (isolated to facial/lingual side only, or involving the interproximal space).
  - Extent of the recession (single tooth, multiple teeth).
- Lack of keratinized/attached gingiva in the absence of deep probing depths:
  - If the lack of attached gingiva is caused by a deep pocket exceeding the width of keratinized gingiva, it is a pocket reduction problem and needs to be treated as such (see Chapter 6).
- Lack of tissue thickness (or thin biotype).
- High frenum attachment.
- Shallow vestibule.
- Discolored tissue.
- Area is highly visible (facial surface anterior maxilla).
- Excessive tissue thickness/bulky gingiva.

Since many mucogingival procedures harvest intraoral soft tissue for grafting purposes, it needs to be determined if:

- The patient would accept a second surgery to harvest soft tissue in the mouth.
- There is a suitable donor site:
  - *Palate for most grafts*: Should be of normal width and depth (>10 mm), covered with healthy, thick tissue near premolars and 1st molar.
  - *Maxillary tuberosity for small connective tissue grafts*: Thick tissue.

Prognosis of Treatment Success

For recession/root coverage, many classification systems have been developed (i.e., Sullivan & Atkins, Miller) to aid with treatment planning and prognosis, but have limitations.[6] In general, the likelihood of gaining root coverage depends on the factors shown in ▶ Table 8.1.

For gaining keratinized gingiva, the likelihood of success depends mostly on surgical and patient factors (▶ Table 8.2).

Gaining tissue thickness is very predictable, and mostly depends on surgical skill of the surgeon and general wound

Table 8.1 Prognostic factors that make root coverage/correction of recession more likely

Factor	Improves prognosis	Worsens prognosis
Location of recession defect	Facial (easiest)/lingual	Interproximal (typically not correctable)
Depth	Shallow (up to mucogingival junction)	Deep (past mucogingival junction; may need multiple procedures)
Width	Narrow	Wide
Number of defects	Single (easiest)	Multiple (more difficult to correct)
Tooth position		Tooth tipped/rotated facially
Root anatomy	Normal Does not protrude out of bone	Contains root defects Root protrudes significantly outside of bone
Restorative factors	No caries No restoration Clean root surface	Root surface restoration (gingiva typically will not cover restorations)
Tissue thickness	Normal/thick gingiva	Thin gingiva
Medical conditions	Healthy	Tobacco use Any condition affecting wound healing
Oral hygiene		Aggressive tooth brushing Poor oral hygiene

Table 8.2 Prognostic factors that make gaining keratinized tissue more likely

Factor	Improves prognosis	Worsens prognosis
If using a grafting procedure, availability of suitable graft		Shallow palate Thin palatal tissue Thin graft
Wound stability	Graft/tissue cannot move after surgery	Excessive muscle activity Restricted access to surgery site Excessive loose tissue at site Cannot fixate graft Poor suturing
Esthetic demand	None	Must match color of surrounding tissue (not possible with conventional grafting)
Medical condition	Good overall health	Tobacco use Any condition affecting wound healing

healing ability of the patient. Similarly, frenectomy and vestibuloplasty procedures are predictable as long as sound surgical skills are used and the patient is able to heal normally.

When to Refer

If the condition is stable based on past records, and not a concern for the patient or treatment, mucogingival conditions can be managed with periodic evaluation, routine periodontal maintenance, and oral hygiene instructions that emphasize on gentle cleaning techniques.

However, definite treatment of mucogingival conditions typically requires surgery and the success of the surgery depends largely on surgical skill. Consequently, referral to a periodontist is usually warranted for most but the simplest procedures. The major prerequisite skill for these surgeries is the ability to raise a split thickness flap, and handle delicate thin tissues that are difficult to suture. Mucogingival surgeries range in difficulty level from relatively easy to difficult in the following way:
- Basic frenectomy of a single, fibrous, well-defined frenum.
- Placing a free gingival graft over a frenectomy site to prevent frenum attachment in a nonesthetic site (i.e., mandibular vestibule apical to central incisors).
- Augmenting a posterior edentulous site with limited keratinized tissue/vestibule prior to implant placement or removable partial denture construction.

- Augmenting thin gingival tissue at a posterior tooth with a connective tissue graft.
- Complex grafting involving multiple teeth or a combination of procedures.

8.4.3 Treatment Planning

Planning surgical correction of mucogingival defects can be complicated and it is dependent on a particular surgeon's preference for a given technique. In general, treatment planning begins with identifying the nature of the mucogingival problem(s) and selecting the procedure that addresses the problem(s) best. Sometimes, it is possible that several surgeries have to be combined in sequence to achieve the desired effect (▶Table 8.3).

Increasing Root Coverage/improving Recession

While there are many techniques that can improve root coverage, the go-to method for improving recession or gaining root coverage is a connective tissue graft procedure. With this procedure, a piece of connective tissue (or a matrix resembling connective tissue) is applied to the root surface that needs to be covered (see connective tissue grafting in Section 8.5.3 of this chapter). The connective tissue piece used in this procedure is

Table 8.3 Surgical treatment planning for mucogingival problems

Surgery	Desired outcome/requirement									
	Gain root coverage/improve	Multiple adjacent sites	Requires donor site	Gain keratinized tissue	Increase tissue thickness	Remove frenum	Deepen vestibule	Remove discoloration*	Must color match	Remove thick/bulky
Split Apical positioned flap	×	✓	×	✓	×	•	✓	×	✓	×
Pedicle flap	✓	×		•	×	×	0	×	✓	×
Connective tissue (CT) graft	✓	✓	✓	•	✓	×	×	✓	✓	–
Nonautogenous CT graft	✓	✓	×	×	✓	×	×	✓	✓	–
Free gingival graft	•	✓	✓	✓	✓	✓	✓	–	×	×
Coronally positioned flap	✓	✓	×	×	×	–	–	×	✓	×
Frenectomy	•	✓	×	×	×	✓	•	0	0	•
Vestibuloplasty	0	✓	×	•	×	•	✓	×	0	×
Guided tissue regeneration	✓	✓	×	0	✓	×	×	×	✓	–
Gingivectomy/gingival flap	–	✓	×	–	–	×	×	✓	✓	✓

Select surgery that matches most closely the relevant components of the mucogingival problem:

✓ Surgery likely will achieve this goal.

• Surgery may produce minor improvement.

0: Surgery has no effect.

× Surgery will not achieve this goal.

– Surgery will produce opposite effect.

* Submit excised gingiva to oral pathology lab if cause of discoloration or excess is unknown.

commonly obtained during the same surgery from the same patient's palate, and is usually billed for each tooth that needs root coverage. If several sites adjacent to each other needing connective tissue grafting, surgeons will typically provide a discount for these additional sites to aid case acceptance.

If there is no suitable intraoral donor site, or the patient objects to harvesting tissue, it is possible to use allodermal matrix derivative from a tissue bank as a substitute graft material. It may also not be feasible to use autogenous connective tissue if a patient has many large recession defects or has a shallow palate, and using allograft materials may be a preferable alternative to excessive tissue removal from the palate. Some surgeons also use resorbable collagen membranes in place of a connective tissue graft for root coverage with acceptable results. In any of these instances, patients are typically billed for nonautogenous connective tissue grafts for each tooth.

An alternative to connective tissue grafts are pedicle flaps (including double pedicle flaps) that rotate adjacent gingiva onto the defect. The advantage of this procedure, compared to an autogenous connective tissue graft, is that no palatal surgery is required, but it does require sufficient gingiva and vestibule depth in the area surrounding the recession defect. As this procedure takes tissue from the adjacent gingiva, this procedure is best suited for a single, isolated recession defect. As with connective tissue grafts, they are billed by tooth.

An alternative to both connective tissue grafting and pedicle flaps, the coronally positioned flap can achieve root coverage on multiple adjacent teeth by moving the gingival margin coronally. This procedure is usually charged as a gingival flap procedure for each quadrant. The disadvantage of this procedure is that it does not enhance tissue thickness or keratinization, and decreases vestibular depth.

Increasing the Amount of Keratinized Tissue

Although connective tissue grafts can enhance thickness and toughness of the tissue surrounding teeth, the typical method for increasing keratinized tissue is the free gingival graft procedure, which again is billed by tooth. Here, a piece of tissue with surface epithelium is harvested and applied to the site lacking keratinized tissue. Typically, the harvesting is done during the grafting procedure using the patient's palate, but this usually produces a lighter-colored gingival patch at the recipient site and possible significant pain. To overcome these limitations, tissue-engineered tissue grafts grown from the patient's own gingival cells (Gintuit) or 3D-printed collagen matrixes mimicking tissue (Mucograft) are becoming available that may eventually replace the autogenous grafts. As with connective tissue grafting, surgeons may provide a discount for additional adjacent teeth to aid case acceptance.

An alternative to free gingival grafts that avoids the need for a palatal donor site and the "tire patch" appearance of a gingival graft is a split thickness variant of the apical positioned flap, which is billed by quadrant. The apically positioned flap used in this context does not aim to reduce pocketing, but splits the limited amount of keratinized gingiva and repositions the apical portion so that the gingival epithelium from both sides of the incision line will fill in the open wound and create new additional keratinized tissue. The downside of this procedure is that it may be more technique sensitive and less predictable than the free gingival graft procedure.

Correcting Combined Defects Featuring Recession and Lack of Keratinized Tissue

A special mucogingival problem exists if a recession defect exceeds the width of keratinized tissue producing both a root coverage and lack of keratinized tissue concern. This may also be combined with a frenum that attaches at the base of the recession defect. Usually, this occurs at mandibular central incisors or at the facial roots of molars. An effective method dealing with this problem is a two-step approach. In the first step, a free gingival graft procedure increases keratinized tissue and deepens the vestibule while removing any frenum attachment from the recession defect base. After several months of healing, a second surgery is then used to coronally position this new tissue on to root surface, resolving the recession defect.

While this approach can be used most of the time, it is of limited use in highly visible sites (if the patient will not accept anything but perfect color match) or if free gingival graft surgery is not possible. In this case, a connective tissue graft or nonautogenous connective tissue graft in combination with a double pedicle flap can produce root coverage, although it may not produce keratinized tissue.

Yet another alternative may also be a guided tissue regeneration procedure, which can also be used to produce root coverage.

Increasing Tissue Thickness

Tissue thickness is best produced by inserting a connective tissue graft into the existing gingiva. Alternatively, a nonautogenous graft or collagen membrane can be used as well, although these materials tend to produce less tissue thickness than an autogenous graft.

Removing Frenum Attachments/improving Vestibular Depth

A frenum can be removed using a basic frenulectomy procedure, but a free gingival graft may be more effective if the frenum is wide and the area is generally lacking in keratinized tissue.

A free gingiva graft can locally increase the vestibule, but for large-scale vestibule depth increase, vestibuloplasty is needed.

8.5 Describe Surgical Strategies that Augment Gingival Tissues

8.5.1 Instrumentation

Gingival tissue augmentation procedures can be done with a typical infection control setup for dental procedures and a basic periodontal surgery setup that includes the following:
- Local anesthesia instruments and supplies.
- Mirror and periodontal probe.
- Scalpel and several blades (no. 15c is suitable for traditional augmentation surgery).
  - Some surgeons may use microsurgical blades and other specialized instruments to minimize incisions and shorten healing time.
  - A double-bladed scalpel holding two no. 15c blades spaced 1.5-mm apart can be useful for harvesting soft tissue, but not essential to this type of surgery.

○ A variety of palatal soft tissue harvesters that harvest connective tissue or epithelial tissue that are available commercially, but not essential to this type of surgery.
- Scalers and curettes for root planning.
- Small tissue forceps.
- Sterile wooden tongue depressor.
- Hemostat.
- Sterile saline (or extra local anesthesia solution).
- Suturing supplies (i.e., 6 to 0 resorbable sutures, i.e., PGA—with a reverse cutting half-circle or 3/8 circle needle), needle holder (i.e., Castroviejo), and suture scissors.
- Tissue glue (i.e., Glustitch), a medical grade cyanoacrylate solution.
- Oxidized cellulose (or other hemostatic, resorbable agent that can be placed into wounds).
- Sterile 2 × 2 gauze.
- Surgical suction tip.
- *Optional:* A small cotton pellet, root conditioning agent (i.e., content of a 250-mg tetracycline HCl capsule, citric acid, ethylenediaminetetraacetic acid (EDTA) mixed with sterile saline to saturation).

As with most periodontal surgery, this technique can be accomplished using local infiltration anesthesia with 2% lidocaine and 1:100,000 epinephrine. Local infiltration, with 2% lidocaine and 1:50,000 epinephrine, is useful to produce a drier surgical field, and 0.5% bupivacaine and 1:100,000 epinephrine (i.e., Marcaine) is useful for prolonged anesthesia after surgery.

8.5.2 Patient Preoperative Preparation

The most common postoperative complications of mucogingival surgery—bleeding, pain, and swelling—can be minimized with good preoperative patient preparation. The following steps will empower the patient to improve the healing process and lead to a good postoperative experience:
- Educate the patient that there will be some pain and bleeding and that this is a normal part of the healing process after surgery. The patient should expect pain to be worst right after the anesthesia wears off and slowly decreasing thereafter, and that pain medication will be given.
- Prior to mucogingival surgery using tissue from the palate, create a surgical stent:
  ○ Treatment plan the stent as it requires a laboratory procedure. For example, the ADA CDT code D4999 (Unspecified Periodontal Procedure by Report) can be used along with a narrative (i.e., Fabrication of a surgical stent to protect donor site during wound healing after gingival grafting procedure) for billing purposes.
  ○ Take an alginate impression of the palate.
  ○ Create or have a laboratory fabricate a stent. This stent needs to have a rigid resin base that covers the palate and reaches interproximally similar to an interim removable partial denture base. This stent should have a relieved surface (about 1-mm deep) over the planned donor site. This area can be filled with soft tissue liner just prior to insertion for increased comfort.
  ○ Adjust the stent prior to surgery so that it will fit snug against the palate and holds firmly on to the teeth.
  ○ It is important that the stent fits tightly against the palate as it will apply pressure to the palatal wound at the donor site and aid with stopping bleeding and swelling after the surgery. It also will act as a rigid barrier to

protect the wound after surgery, speed up healing, and greatly limit pain.
- Instruct the patient to take the patient's preferred over-the-counter analgesic just before the surgery (i.e., 2 to 3 × 200-mg Ibuprofen, 325-mg Aspirin, or 500-mg Acetaminophen), and have the patient keep taking this dose every 4 to 6 hours after the surgery, as long as needed. Make sure the patient understands the maximum dose of the analgesic, and that the analgesic will dull but not eliminate the pain.
- If the patient has a history of significant soft tissue swelling after injury, consider prescribing a short course of low-dose steroid (i.e., 0.25-mg dexamethasone) every 6 hours starting just before the surgery for the first 3 days after surgery. Significant tissue swelling in the palate can cause significant pain as the edema will stretch the dense connective tissue of the palate, and the steroid will decrease development edema-related pain.
- Prescribe a short course of short-acting opioid for the first 2 days after the surgery that the patient can take in addition to the antiinflammatory analgesic. For example, 5-mg Oxycodone HCl every 4 to 6 hours in an opioid-naïve patient, or prescribe an appropriate analgesic-opioid combination (i.e., 5-mg Hydrocodone bitartrate and 325-mg acetaminophen; 7.5-mg Hydrocodone bitartrate and 200-mg Ibuprofen). Make sure to comply with any local regulations concerning opioid use, and educate patient on addiction risk and proper disposal.
- Instruct the patient to control pain after surgery by applying ice. For the usual buccal recipient site, ice in the form of a towel-wrapped ice bag gently applied to the facial skin overlying the surgery area is effective in controlling pain. Ice chips or popsicles are effective in applying cold to the palatal donor site and providing pain relief there.
- Instruct the patient to use warm salt water rinses starting several days after the surgery, which tends to improve the feeling of the surgery site.

8.5.3 Connective Tissue Grafting

An established, very common and versatile method for gaining root coverage and increasing soft tissue thickness is the subepithelial connective tissue graft covered by a coronally advanced flap. There are many variations of this procedure based on the type and how the connective tissue graft is obtained, and the incision design for the recipient site. The following procedure closely resembles Dr. Langer's original description of grafting, and is one of the easier connective tissue grafting procedures to learn.

Subepithelial Connective Tissue Graft Combined with Coronally Advanced Flap

Begin with a buccal infiltration anesthesia for the area surrounding the recipient site, and performing a greater palatal nerve block for the donor site.

Prepare the Recipient Site

The traditional approach uses a pouch incision for the recipient site (▶ Fig. 8.2).
- Evaluate the recipient site, which is the recession defect and the adjacent papillae. Look for the position of the cementoenamel junction (CEJ) on the exposed root, and the position of the mucogingival junction.

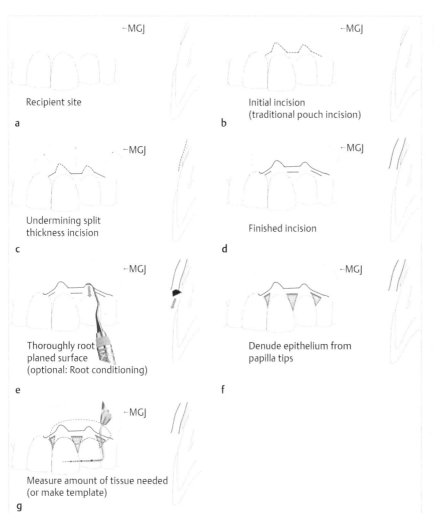

- Begin the split thickness incision with an intrasulcular incision for the apical half of the recession defect, aiming the scalpel toward the alveolar crest. Advance the blade until it contacts the bone crest covering the facial root surface.
- While near the bone, slide the blade slightly to the facial so that the edge of the bone can be felt. Carefully advance the blade under the tissue, making sure not to perforate the gingiva.
- Advance and sweep the blade across the bone, keeping most of the gingiva facial to the bone, creating a semicircular pouch under the gingiva facial to the tooth.
- Advance past the mucogingival junction as evidenced by the insertion depth of the blade. Some limited bleeding may occur after this point.
- Carefully advance the blade coronally along the side of the defect, making sure that the majority of the gingiva stays on the facial side of the blade while the lingual side of the blade touches the alveolar bone surface covered by a thin layer of connective tissue. Proceed until the tip of the interproximal alveolar crest is reached, which will be near the facial zenith of the CEJ.
- Continue to advance the blade along the side of the interproximal bone until the sulcus of the adjacent teeth is reached. This should completely undermine and separate the gingiva from the adjacent teeth to the base of the interproximal papilla to some distance past the mucogingival junction.
- At the coronal end of the interproximal undermining effort, make a linear, straight incision across the papilla from a point

slightly coronal to the point where the gingival margin meets the exposed CEJ and connect this horizontally to the adjacent tooth. Do this on both sides of the recession defect. As a result, this will open a large pouch of diffusely bleeding tissue.
- Denude the papilla by shaving off the epithelial tissue with the scalpel. This can be done by placing the scalpel on the facial surface of the root along the long axis of the tooth, and following the tooth contour the inteproximal bone. Once on the interproximal bone, follow the facial surface of the interproximal bone to the adjacent tooth, while keeping the same apio-coronal orientation of the blade. This should remove the facial epithelium on the papilla revealing lighter pink tissue with small bleeding capillaries.
- Aggressively scale and root plane the root surface with scalers and curettes. This produces a clean, hard, glassy smooth surface that is slightly flattened. Remove any root surface restorations or caries at this point.
- Make a template for the tissue graft using a clean, preferably sterile piece of cardboard or foil (i.e., the brown cardboard insert protecting the blade inside most scalpel blade wrapper) and cut it to size using suture scissors. Cut the template into a form that covers the root surface apical to the CEJ and about 3 to 4 mm of the bone/periosteum surrounding the defect.
- *Optional, some studies suggest a beneficial effect of root conditioning while others do not*: Using a hemostat, pick up a cotton pellet, soak it with root condition agent (i.e., EDTA,

citric acid, and tetracycline) and burnish the root conditioning agent into the root surface for about a minute.
- Cover the recipient site with wet sterile gauze.

Harvest the Donor Tissue

While there are many variations of palatal tissue harvesting, here the double, paralleling incision may be the easiest to perform by inexperienced providers (▶ Fig. 8.3):
- Evaluate the palate, note the area of increased tissue thickness near the premolars and note the location of the soft tissue thickening on the floor of the palate near the 2nd molar marking the greater palatal foramen.
- Apply the template on the thick palatal tissue near the premolars. The border of the template should be 3 mm from the gingival margin of the teeth. The apical border of the template should be well clear off the palatal floor. Rotate the template to see which orientation covers thick palatal tissue best. Mark the corners of template with a periodontal probe by piecing the underlying soft tissue.
- With a new scalpel blade, make a straight, linear, full thickness incision aiming toward the bone using the template dots as a guide. Make sure not to infringe on the gingival margin of the adjacent teeth. This will be the coronal end of the connective tissue graft.
  - *Variation*: With a double-bladed scalpel blade, make a linear incision following the coronal template marks, but aim the blades parallel to the bone surface and making sure

that the blade does not perforate the epithelium. This will instantly create a uniformly thick slice of connective tissue.
- At the mesial and distal ends of this linear incision, create two full thickness vertical incisions that stop at the apical border of the template. Make sure not to advance toward the palatal floor as this may sever the greater palatine artery and cause severe bleeding. Some bleeding will occur nevertheless from the distal vertical incision.
  - If a double-bladed scalpel has been used, this will create two flap edges similar to book pages. The middle "page" is the connective tissue that can now be cut off at the base with scalpel, and the outer "page" of epithelium can now be sutured to the surrounding tissue to cover the donor site.
- With a tissue forceps, push back the coronal flap edge, and begin dissecting away the epithelial layer 1.5 to 2 mm from the flap surface by moving the scalpel with light pressure mesial and distal across the flap edge. Continue this until the underlying connective tissue is completely uncovered while not perforating or ripping the epithelial flap.
- Grab the coronal edge of the connective tissue with a tissue forceps and dissect if off the underlying bone with a scalpel. This should give a spongy, yellow-pink sheet of tissue with area of bleeding. Applying intermittent pressure with sterile gauze and infiltration with epinephrine-containing anesthetic greatly reduces bleeding during this procedure. The goal of this step is to harvest a piece of connective tissue shaped like the template and possessing a width of about 1.5 mm.

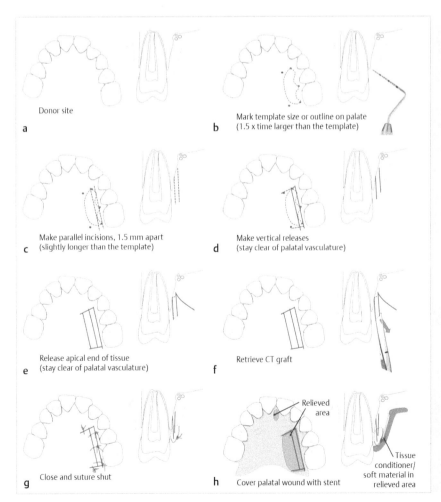

a Donor site

b Mark template size or outline on palate (1.5 x time larger than the template)

c Make parallel incisions, 1.5 mm apart (slightly longer than the template)

d Make vertical releases (stay clear of palatal vasculature)

e Release apical end of tissue (stay clear of palatal vasculature)

f Retrieve CT graft

g Close and suture shut

h Cover palatal wound with stent — Relieved area — Tissue conditioner/ soft material in relieved area

Fig. 8.3 (a–h) Harvesting a connective tissue graft from the palate using a parallel incision design. This is the easiest method if a double-bladed scalpel is used.

- Once the end of the soft tissue area is reached, free the soft tissue graft by cutting the apical end with a scalpel, aiming it toward the bone and on the palatal wall (and not the palatal floor).
- Transfer the soft tissue graft to the sterile tongue depressor and drip a few drops of sterile saline (or anesthetic) on it to keep it moist.
- Take the epithelial flap and firmly press it against the underlying bone/connective tissue of the now empty donor site for a few minutes. This achieves hemostasis and allows suturing of the flap to the surrounding tissue with a series of simple interrupted sutures. Once sutured, cover the site with wet gauze and have an assistant apply pressure again until hemostasis is achieved.
- Apply the surgical stent (if one was made).
- As the graft gently adheres to the tongue depressor, it can easily be cleaned and trimmed with a scalpel. Inspect the graft. Excise any glandular tissue, which are dark pink dense nodules. Adipose tissue will appear yellow against the pale pink connective tissue. While some adipose tissue is acceptable, try to trim off areas of pure yellow tissue with a scalpel while keeping the graft intact. Gently rinse off large red blood clots from the graft. If the graft contains a dark pink edge in the form of palatal epithelium, cut off this edge from the remaining graft.

Apply Connective Tissue Graft to Recipient Site

After a connective graft has been obtained, it needs to be placed as soon as possible (▶ Fig. 8.4):
- Insert the graft into the recipient pouch. If the graft does not completely fit in the pouch, enlarge it with more split thickness dissection until it fits.
- Secure the coronal mesial and distal graft edges to the denuded interproximal tissue with simple interrupted sutures using a fine resorbable material. Do not over-tighten the suture as it may rip the graft. The graft just needs to drape across the root surface.
- *Optional:* If there is enough tissue attached to the bone and good surgical access, secure the apical border of the graft to the underlying periosteum. This will not always be possible as suturing may be difficult.
- Take the recipient site flap edge and secure it over the graft using a sling suture in the mid-facial area and simple interrupted sutures interproximally. The recipient site flap

edge should completely cover the graft and the root surface like a blanket.
- Apply pressure for 5 minutes to induce hemostasis and eliminate any blood accumulation around the graft. Make sure to apply pressure evenly and perpendicular to the graft site in order not to dislodge the graft.
- Provide typical postoperative instruction similar to any oral surgery and repeat instructions regarding pain control.

Variations of Connective Tissue Augmentation

While the above surgery is somewhat traditional, many variations of this surgery exist for various purposes such as decreased pain, surgery time, access solutions, and so on. Many of these are effective and produce similar outcomes.

Variations in the Source of Connective Tissue

Although the palate is the most common source of autogenous connective tissue for recession treatment, anesthesia and postoperative pain are always a concern with palatal harvest sites. It is also possible to obtain soft tissue for root coverage from the maxillary tuberosity, although this depends on the presence of a sufficiently developed tuberosity.

Situations may arise where the amount of connective tissue needed to correct multiple recession defects exceeds the available amount of autogenous soft tissue. In these cases, acellular dermal matrix, a thick collagen matrix derived from dermis of organ donor skins, can be used to treat recession as substitute for palatal tissue. Dermal matrix is supplied as thick, white felt-like strip in a sterile envelope similar to regenerative membrane, and it needs to be reconstituted prior to use by placing it several times in sterile saline. After these rinses, the now hydrated membrane can be used like a subepithelial connective tissue graft. Care has to be taken to place the side with the holes toward the recipient site flap as this side contains the basement membrane, which then supposedly drives epithelial tissue growth. A problem with acellular dermal matrix grafts is that results vary widely, and that the amount of root coverage is generally less than that obtained with autogenous grafts.[7] A new alternative to acellular matrix grafts are 3d-printed collagen sponges mimicking the dermal collagen structures (Mucograft), but it is unknown yet how effective these materials are.

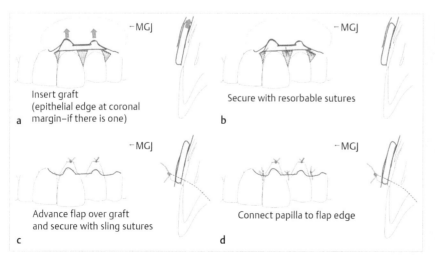

a Insert graft (epithelial edge at coronal margin–if there is one)

b Secure with resorbable sutures

c Advance flap over graft and secure with sling sutures

d Connect papilla to flap edge

Fig. 8.4 (a–d) Application of connective tissue graft into pouch.

Another alternative to using palatal tissue for recession treatment is guided tissue regeneration. Here, either resorbable or nonresorbable membranes are used to redevelop periodontal supporting tissue over the denuded root surface, although it can be challenging to cover the membrane with the receded gingival tissue.

Variations in Donor Site Incision Design

The trap door approach presented here is part of the original subepithelial connective tissue graft procedure and relatively easy to perform. However, the connective tissue can also be harvested through a single access incision, which seems to improve healing and produce less postoperative pain than the traditional trap-door approach.[8] Another approach is using parallel incisions and eliminating the vertical releases, resulting in a smaller wound size and less pain (see ▶Fig. 8.5a, for the comparison of incision designs). Harvesting can be made easier with specialized instruments such as the double-bladed scalpel or palatal tissue harvesters (i.e., Unigraft knife).

Variations in Recipient Site Incision Design

Surgeons have developed many different incision designs for the recipient site in order to improve upon the original connective tissue grafting concept. Most of these innovations aim to reduce postoperative pain and healing time by minimizing the incision area and avoiding external incisions. Some examples of these variations include the following (▶Fig. 8.5b):
- The tunnel subepithelial connective tissue graft, where the graft is inserted into a tunnel of undermined facial gingival tissue between several teeth.
- A variation of the tunnel technique where the graft is inserted from the side through a vertical incision.
- The vestibular incision subperiosteal tunnel access (VISTA) where graft material is inserted from the vestibule.[9]
- The pinhole surgical technique that inserts collagen membranes through a small access hole near the recession defect.[10]

8.5.4 Gingival Grafting

Unlike with connective tissue grafting, there are fewer variations on augmenting keratinized tissue, as free gingival graft surgery is the most predictable method of gaining keratinized gingiva.[7] Current techniques are still similar to the original description by Dr Bjorn in 1963. The procedure is also similar to the connective tissue grafting procedure presented in this chapter, except that the graft is a block of epithelium and connective tissue, and that the graft is placed on top of denuded tissue.

Free Gingival Graft Procedure

For best pain and bleeding control, fabricate a rigid surgical stent that covers the palate prior to surgery. Begin with a buccal infiltration anesthesia for the area surrounding the recipient site, and performing a greater palatal nerve block for the donor site.

Prepare the Recipient Site

The recipient site is prepared as follows (▶Fig. 8.6):
- Evaluate the recipient site, which is the recession defect and the adjacent papillae. Look for the position of the mucogingival junction as this will be where the incision will be placed, and look for any frenum attachments, which need to be removed prior to placing the graft.
- Begin the split thickness incision at the mucogingival junction about 1 tooth distal to the site lacking attached gingiva. Insert the blade 1.5 mm into the tissue, which usually means that the beveled part of the scalpel blade just about disappears into the tissue.
- Make this incision so that it spans the tooth distal and the tooth mesial to the tooth with the mucogingival defect.
- Pull on the lip (or cheek depending on the location of the defect) and apply tension on the mucosa apical to the split incision. Aim the blade into the split thickness incision and parallel to the facial surface of the tooth or the alveolar bone surface.
- Gently dissect the tissue by moving the sharp scalpel blade back and forth across the split thickness incision, leaving a thick layer of red connective tissue on the bone surface. The goal is essentially to peel off the epithelium while keeping the underlying connective tissue intact, as at least 1 mm of connective tissue is needed for securing the graft. Watch as these incisions widen the gap between gingiva and mucosa, producing a pouch.
- Sever any connective tissue or muscle bands of frenum attachments that are encountered and deepen the pouch to double the width of the graft. Make sure not to cut any vital structures such as the mental foramen. Typically, there needs to be about 12-mm space for a 5 to 6 mm wide graft.
- Denude the papilla and gingiva surrounding the mucogingival defect by shaving off the epithelial tissue with the scalpel. This can be done by placing the scalpel on

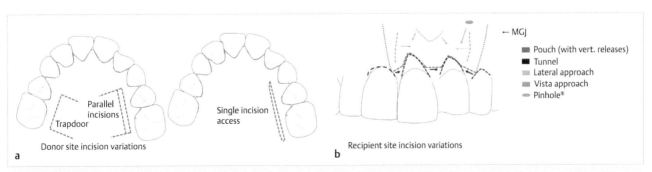

Fig. 8.5 Variations on the connective tissue graft. (a) Variations on palatal connective tissue harvesting through various incision designs. (b) A comparative view of more widely known variations in recipient site incision design.

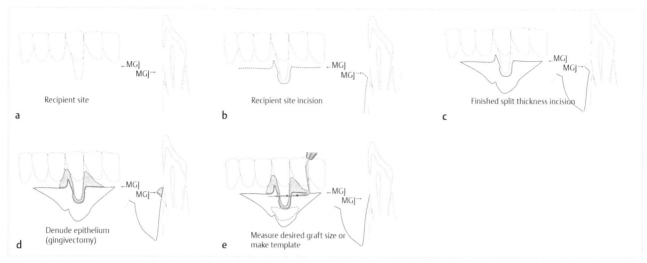

Fig. 8.6 (a–e) Recipient site preparation for a free gingival graft. For improved color match, denude the gingiva coronal to the planned graft by shaving the epithelium off with a sharp scalpel blade until the tissue bleeds slightly (**d**).

the facial surface of the root along the long axis of the tooth, and following the tooth contour the interproximal bone. Once on the interproximal bone, follow the facial surface of the interproximal bone to the adjacent tooth, while keeping the same apio-coronal orientation of the blade. This should remove the facial epithelium on the papilla revealing lighter pink tissue with small bleeding capillaries.

- Scale and root plane the adjacent root and tooth surfaces to produce a healthier healing environment.
- Make a template for the tissue graft using a clean, preferably sterile material (i.e., the protective liner inside the scalpel packet can be used as template material) and cut it to size using suture scissors. Typically, the graft template should be shaped like a shield that covers the area lacking keratinized tissue and about ½ tooth width of the surrounding size as the graft shrinks about 50% as it heals.
- Cover the recipient site with wet sterile gauze until ready to proceed with the next steps (see ▶ Fig. 8.7, for steps).

Harvest the Donor Tissue

There are some variations in harvesting the tissue, but the following method is common (▶ Fig. 8.7):

- Evaluate the palate, note the area of increased tissue thickness near the premolars and note the location of the soft tissue thickening on the floor of the palate near the 2nd molar marking the greater palatal foramen.
- Apply the template on the thick palatal tissue near the premolars. The border of the template should be 3 mm from the gingival margin of the teeth. The apical border of the template should be well clear off the palatal floor. Rotate the template to see which orientation covers thick palatal tissue best. Mark the corners of template with a periodontal probe by piecing the underlying soft tissue.
- With a new scalpel blade, trace the outline of the template with a scalpel, sinking the blade into the tissue about 1.5 mm, which is the width of the bevel on the scalpel blade. Make sure not to infringe on the gingival margin of the adjacent teeth to avoid recession, and avoid the palatal floor with the greater palatine vascular bundle. There will be some bleeding that occurs at this time.

- Pick up a corner of tissue within the incised outline using a tissue forceps, and bend this toward the graft, revealing the tissue side.
- Run the scalpel blade lightly back and forth across the tissue side 1.5 mm from the epithelial surface. Pick up the corner and slowly peel away the epithelial layer from the underlying connective tissue.
- Working toward the center of the graft, increase incision depth slightly so that the graft becomes thicker (about 2.0 mm) and contains a thin layer of dark pink connective tissue.
- Working toward the far side of the graft, decrease incision depth slightly so that the graft becomes thinner (about 1.5 mm).
- Pick up the graft and place it on a sterile tongue depressor. Drip some sterile saline on it to keep it moist.
- Immediately have an assistant apply pressure on the now denuded connective tissue on the palate with a piece of wet gauze for 5 to 10 minutes.
  - If pressure alone does not stop bleeding, place a hemostatic agent, such as oxidized cellulose, on the wound and reapply pressure for 5 to 10 minutes.
  - If there is persistent bleeding from the distoapical corner of the donor site, place a simple interrupted suture through the tissue just distal and apical to the donor site and suture it tightly.
  - Apply 1 to 2 drops of tissue glue on the denuded connective tissue. "Cure" the tissue glue by applying wet gauze on it. Be careful not to drop tissue glue on the patient's tongue, eyes, or on gloves.
- While the assistant applies pressure on the palate, trim the graft. Remove blood clots by gently dabbing the graft with wet gauze. As the graft adheres to the wooden tongue depressor, identify the pale pink epithelium. Remove any larger pieces of yellow adipose tissue from the graft, and any nodular glandular tissue. Trim off any rugae folds from the epithelial surface if there are any. Trim the connective tissue side so that the graft thickness does not exceed 2.0 mm. Trim the mesial, apical, and distal side with a scalpel that there is a 45 degree bevel on the sides of the graft so that the epithelium slightly protrudes over the connective tissue portion of the graft.
- As soon as fair hemostasis has been achieved on the palate, immediately insert the surgical stent.

Apply Free Gingival Graft to Recipient Site

Apply the free gingival graft as soon as possible after harvest (► Fig. 8.7f and ► Fig. 8.7g):

- Visualize the epithelium and insert a suture into the mesial coronal corner of the graft while the graft is still adhering on the wooden tongue depressor. Feed the suture through until most of it has passed through the graft.
- With an assistant's help, transfer the wooden tongue depressor with the graft closely to the patient's mouth. Insert the needle now through the base of the gingiva mesial to the mucogingival defect and have it emerge a few millimeters coronal near the base of the papilla. Tie now the simple interrupted suture knot so that the mesial coronal corner of the graft ends up resting on the former mucogingival junction mesial to the mucogingival defect.
- Suture the distal coronal corner to the mucogingival junction distal to the mucogingival defect using a simple interrupted suture. The graft should now passively rest on the denuded mucosa apical to the mucogingival junction.
- Use an inverting horizontal mattress suture to press the graft against the underlying connective tissue:
  ○ Insert the suture needle mesial to the apical 1/3 of the graft into the underlying connective tissue, and have the needle reemerge mesial to the coronal 1/3 of the graft.
  ○ Insert the suture needle distal to the coronal 1/3 of the graft and have it reemerge distal to the apical 1/3 of the graft.
  ○ Tie a surgical knot. There will now be two horizontal sutures running over the coronal and apical 1/3 of the graft.

- Use a combined horizontal-vertical inverting mattress sutures to further secure the graft:
  ○ Insert the suture needle far apical to the mesial 1/3 of the graft (which also will be apical to the mesial papilla) and have it reemerge just apical to the graft.
  ○ Insert the suture into the base of the gingiva just coronal to the mesial 1/3 of the graft and have it reemerge in the papilla coronal to the mesial 1/3 of the graft.
  ○ Insert the suture into the papilla coronal to the distal 1/3 of the graft, and have it reemerge just coronal to the distal 1/3 of the graft.
  ○ Insert the suture just apical to the distal 1/3 of the graft and have it reemerge far apical to the distal 1/3 of the graft.
  ○ Tie a surgical knot at the base of this tissue pouch. This will delay epithelialization and significantly deepen the vestibule at the graft site. This should create a "#" pattern across the graft that firmly fixates it into place.
- Check if the graft moves at all when aggressively pulling on the lip or cheek. The graft should not move relative to the underlying tissue. If it does move, deepen the pouch around the graft until there is no graft movement. The reason for this step is that graft mobility will make the graft fail.
- Firmly apply pressure with wet gauze on the graft to induce hemostasis and force out any intervening air or blood that may prevent graft survival.
- Provide typical postoperative instruction similar to any oral surgery and repeat instructions regarding pain control.

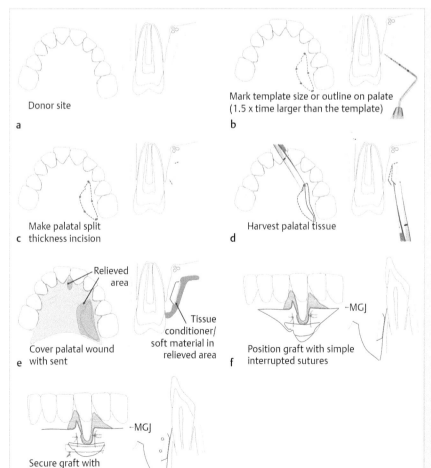

Donor site

a

Mark template size or outline on palate
(1.5 x time larger than the template)

b

Make palatal split
c thickness incision

Harvest palatal tissue

d

Relieved area

Cover palatal wound
e with sent

Tissue conditioner/ soft material in relieved area

MGJ

Position graft with simple
f interrupted sutures

MGJ

Secure graft with
g overlaying sutures

Fig. 8.7 (a–g) Harvesting of a free gingival graft and application of graft to recipient site. (This particular "NMB" stent design was developed by Mr. Nazir, CDT, Dr. Mardirossian, and Dr. Boehm).

Variations

There are only few variations on gingival grafting. One variation involves using a palatal tissue harvester that peels off epithelial tissue similar to a potato peeler. This is useful for harvesting a large strip of palatal tissue.

For improved color matching, some researchers suggest using a free gingival graft that has been partially denuded of the epithelium from the mesial, distal, and apical ends of the graft.[11] For improved effectiveness in achieving root coverage at sites with reduced papillae and lack of keratinized tissue, the "free gingival unit graft" has been proposed that includes marginal and papillary gingiva from the palatal donor site.

Recently, to avoid the pain and color tissue mismatch issues from palatal harvesting, there is a commercially available service that produces tissue engineered gingival grafts from a small amount of patient gingiva (i.e., Gintuit).

Instead of sutures, some researchers proposed using small gingival screws to fixate to graft, or tissue glue, but it is yet unknown if this will replace the conventional suturing techniques.

8.5.5 Apical Positioned Flap Surgery

Apically displaced flaps have been traditionally used to resolve pockets while preserving the existing keratinized gingiva. A split thickness version of this procedure has been used for many years to gain keratinized tissue by apical positioning of the mucogingival junction. Contemporary versions of this procedure split the keratinized tissue with an incision into a coronal portion including the gingival margin, and an apical portion that is mobilized with a split thickness incision and repositioned apically. The resulting shallow, slit-like open wound fills with granulation tissue and is overgrown by keratin-producing epithelial cells from both coronal end apical sides of the incision, which then becomes new keratinized gingiva. This procedure is particularly useful for implant therapy as implant sites often have reduced amounts of keratinized gingiva. For sites with teeth, this method also presents an alternative to free gingival grafting as it can create additional keratinized gingiva over a long distance with good color match. However, a major limitation of this procedure is that it requires at least some preexisting keratinized gingiva, and is extremely difficult to perform successfully in a patient with thin gingival biotype. Although it often produces a good color match, it can also produce a prominent white scar at the apical edge of the incision.

While many variations of this surgery are possible depending on the demands of a given case and a surgeon's preference, a simple method follows these steps:
- Evaluate the site first, determine the site of the mucogingival junction and the amount of keratinized gingiva. Determine the area that has minimal keratinized gingiva and extend it by two teeth on the mesial and distal side, which is the incision site. Check that the gingival tissue at the site of incision is thick and healthy, as thin, friable and inflamed tissue will likely rip during the surgery and produce subpar results.
- Provide ample local infiltration anesthesia in the vestibule and facial mucosa of the sextant receiving the surgery.

Finish infiltration with 2% lidocaine/1:50,000 epinephrine in the facial mucosa, few drops at a time.
- Make a linear, straight split-thickness incision distal to mesial at the half-way point between the mucogingival junction and the lowest gingival margin. The scalpel blade should be about 1.5 mm (the width of the scalpel bevel) into the tissue.
- Apply apical and lateral tension on the vestibular mucosa by either pulling on the lip (or cheek) or placing a mirror handle into the vestibule. The tension should make the original incision gape.
- With continued tension on the vestibule, insert the scalpel blade into the incision, angling it parallel to the teeth and the facial alveolar bone surface. Gently run the blade back and forth within the incision, which will release the apical incision margin and widen the gash in the tissue. Intermittently, apply firm pressure with sterile gauze to control bleeding.
- Continue the sharp dissection of the gingiva, passing under the mucogingival junction while leaving a substantial layer of soft tissue on the bone surface. Make sure not to perforate through the buccal flap as there sometimes is an undercut in the alveolar ridge at the level of the mucogingival junction. Continue the incision until there is a 4 to 5 mm wide gap between coronal and apical incision edges.
- Tack the apical incision edge to the underlying connective tissue at the new apical position with tacking sutures: for each area apical to a papilla, insert the suture needle 3-mm apical to the apical incision edge so that it engages a good amount of periosteum and emerges near the vestibular floor. Tie a surgical knot so that the tissue is firmly held in an apical position against the underlying connective tissue, but avoid tightening the knot to the point that the tissue blanches.
- With sterile gauze, apply firm pressure toward the bone and vestibule on the incision site to induce hemostasis. There should now be a shallow linear gap in the gingiva exposing a few millimeters of bare connective tissue. This will fill in with epithelium over the next 1 to 2 weeks and produce about half of the area in new gingiva.
- Provide the usual postoperative instructions.

8.5.6 Pedicle Flap Surgeries

A traditional method that can produce root coverage and increase keratinized tissue at the same time at a single isolated facial or lingual gingival recession defect is the pedicle flap. These are also called lateral positioned flaps as they mobilize an area of gingiva and rotate it mesially or distally over a denuded root surface. As stated, the advantage of this procedure is that this surgery can achieve both increased root coverage and gain of keratinized tissue while maintaining excellent color match. However, the main limiting factor is that requires sufficient keratinized gingiva adjacent to it, a thick or normal gingival biotype, and sufficient vestibular depth for flap movement. The procedure typically is done as follows (▶ Fig. 8.8):
- Evaluate the site with the recession defect and adjacent gingival area. Visualize the size of the recession defect and see if there is twice as much keratinized gingiva adjacent to it. Decide which side of the defect will be rotated into the defect, which will be the donor side. The other side will be the recipient side, and serve as anchor point for the pedicle. Ensure that the recipient site consists of thick gingiva. Ensure also that the donor site is thick, and has healthy

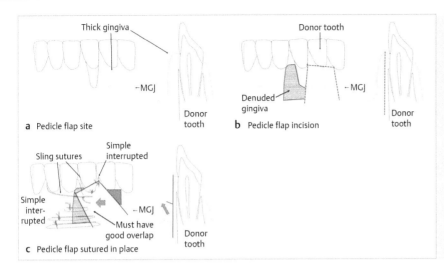

Fig. 8.8 (a–c) Pedicle flap surgery. For the pedicle flap to work, it is important that the connective tissue at the donor site is thick and that a large area of epithelium is denuded so that there is blood supply for the repositioned pedicle flap. For suturing, it is important that the pedicle is held in a position where it overlaps a large area of denuded tissue while not being stretched too much. The denuded areas will fill in with the surrounding gingiva.

tissue. Evaluate the vestibule and check that the vestibule is deep enough to accommodate a rotated pedicle.
- Provide ample infiltration anesthesia.
- Take a new scalpel blade, and shave off the epithelium from the recipient site, exposing a strip of about 4 to 5 mm wide connective tissue in mesio-distal direction.
- Insert the scalpel blade into the sulcus at the base of the gingival defect adjacent to the donor site, keeping it angled parallel to the alveolar bone surface in a mesial-distal direction. Advance the blade until it is immersed in tissue for twice the width of the recession defect. Stay close to the alveolar bone, and move the blade coronally up to a point 2-mm coronal to the CEJ. The goal of this is to produce a flap that is almost as thick as a full thickness flap, but with a small amount of tissue still covering the bone.
- Reinsert the scalpel blade into the sulcus at the base of the gingival defect, and further separate the donor tissue by moving the blade apically along the surface of the bone and further undermining the donor site past the mucogingival junction.
- Now create the free pedicle flap by making a full thickness, straight, and linear incision at the donor site gingival margin from 2-mm coronal to the CEJ in mesial-distal direction until a point is reached that is twice as far as the recession defect's width.
- From this point, make a slightly slanted vertical release to the depth of the vestibule so that the base of the flap is wider than the coronal end. This should create a loose trapezoidal tag of gingival tissue or the pedicle flap.
- Scale and root plane the denuded root surface thoroughly.
- *Optional*: Apply root-conditioning agent (i.e., citric acid, EDTA) and wash the root surface.
- *Create a sling suture to hold the tissue over the recession defect*: Insert the suture needle into the center of the coronal 1/3 of the pedicle flap and retrieve the needle from the underside of the flap. Insert the needle again into the interproximal papilla base from the defect side so that the needle reemerges under the contact point on the opposite side of the tooth with the recession defect. Wrap the suture around the tooth on the far side of the recipient site and back under the contact point. Tie the suture knot so that the tissue is held over the denuded root surface.
- With very fine suturing material connect and tack down the flap on the recipient site with a series of simple interrupted

sutures, one suture for every 3-mm pedicle length in apico-coronal direction, and 3 mm from the flap edge. At the end of this, root coverage and adjacent soft tissue should be completely covered with pink soft tissue. At the donor site, there is exposed red connective tissue.
- Apply firm pressure with wet gauze against the pedicle flap overlying the root surface to achieve hemostasis.
- Provide typical postoperative instructions.

8.5.7 Variant: Double Pedicle Flap and Double Pedicle Flap Combined with Connective Tissue Graft

A variant of the pedicle flap is the double pedicle flap that uses gingiva from both sides of the recession defect to cover a root surface. The benefit of this procedure is that it requires less gingiva and less flap movement that could compromise blood supply, and is often possible to perform when there is not enough adjacent gingival tissue for a single pedicle flap. This procedure is useful for repair of single, narrow gingival recession defects such as Stillman's clefts. Although surgically demanding, requiring many fine sutures to link the two pedicles together, it can be combined with a connective tissue graft for predictably increased root coverage and tissue thickness.

8.6 Describe Surgical Strategies that Reposition Gingiva and Vestibular Mucosa

At times, it may also be necessary to reposition gingiva or vestibular mucosa to have mucogingival architecture that is conducive to oral health.

8.6.1 Coronally Positioned Flap

A coronal positioned flap may provide root coverage for multiple shallow gingival recession defects where connective tissue grafting is not feasible. A coronally positioned flap can reposition a free gingival graft that was originally placed to correct a lack of keratinized gingiva at a site that lacked both keratinized tissue and root coverage.

There are many different ways of coronally positioning tissue. One method is to create a split thickness flap and coronally advance it onto the tooth, as seen with the connective tissue graft procedure earlier in this chapter. One simple and effective way of improving root coverage with little postoperative pain is the semilunar coronally positioned flap (▶ Fig. 8.9), as long as the tissue is healthy with minimal probing depth:

- Provide ample infiltration anesthesia for the area and adjacent teeth.
- Root plane exposed root surface.
- Create the semilunar incision:
  ○ Insert the scalpel into the sulcus at the gingival defect base roughly parallel to the tooth surface and aiming at the facial bone surface of the alveolar bone.
  ○ Advance the blade on the facial bone surface until reaching a depth past the gingival margin that is somewhat greater than the depth of the recession defect.
  ○ Sweep the blade mesially and distally from this position, following the gingival margin contour. Stop at least 2-mm shy of the papilla tip as this area will supply the flap with blood. This should create a sizeable pouch of gingiva.
  ○ Reinsert the blade into this pouch, and change the angulation of the blade away from the bone surface. Insert the blade deeper, and penetrate the gingiva or mucosa at a depth that quite exceeds the depth of the recession defect. Seep the blade mesially and distally to create a crescent-shaped incision line. There should now be a wide bridge of gingiva overlying the root surface, and beginning to creep over the exposed root surface as the tissue's elasticity pulls it coronally.
- With wet gauze, move the bridge of gingiva on to the exposed root surface and hold it there for 5 minutes until coagulation secures the graft in the new position. Frequently, no suturing is necessary.
- Inspect the tissue. There should not be any exposed hard tissue at the apical crescent-shaped incision. If there is, either press the tissue back apically and suture the incision, or harvest and place a free gingival graft over the fenestration.
- Once hemostasis has been achieved, provide typical postoperative instructions.

8.6.2 Frenectomy

Basic frenectomy is a simple procedure that eliminates frenum pull. This procedure can not only easily be done with electrosurgery or soft tissue lasers, but can also be quickly done with traditional scalpel surgery. A well-defined, fibrous frenum can be removed in the following way (see ▶ Fig. 8.10):

- Provide ample infiltration anesthesia in the area of the frenum to be excised.

- Pull on the lip (or cheek) in order to activate the frenum and make it stand out.
- Take a hemostat and grab the frenum near the gingiva.
- With either tissue scissors or a scalpel, cut through the frenum base on the gingiva and around the hemostat.
- With either tissue scissors or a scalpel, cut off the frenum base from the surface of the vestibular mucosa.
- This creates a diamond-shaped wound where the frenum used to be. To reduce the chance of re-attachment, place a series of nonresorbable sutures (i.e., simple interrupted) into the open wound. The goal of suturing here is not to obtain wound closure, but to place a foreign body and irritant into the wound. This will delay wound healing, favor healing by secondary intention and discourage frenum re-attachment. (▶ Fig. 8.10d).
- Apply pressure with wet gauze until hemostasis occurs.
- Provide basic postoperative instructions.

For wide frenum attachments, there is a larger risk of frenum attachment. A variant of frenectomy includes addition of a free gingival graft over the frenum excision site, which is an effective method in preventing frenum re-attachment.

8.6.3 Vestibuloplasty Procedures

While vestibuloplasty is usually considered in the context of preprosthetic oral maxillofacial surgery, there are periodontal scenarios where a shallow vestibule combined with a low amount of keratinized gingiva makes oral hygiene difficult. This usually occurs in the anterior mandible and neither a free gingival graft nor frenectomy procedure covers enough of an area to be effective in this scenario. A solution for this is the Edlan-Mejchar vestibuloplasty technique. This technique uses a split thickness incision in vestibular mucosa to reposition mucosa as a nonmobile, pseudo-attached gingiva on the alveolar ridge and create new mucosa by secondary intention healing. For large areas of shallow vestibule and low keratinized tissue, this method has been shown to improve oral health by allowing better plaque control.

The vestibuloplasty can be achieved with the following steps:

- Evaluate the vestibule and determine the mucogingival junction. Visualize how much "attached" gingiva needs to be achieved, and how deep the vestibule should be. Usually, the aim is to achieve 5 mm of "attached" gingiva from the gingival margin, and a vestibular depth of 10 mm from the gingival margin. Typically, this is the tissue 10-mm apical/facial to the gingival margin, which is the incision site. Visualize the location of vital structures such as the mental foramen, and check the vestibular mucosa for the presence of any abnormal large blood vessels (>1 mm in width). If there are large blood vessels, consider referral

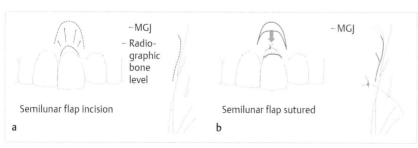

Fig. 8.9 (a–b) Steps for creating a semilunar flap. An undermining split thickness incision is made from the gingival sulcus to some point beyond the mucogingival junction, creating a bridge of epithelium that tends to slide coronally and cover a shallow recession defect. Often, no suturing is required, but a sling suture can secure the tissue in a more coronal position.

Semilunar flap incision

a

Semilunar flap sutured

b

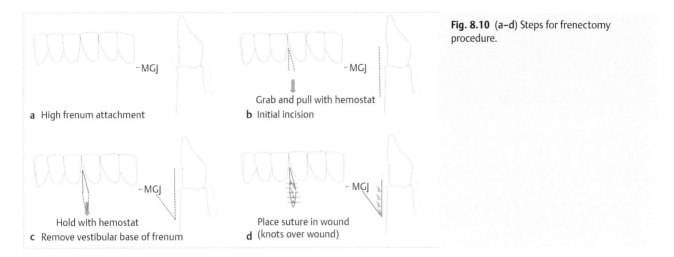

Fig. 8.10 (a–d) Steps for frenectomy procedure.

a High frenum attachment

b Initial incision — Grab and pull with hemostat

c Remove vestibular base of frenum — Hold with hemostat

d Place suture in wound (knots over wound)

to an experienced surgeon for coagulation and removal of these vessels.

- Apply ample buccal infiltration into facial mucosa and vestibular mucosa. Make sure to infiltrate deeply in the vestibule. Finish with small infiltrations of 2% lidocaine and 1:50,000 epinephrine.
- Aggressively pull on the lip to stretch the vestibular mucosa away from the mucogingival junction. With a sharp scalpel, incise the mucosa at the desired distance from the gingival margin, which will become the floor of the new vestibule. Carry this from canine to canine in a smooth slightly curved incision. The blade only needs to penetrate the mucosa by about 0.5 mm, at which point the incisal edge of the flap will start to separate.
- Aim the scalpel blade under the coronal flap edge now, and work toward the bone by running the scalpel blade back and forth over the exposed soft tissue fibers. With continued cutting, the lip tissue will become more mobile and the mucosa at the coronal incision side will collapse toward the alveolar ridge. Continue this process, aiming to achieve a tissue thickness of about 1 to 2 mm, avoiding vital structures and working toward the alveolar bone until the scalpel tissue contacts hard tissue.
- From there, continue sharp dissection along the surface of the alveolar bone until the desired vestibular depth is reached.
- Drape the mucosa of the coronal incision edge over the alveolar bone and press it firmly into place with wet gauze. Use tacking sutures if necessary to hold the tissue in the new position, but usually this is not needed as the mucosa will readily adhere to the periosteum.
- Place wet gauze in the deepened vestibule and press the lip against it until hemostasis has been achieved.
- Provide usual postoperative instructions. Even though dramatic, the large open wound in the vestibule will readily granulate and fill in with new epithelium within 2 weeks.

8.7 Key Takeaways

- Recognizing soft tissue deficiencies is an important part of comprehensive periodontal therapy, and is often overlooked. Early recognition and treatment enhances predictability and treatment success.
- Periodontal therapy, for gingival recession, is often a compromise between pocket reduction versus increased recession.
- Generally, 2 mm of keratinized mucosa is needed for gingival health in teeth and implants.
- Multiple strategies exist for root coverage and correcting mucogingival deficiencies but all rely on identifying the problem, controlling contributing factors and choosing the proper surgical procedure(s).
- Premedication with analgesics, surgical stents, and setting correct patient expectations greatly reduces postoperative complications with mucogingival surgery.

8.8 Review Questions

A 56-year old Hispanic female presents to you complaining about a loose partial denture and concerned about the teeth getting longer in the front. Other than missing teeth, she is physically healthy and was seen for a physical 2 weeks ago. She does not take any medication or supplement, and denies ever having used tobacco. She reports that she had the partial denture made 9 years ago, which was the last time she has seen a dentist. The denture originally fit well, but over time has starting to become loose and she took it out for the photographs.

Blood pressure is 120/59 mm Hg and pulse is 65/min.

The extraoral exam did not reveal any significant findings as skin, lymph nodes muscle, temporomandibular joint (TMJ) area appeared and felt normal. Intraoral exam revealed shallow caries on a number of occlusal and interproximal surfaces (nos. 2 O, 3 M, 6 M+D, 12 M+D, 14 DO, 15 O, 19 OB, 20 O, and 29 O). As these were pointed out to the patient, she mentions that the teeth sometimes were sensitive toward cold or juice. Several wear facets and abfraction type lesions (nos. 2, 20 to 26, 28, and 29) were also seen, and the patient reports that she does clench her teeth during tasks she focuses on such as driving. Oral cancer screening did not identify any lesions or salivary gland abnormalities. The palate is 15 to 20 mm deep and covered with healthy thick gingiva, especially near the premolars. However, there were signs of periodontal disease including isolated 5 to 6 mm pocketing and significant facial and interproximal recession.

The patient's clinical presentation (▶ Fig. 8.11) and radiographs (▶ Fig. 8.12) are shown in these figures.

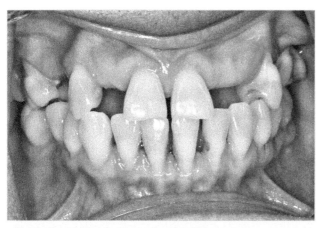

Fig. 8.11 Initial facial presentation of review case.

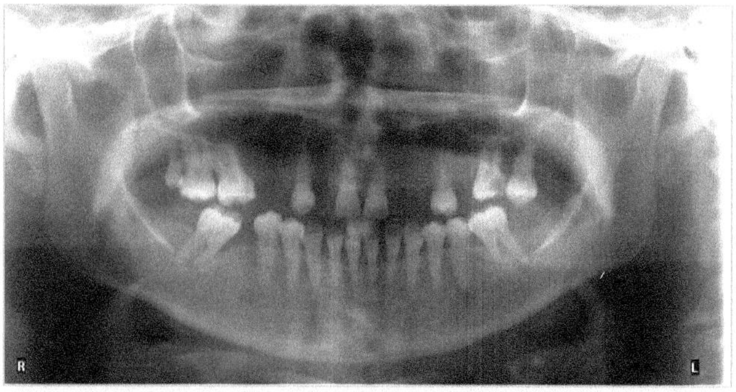

Fig. 8.12 Panoramic radiograph at initial exam.

Findings in the periodontal chart are as follows:

Maxilla facial		1	2	3	4	5	6	7	8	9	10	11	12	13	14	15	16
	PD	333	322	226			323		323	333			433		533	433	
	BOP																
	CAL	2	3	6			2		2	2			5		5	5	
	GR		12	344			11						233		233	342	
	MGJ	999	989	855			969		989	988			877		656	768	
	Furc			2											1	1	
	PLQ																
Maxilla lingual	PD	223	323	323			323		323	323			423		525	523	
	BOP																
	CAL												3		24	3	
	GR												2			11	
	Furc		1	1											2	1	
	Mobil																
	PLQ																

Mandible lingual		32	31	30	29	28	27	26	25	24	23	22	21	20	19	18	17
	PD		324		222	222	222	322	223	222	223	323	222	322	422		
	BOP																
	CAL		4		5	3	3	5	6	5	5	4	3	2	6		
	GR		233		233		2	343	344	334	333	321	1	111	433		
	MGJ		433		569	768	669	655	656	756	666	879	999	989	989		
	Furc		2												2		
	PLQ																
Mandible facial	PD		335		222	322	222	222	222	222	222	222	222	222	323		
	BOP																
	CAL		3		6	3	2	4	5	5	5	4	5	4	3		
	GR				654	222		2	232	243	333	2	243	42	23		
	MGJ		766		447	857	989	757	748	858	969	999	769	979	866		
	Furc														1		
	Mobil																
	PLQ																

Abbreviations: BOP, bleeding on probing (1), suppuration (2); CAL, clinical attachment level; Furc, furcation involvement (Glickman class); GR, gingival recession; MGJ, position of mucogingival junction from margin; Mobil, tooth mobility (Miller grade); PD, probing depths; PLQ, plaque level (0 = none, 5 = heavy).

Oral hygiene instruction was given and scaling and root planing performed for all quadrants with pockets of 5 or more millimeters depth. Carious lesions were removed and restored with direct composite restorations. At the reevaluation visit, probing depths were now 2 to 3 mm with no bleeding on probing, but recession (AGR)/keratinized gingiva (MGJ) essentially was the same. The exception was tooth no. 21, where there is a high frenum attachment inserting close to the mesiobuccal line angle of the tooth. At this position, there is only 1-mm keratinized gingiva while the probing depth is almost 2 mm. Before the construction of a new maxillary partial denture, you evaluate the patient's gingiva, and are wondering if the mucogingival conditions can be improved.

Learning Objective: Recognize indications for mucogingival surgery.

1. What are the causes and contributing factors of the patient's gingival recession? (Select all that apply)
   A. Periodontitis
   B. Tobacco use
   C. Orthodontics
   D. Occlusal trauma

2. Evaluate the following statements.
   Statement 1: If you want to close the diastema between teeth nos. 8 and 9, you should consider frenectomy at this site.
   Statement 2: At tooth no. 21, the frenum attachment likely is a contributing factor to the recession seen at this tooth.
   A. Both statements are correct
   B. Neither statement is correct
   C. Only the first statement is correct
   D. Only the second statement is correct

3. If you were a general dentist managing this patient's recession, what would be a key deciding factor for referring this patient to a periodontal specialist?
   A. Complex medical history
   B. Extent of recession
   C. Need for large-scale vestibuloplasty
   D. Severe periodontal disease

Learning Objective: Create treatment plans that prevent, manage, or correct mucogingival problems.

4. The patient in this case currently uses a medium brush and whitening toothpaste. If you observed the patient while she is brushing her teeth, which motion would be MOST likely to worsen her gingival recession?
   A. Sweeping the brush from the gums to the teeth
   B. Wiggling the brush head while it is pointed at the sulcus
   C. Scrubbing across the facial tooth surfaces
   D. Making big circles over teeth and gingiva

5. Evaluate the gingival area around the mandibular incisors. Which of the following mucogingival conditions are present?
   a) Facial gingival recession
   b) No attached gingiva
   c) Interproximal gingival recession
   d) Thin gingiva
   e) Shallow vestibule
   A. a, b, d
   B. b, c, e
   C. b, d, e
   D. a, c, d

6. Evaluate the following statements.
   Statement 1: Increasing root coverage is not at all possible for the mandibular incisors.
   Statement 2: Because the interdental papillae have been reduced in height.
   A. Both the statement and the reason are correct and related
   B. Both the statement and the reason are correct but NOT related
   C. The statement is correct, but the reason is NOT
   D. The statement is NOT correct, but the reason is correct
   E. NEITHER the statement NOR the reason is correct

7. If your goal is to increase root coverage and thicken the facial gingiva overlaying the mandibular incisors, you would need to treatment plan a?
   A. Free gingival graft
   B. Connective tissue graft
   C. Apically positioned flap
   D. Gingival flap (for coronal repositioning)

Learning Objective: Describe surgical strategies that augment gingival tissues.

8. What is the defining element common to nearly all mucogingival surgery techniques?
   A. Split-thickness incisions
   B. Use of collagen membranes
   C. Palatal tissue harvest
   D. Tissue elevation past the mucogingival junction

9. Evaluate the following statements.
   Statement 1: A palatal graft for the free gingival graft procedure contains epithelium.
   Statement 2: The recipient site incision for both gingival graft and connective tissue grafting are exactly the same.
   A. Both statements are true
   B. Both statements are false
   C. The first statement is true, the second is false
   D. The first statement is false, the second is true

10. In this case, what would make connective tissue grafting for the mandibular incisor site challenging?
    A. Shallow palate
    B. Thin tissue at recipient site
    C. Medical history
    D. Shallow vestibule

Learning Objective: Describe surgical strategies that reposition gingiva and vestibular mucosa.

11. Evaluate the following statements.
    Statement 1: For tooth no. 21, placement of a free gingival graft also needs to include a frenectomy.

Statement 2: For tooth no. 21, a placed free gingival graft can be later repositioned coronally.
A. Both statements are true
B. Both statements are false
C. The first statement is true, the second is false
D. The first statement is false, the second is true

12. After the Edlan-Mejchar vestibuloplasty procedure, there is …
A. A large ulcer on the alveolar ridge
B. Exposed alveolar bone
C. A free gingival graft in the vestibule
D. Vestibular mucosa covering the alveolar ridge

8.9 Answers

1. **A** and **D**. The interproximal loss of tissue is best explained by the patient's history of generalized periodontitis as evidenced mostly by the interproximal bone loss. The facial recession seems to be associated mostly with abfraction type lesions that are in turn associated with occlusal trauma, maybe from the patient's clenching habit and loss of teeth. The patient denied using tobacco, and the tooth staining may also have been from caries or certain foods. The patient did not report having orthodontic treatment done, and the patient's somewhat irregular occlusal plane and lack of root alterations suggest that this is true. Not an answer choice, but possible contributing factor is the patient's anatomy as the incisors are tipped forward and the patient seems to have a thin gingival biotype. This is suggested by the mandibular incisors where the root surface or underlying bone seems to show through the gingiva.

2. **A.** As seen on the case photograph, there is a wide frenum attachment at the interproximal papilla between teeth nos. 8 and 9, and this site also has a diastema. Orthodontic treatment could close the space, but the frenum would likely cause relapse without a permanent wire retainer. What makes the recession worrisome at tooth no. 21 is that there is inflammation as evidenced by the erythema seen in the case photograph, and a high frenum attachment, which likely will worsen the recession that is there already.

3. **B.** This patient is healthy, so medical complexity is not an issue in this case. In other cases, patients with complex medical history may benefit from collaboration with a periodontal specialist. Even though the patient has several prominent frena, vestibuloplasty is not indicated as the vestibule space seen in the photographs is quite large. Even though the patient has moderate bone loss and isolated severe facial attachment loss, it seems that the patient's periodontal condition can be stabilized given the low amount of pocketing seen at the reevaluation visit. So, the main reason for referral may be the number of recession sites, which includes almost every tooth seen on the case photographs.

4. **C.** Out of the techniques listed here, scrubbing is the most aggressive method as the bristles will sweep across the gingival margin. Choice **B** describes the modified Bass technique, which is less aggressive as there is little unidirectional bristle movement. Choice **A** (Stillman's technique) and Choice **D** (Fones' technique) are least likely to cause tissue damage at the gingival margin as the force of the bristles is not directed against the gingival margin.

5. **D.** The vestibule is likely deep enough to accommodate the tip of a tooth brush head, given the appearance on the photograph. There is sufficient attached gingiva as the data indicates a 5-mm width of the keratinized tissue (MGJ) and there is 2 to 3 mm probing depth at the facial margin, which produces a zone of attached gingiva of 2 to 3 mm. Generally, the attached gingiva of 2 mm or larger width is considered sufficient. The patient does however have gingiva recession as seen on photographs and periodontal charting, both facially and interproximally. The tooth roots seem to shine through the tissue, likely indicating thin gingiva tissue.

6. **D.** The reason is correct in that the height of the interproximal papillae is one of the main limiting factors for root coverage. If in this case, the papillae were healthy with complete interproximal fill and sound bone support, complete root coverage would be likely. However, complete root coverage is not possible as at the level of the CEJ there is no interdental tissue that could provide blood supply and progenitor cells. Although the interproximal tissue is compromised, limited root coverage is still possible as the deep facial recession defects are still surrounded by soft tissue.

7. **B.** From these choices, only connective tissue grafts (either autogenous or other sources) can increase root coverage and thicken the tissue. A free gingival graft will increase keratinized tissue, but not increase root coverage unless combined with a second coronally positioned flap. A coronally positioned flap by itself may increase root coverage, but it will not increase tissue thickness, which is also desired here. An apically positioned flap is the worst choice for this scenario as it can increase keratinized tissue, but will not result in root coverage or increased tissue thickness.

8. **A.** Virtually any mucogingival surgery uses split thickness incisions at some point as these are required to either mobilize tissue flaps or create recipient beds that can receive soft tissue graft material. Collagen membranes only have limited use in mucogingival surgery and are used mainly for guided tissue regeneration. Palatal harvesting is commonly done for autogenous connective tissue grafts and free gingival grafts, but are not used for any basic pedicle or repositioned flap, so it is a stretch to say that they are used for every mucogingival surgery. There also is the alternative of allograft material that can be used instead of palatal tissue. Tissue elevation past the mucogingival junction is a concept more useful for full thickness flaps for surgeries that require access to bone. For mucogingival surgeries, tissue often, but not always, gets incised past or near the mucogingival junction to allow for the movement of a flap edge or pedicle.

9. **C.** While both free gingival graft and connective tissue graft procedures typically use palatal tissue, the incision differs. The free gingival graft incision for the recipient site usually begins at the mucogingival junction and extends apically, whereas the connective tissue graft procedure typically incorporates some gingiva into the incision design.

10. **B.** While all these conditions are potential obstacles to connective tissue harvesting, only the thinness of the soft tissue is evident in this case. The palate according to the

case description is 15 to 20 mm deep with thick tissue near the premolars, which should provide sufficient connective tissue for grafting. While coagulation disorders and connective tissue disorders can complicate grafting procedures, this patient is healthy. A shallow vestibule can complicate coronally positioned flap surgery, but is not present here.

11. **A.** The frenum needs to be removed either prior or as part of the free gingival graft that is planned for this site as the frenum would likely dislodge the graft during healing. For sites with recession and lacking keratinized tissue, a two-step procedure using first a free gingival graft to augment the tissue and then repositioning it can increase root coverage.

12. **D.** The Edlan-Mejchar vestibuloplasty takes the original mucosa from the alveolar ridge, vestibule, and lip, and repositions it on the alveolar ridge while leaving an area of lip connective tissue exposed. There is no bone exposure, which results in quick healing with relatively little pain. A free gingival graft is not used in this type of vestibuloplasty.

8.10 Evidence-based Activities

- Find studies that evaluate or report mucogingival procedures and techniques not described in detail in this chapter (see surgery variations). Also, debate their merit.
- Obtain a clinical case from your instructor/institution or the internet and discuss what surgical treatment may be most suitable for it. Have your instructor (or mentor) provide insights on his or her experience with these treatments.
- Critically evaluate the surgical cases presented in this chapter and debate how the surgical technique can be improved. Have your instructor (or mentor) describe how he or she performs mucogingival surgeries and compare his or her method with the methods presented here. If possible, compare it with other periodontists you have contact with and see how methods compare or differ.
- Go to the University of Texas Health Science Center School of Dentistry at San Antonio's library of critically appraised topics (CAT) at https://cats.uthscsa.edu/ and search for a review

on gingival grafts. Read any CAT you can find, and debate if the conclusion is still correct based on current literature.
- Create a CAT on using Emdogain, regeneration, tissue engineered grafts or growth factors in treating mucogingival conditions (or any other topic for which a CAT is not available) following the outline provided by Sauve S, et al in "The critically appraised topic: a practical approach to learning critical appraisal" (Ann R Coll: Physicians Surg Can; 1995; 28:396–398).

References

[1] Chrysanthakopoulos NA. Prevalence and associated factors of gingival recession in Greek adults. J Investig Clin Dent 2013;4(3):178–185

[2] Heasman PA, Holliday R, Bryant A, Preshaw PM. Evidence for the occurrence of gingival recession and non-carious cervical lesions as a consequence of traumatic toothbrushing. J Clin Periodontol 2015;42(Suppl 16):S237–S255

[3] Ueno D, Nagano T, Watanabe T, Shirakawa S, Yashima A, Gomi K. Effect of the keratinized mucosa width on the health status of periimplant and contralateral periodontal tissues: A cross-sectional study. Implant Dent 2016;25(6):796–801

[4] Halperin-Sternfeld M, Zigdon-Giladi H, Machtei EE. The association between shallow vestibular depth and peri-implant parameters: a retrospective 6 years longitudinal study. J Clin Periodontol 2016;43(3):305–310

[5] Dörfer CE, Staehle HJ, Wolff D. Three-year randomized study of manual and power toothbrush effects on pre-existing gingival recession. J Clin Periodontol 2016;43(6):512–519

[6] Pini-Prato G. The Miller classification of gingival recession: limits and drawbacks. J Clin Periodontol 2011;38(3):243–245

[7] Tonetti MS, Jepsen S; Working Group 2 of the European Workshop on Periodontology. Clinical efficacy of periodontal plastic surgery procedures: consensus report of Group 2 of the 10th European Workshop on Periodontology. J Clin Periodontol 2014;41(Suppl 15):S36–S43

[8] Fickl S, Fischer KR, Jockel-Schneider Y, Stappert CF, Schlagenhauf U, Kebschull M. Early wound healing and patient morbidity after single-incision vs. trapdoor graft harvesting from the palate—a clinical study. Clin Oral Investig 2014;18(9):2213–2219

[9] Zadeh HH. Minimally invasive treatment of maxillary anterior gingival recession defects by vestibular incision subperiosteal tunnel access and platelet-derived growth factor BB. Int J Periodontics Restorative Dent 2011;31(6):653–660

[10] Chao JC. A novel approach to root coverage: the pinhole surgical technique. Int J Periodontics Restorative Dent 2012;32(5):521–531

[11] Cortellini P, Tonetti M, Prato GP. The partly epithelialized free gingival graft (pe-fgg) at lower incisors. A pilot study with implications for alignment of the mucogingival junction. J Clin Periodontol 2012;39(7):674–680

9 Managing Tooth Mobility

Abstract

One of the most immediate dental concerns linked to periodontal disease is tooth mobility, and unlike pocket depth or attachment level, tooth mobility is easily understood by patients. But, what can be done about tooth mobility? Unlike plaque, bleeding on probing, and pocketing, this clinical measure rarely changes with scaling and root planing. This chapter describes the causes of tooth mobility and how it is related to occlusal trauma. While occlusal treatment is a very large topic worthy of its own textbooks and courses, this chapter aims to provide a basic understanding on how tooth mobility develops, the relationship of occlusal trauma to tooth mobility, and how it is related to periodontal disease. This chapter also provides instructions on how to identify occlusal trauma, analyze occlusion, treat minor occlusal discrepancies, and alleviate tooth mobility.

Keywords: mobility, occlusal adjustment, splint

9.1 Learning Objectives

- Recognize causes of tooth mobility.
- Identify occlusal trauma.
- Correct occlusal trauma.
- Alleviate tooth mobility.

9.2 Case

A 62-year old Caucasian male presented to get "everything taken care of" since he complains of several chipped teeth and last had dental treatment 7 years ago.

He has smoked about two packs of cigarettes each day for the last 20 years, and has thought about quitting, but has not done so. He has chronic back pain for which he takes 10-mg Norco as needed, and has hypertension, which is treated with 50-mg Atenolol and 50-mg Nortriptyline once daily. He also takes folic acid 1 mg/day, and has received two IV injection of Denosumab (Prolia) about 2 years and 2 and half years ago for "low bone density."

Blood pressure is 147/85 mm Hg and pulse is 69/minute.

Extraoral exam findings revealed no abnormal findings for the facial skin, lymph nodes, thyroid gland, cranial nerves, salivary glands, masticatory muscles, and temporomandibular joint other than solar elastosis on his facial skin from his previous work as a construction worker. Intraorally, no mucosal pathology was apparent other than periodontal disease and mild nicotine stomatitis near the soft palate. Several fractured teeth and restorations (teeth nos. 3, 13, 14, and 30) are present along with generalized abfractions (teeth nos. 3, 6, 7, 10 to 12, 19 to 25, and 27 to 30) and moderate attrition. Group function was observed in this Angle Class II Division 1 occlusion. Facial profile is convex. Overjet is 5 mm and overbite is about 50%. The patient reports that his wife told him that he grinds his teeth while he sleeps.

For clinical appearance and radiographs (see ▸ Fig. 9.1 and ▸ Fig. 9.2) Findings in the periodontal chart are as follows.

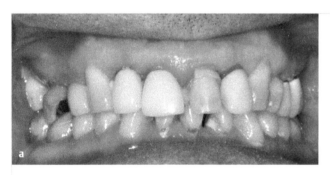
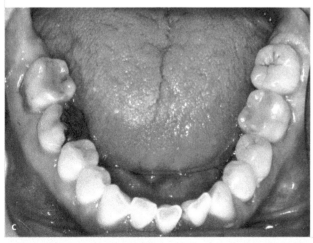
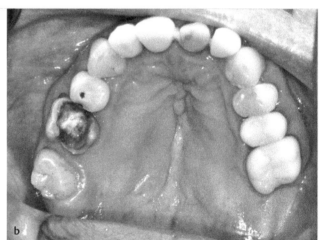

Fig. 9.1 (a–c) Facial and occlusal views.

Maxilla

		1	2	3	4	5	6	7	8	9	10	11	12	13	14	15	16
Maxilla facial	PD	537		765	735		423	323	324	325	523	325	323	433	363		
	BOP				1 1					1	1 1						
	CAL	5		6	3					1	2				5		
	GR																
	MGJ	345	656	656	655	565	589	999	995	599	888	886	556	656	656		
	Furc	1		3											3		
	PLQ	1		1											2		
Maxilla lingual	PD	657		546	997		424	525	524	435	535	534	777	546	333		
	BOP			1					1					1			
	CAL																
	GR																
	Furc	2 2		2 3											3 2		
	Mobil			1				1	1		1		1	1	1		
	PLQ	2		2			1	1	1	1	1	1	1	1	2		

Mandible

		32	31	30	29	28	27	26	25	24	23	22	21	20	19	18	17
Mandible lingual	PD		634	455	443	323	312	323	324		323	222	323	346		623	323
	BOP			5										5		5	4
	CAL																
	GR																
	MGJ		888	888	777	666	555	555	555	555	555	555	666	777		889	999
	Furc		3	1													2
	PLQ		1	1	1	1	2	4	4		4	4	2	2		3	3
Mandible facial	PD		753	423	323	323	233	324	325		323	323	323	323		623	323
	BOP																
	CAL		8		23	23	2	4	4		4	3	4	4			
	GR																
	MGJ		555	666	555	544	555	666	665		665	555	455	555		555	543
	Furc		3	2												1	
	Mobil			1	1												
	PLQ		2	1			3	3			3					1	1

Abbreviations: BOP, bleeding on probing (1), suppuration (2); CAL, clinical attachment level; Furc, furcation involvement (Glickman class); GR, gingival recession; MGJ, position of mucogingival junction from margin; Mobil, tooth mobility (Miller grade); PD, probing depths; PLQ, plaque level (0 = none, 5 = heavy).

After scaling, root planing, and extractions, probing depths were as follows:

		1	2	3	4	5	6	7	8	9	10	11	12	13	14	15	16
Facial	PD	433		565			433	333	323	325	323	323	423	434	346		
	BOP																
Lingual	PD	566		536			423	533	434	325	533	323	573	334	334		
	BOP																

		32	31	30	29	28	27	26	25	24	23	22	21	20	19	18	17
Lingual	PD		333	333	333	323	222	222	222		222	223	323	333		333	333
	BOP																
Facial	PD		653	423	323	323	223	222	215		222	223	323	323		323	323
	BOP																

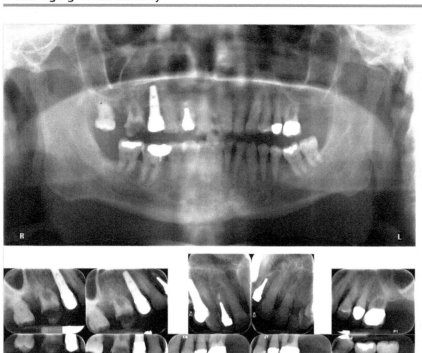

Fig. 9.2 Radiographic series.

What can be learned from this case?

What stands out in this case are the signs of occlusal trauma at his initial presentation. In the facial photograph, notice the uneven plane of occlusion with teeth nos. 3, 9, 10, 11, 13, and 14 protruding past the occlusal plane. Also, notice the deep overbite, and that tooth no. 9 is missing a restoration and has a fractured preparation margin at the mesiofacial line angle. Tooth no. 3 is missing a restoration, had recurrent caries, and appears fractured. Multiple teeth have abfraction lesions on the facial surface near the gingival margin, such as teeth nos. 3, 8, 10, 11, 12, 13, possibly nos. 14, 20, 21, 22, 23, 24, 25, 26, 29, and 30. On the occlusal surfaces of maxillary teeth, notice the wear facets that have exposed dentin at teeth nos. 6, 11, 12, and the worn-through porcelain at tooth no. 4. Worn-through occlusal porcelain is significant as this suggests an extreme level of parafunctional chewing movement capable of wearing through a thick layer of durable and otherwise wear-resistant ceramic. Severe attrition is visible on the incisal surfaces of the anterior teeth, which exposes reparative dentin.

Radiographically, the uneven alveolar crest level parallels the uneven occlusal plane, and there are small, funnel-shaped bone defects at teeth nos. 8, 9, 19, 20, 21, and 30. The periodontal ligament is widened at teeth nos. 12, 13, 28, and 29. There may be a fracture line from the post in the mesial root canal extending to the furcation at tooth no. 30.

There are also obvious signs of periodontal disease such as the deep pocketing, bleeding on probing, and the generalized bone/attachment loss. There are also vertical bone defects associated with local factors such as the furcation entrances of teeth nos. 2, 3, 14, 30, and 31; and the radiographic calculus with defect at the distal of tooth no. 31. The implant at the no. 4 site shows signs of bone loss due to periimplant disease, and there are periapical radiolucencies at teeth nos. 7 and 9 suggesting endodontic infections.

All these suggest a compromised dentition that is difficult to restore to health as many teeth show signs of tooth mobility. Moreover, scaling and root planing (SRP), along with tobacco cessation, did not completely resolve the pockets and did not at all change tooth mobility.

The residual pockets at nos. 1, 3, and 14 are most likely due to the deep furcation involvement of these teeth, and the pocketing around nos. 7, 9, and 10 due to rough tooth surfaces and recurrent caries. The pocketing around tooth no. 31 is most likely due to furcation involvement and deep subgingival calculus. Pocketing around no. 12 is due to mesial root concavity and associated bone defect.

The reason for the tooth mobility is that most teeth have short roots, and severe periodontitis (Stage III, grade C) reduced bone support further. This poor bone support is not changed by SRP, which explains why the tooth mobility has not improved. Given that the patient has a history of bruxing, which produces excessive forces on the teeth, this explains the signs of occlusal trauma and the tooth mobility in this patient.

9.3 Recognizing Causes of Tooth Mobility

Tooth mobility is probably the most difficult and intractable periodontal problem, and typically cannot be solved without an interdisciplinary approach. This is because tooth mobility may be caused by other processes than periodontal disease.

9.3.1 Causes of Tooth Mobility

Teeth derive most of their support by periodontal ligament fibers anchored in the surrounding alveolar bone in most patients. The exception to this are patients with severe alveolar bone loss or severely resorbed roots, where a significant amount of tooth support comes from gingival fibers. This then explains the three general causes of tooth mobility (▶Fig. 9.3).

Periapical/Periodontal Inflammation

Inflammation produces edema and tissue swelling. With periodontal ligament, severe inflammation caused by certain combinations of pathogenic microorganisms and local factors will cause the periodontal ligament to swell while destroying collagen fibers. Likewise, an endodontic infection will destroy the apical fibers of the periodontal ligament and the fluid-buildup in the periapical tissues will force the tooth slightly coronally as it stretched the other periodontal ligament fibers. In both cases, the loss of fiber support and swelling of the periodontal ligament will allow more tooth movement and occasionally produce the clinical appearance of tooth mobility (▶Fig. 9.3—damaged periodontium on right).

Reduced Bone Support

This is the cause of tooth mobility seen in patients with severe periodontitis. Consistent periodontal inflammation destroys collagen fibers of the periodontal ligament while a trend toward bone resorption leads to gradual loss of bone covering the tooth roots. At some point, there will be not enough fibers connecting the tooth to the underlying bone to prevent visible tooth movement (▶Fig. 9.3—reduced periodontium). The point at which this occurs is different for each tooth and depends on root surface morphology. Any root surface feature that increases the root surface area and the number of attached fibers will delay the onset of tooth mobility.

For example, for maxillary central incisors with conical roots, this occurs after about 60% bone loss, but it requires near complete bone loss on maxillary molars for development of noticeable tooth mobility. Also consider that minor tooth mobility is common in mandibular incisors even without periodontal bone loss, mainly because of the narrow size of the tooth roots and thin nature of surrounding alveolar bone.

Occlusal Trauma

It is possible to have tooth mobility in the absence of periodontal or endodontic infection if excessive mechanical forces on the tooth damage the periodontal tissues. In this case, excessive force either ruptures or crushes ligament fibers, leading to immediate loss of fiber support. Or more commonly, continued exposure to excessive forces will trigger remodeling of the periodontal ligament, leading to bone resorption away from the source of occlusal trauma and increased fiber length. Both will allow the tooth to move in response to the excessive force, leading to clinical tooth mobility.

9.3.2 How to Diagnose Causes of Tooth Mobility?

Besides being able to measure tooth mobility, diagnosis of tooth mobility requires evaluation on how inflammation, excessive

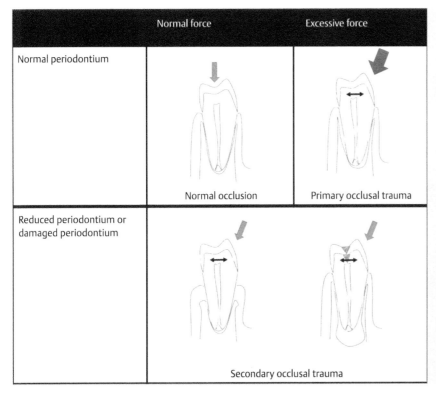

Fig. 9.3 Causes of tooth mobility and occlusal trauma. With a normal periodontium and normal occlusal forces directed along the long axis of the tooth, there will be little clinically observable tooth mobility. Repeated excessive occlusal forces will cause the periodontal ligament and bone to remodel so that the periodontium can absorb the force. This usually results in a widened periodontal ligament, which allows tooth mobility so that the tooth can move away from the excessive force. Usually, this is seen if there is an interference contact resulting in a sideway force against the tooth. If the periodontium is of normal size, this is called primary occlusal trauma. If periodontal disease has sufficiently reduced the periodontium, even normal forces will cause tooth mobility as there is not enough support to resist movement. This is called secondary occlusal trauma. If there is severe inflammation in the periodontium such as caused by an endodontic infection, the periodontium will widen considerably and allow tooth movement.

occlusal force, and loss of support contribute to the observed tooth mobility.

Loss of supporting bone is the simplest identifiable cause of tooth mobility. If there is severe radiographic bone loss that results in a poor crown-to-root ratio worse than 1:1 then some of the observed tooth mobility is likely due to reduced bone support. Usually, incisors will begin to display significant mobility if more than half of bone is lost, whereas maxillary molars require almost complete bone loss to show mobility greater than Miller grade I. Generally, severe tooth mobility (i.e., Miller grade III) is almost always caused by near complete bone loss.

Relatively simple to diagnose is inflammation as a cause of tooth mobility. Swelling in the periodontal ligament due to severe inflammation can cause minor tooth mobility (grade I), and should be suspected for teeth surrounded by severely swollen, red gingiva that bleeds profusely when probed with little pressure. Alternatively, minor tooth mobility may be caused by periapical inflammation in response to endodontic disease, which will become apparent in the form of a periapical radiolucency or radiographic widening of the apical periodontal ligament on fully erupted teeth. The ultimate test of inflammation as a source of tooth mobility is treating the inflammation (i.e., SRP and root canal treatment) and observing a reduction in tooth mobility.

Excessive occlusal force as a source of tooth mobility is more difficult to diagnose as it involves some degree of occlusal analysis and close observation of teeth and radiographs for signs of occlusal trauma (see Section 9.4.4 on how to identify occlusal trauma).

Typically, occlusal trauma in the absence of periodontal inflammation and bone loss produces minor tooth mobility (Miller grade I).

9.3.3 How to Treat Tooth Mobility?

Treating tooth mobility depends on the initial diagnosis of the three causes of tooth mobility (▶ Fig. 9.4). In general, if there is any significant periodontal or endodontic inflammation, it must be treated first.

Once periodontal and endodontic inflammation has been diminished with treatment, tooth mobility needs to be evaluated again. Often, minor tooth mobility (Miller grade I) connected to severe periodontal inflammation connected with heavy plaque and calculus deposits in a patient with mild periodontal disease and no occlusal trauma resolves completely with thorough SRP.

However, tooth mobility is most often caused by a combination of reduced bone support and excessive occlusal force. Since it is often easier to accomplish, the focus is on eliminating any occlusal trauma. Occlusal analysis can suggest ways to eliminate occlusal trauma on a mounted model, and if feasible, this can then be replicated in a patient's mouth through occlusal adjustment. Occlusal adjustment may be as simple as removing a few tenths of millimeters of enamel or restorative material from a few "high" occlusal spots in limited occlusal adjustment, or may require the complete reshaping of most occlusal surfaces with a complete occlusal adjustment (see Section 9.5.2 on how to perform an occlusal analysis and adjustment).

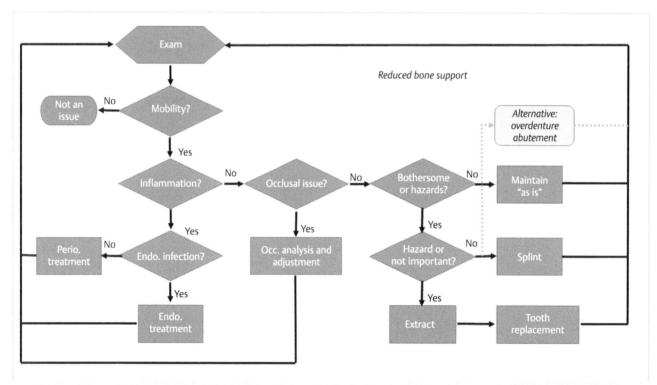

Fig. 9.4 Treatment of tooth mobility. If a tooth is found to be mobile during the exam, check first if there is either periodontal or endodontic inflammation, and treat this with appropriate treatment. If mobility persists and there is evidence of occlusal issues, analyze the occlusion and adjust where necessary. If tooth mobility persists because of reduced bone support, a decision has to be made based on patient comfort, the risk and importance of the problematic tooth. If the tooth is neither a treatment hazard or bothersome, it can be maintained as is, as mobility will not get worse in absence of inflammation or occlusal trauma. If the tooth is bothersome, the symptom of tooth mobility can be removed with a splint as long as the tooth is not a hazard and the patient wants to hold on the tooth. Alternatively, if a patient is receiving a partial or complete denture, bone support can be improved by severely shortening the tooth and using the remaining "stump" as an overdenture abutment where it provides added denture support. For all other situations, the most predictable treatment for mobile teeth is removing them and replacing them with a prosthesis. Endo, Endodontic; Occ, Occlusal; Perio, Periodontal.

It is possible that occlusal adjustment will not eliminate tooth mobility since there is either loss of bone or poor root surface morphology (i.e., a short, thin, and conical tooth root). In this case, it may be decided to leave the tooth "as is" if the patient is not bothered by tooth mobility and the tooth does not present an acute hazard to the patient. A tooth should not be removed simply because of tooth mobility, unless restoration is not possible or there is caries or periodontal infection that is not treatable. If the patient is bothered by tooth mobility and there is no other reason to remove the offending tooth, splinting can relieve the discomfort associated with tooth mobility while maintaining the tooth. A splint connects a mobile tooth or teeth to surrounding teeth that are not mobile, which then eliminates the feeling of tooth mobility if done correctly.

9.4 Identifying Occlusal Trauma

Any periodontal exam should include checking a patient's dentition for signs of occlusal trauma.[1]

9.4.1 Signs of Occlusal Trauma

What are the signs of occlusal trauma? Clinical signs of occlusal trauma include the following:
- Fremitus means tooth movement that can either be observed or felt as a patient occludes. Presence of fremitus is diagnostic for occlusal trauma, and fremitus needs to be eliminated as part of initial, nonsurgical periodontal treatment.
- Tooth mobility not explainable by inflammatory processes or loss of bone support.
- Percussion sensitivity in the absence of pulpal disease. Percussion sensitivity usually indicates inflamed periapical tissue, which may be caused by pulpal disease, and also by irritation triggered by excessive occlusal force.
- Wear facets and attrition, which is excessive for a patient's age and diet pattern, may suggest the presence of occlusal trauma. Some loss of enamel is typical with increasing age, but occlusal dentin should not appear in nongeriatric patients eating mostly soft, cooked, and processed foods. Wear and attrition should not be confused with erosion caused by acidic foods and medical conditions. Erosion can be distinguished

from attrition if the erosion process leaves restorative margins higher than the surrounding tooth structure.
- Abfractions may suggest occlusal trauma. Abfractions are wedge-shaped noncarious cervical lesions that may be caused by high occlusal loads.[2] When evaluating abfractions, it is important to check how the patient uses a toothbrush on this tooth as brushing can cause abfraction-type lesions as well. Similarly, abfraction should not be confused with abrasion, where a mechanical agent such as a gritty dentifrice or smokeless tobacco wears away exposed dentin.
- Tooth and restoration fracture may suggest occlusal trauma, although these can also be related to predisposing restorative factors such as root canal treatment or the presence of large direct restorations.[3]
- Development of exostoses, although other factors such as genetics can also favor the development of exostoses.
- A history of bruxism (tooth grinding) or clenching may suggest the presence of occlusal trauma if there are signs of damage to teeth such as fractures and significant attrition.

Radiographic signs of occlusal trauma include the following:
- Cemental tears.
- Vertical bone defects not attributable to other factors such as furcation entrances and calculus. Usually, these defects will appear as narrow, funnel-shaped bone defects on teeth with significant occlusal wear.
- Widened periodontal ligament near the alveolar crest.[4] A widened periodontal ligament due to occlusal trauma should correspond to clinically observable tooth mobility. Since a widened periodontal ligament can also be caused by rare medical conditions such as scleroderma and osteosarcomas,[5] thorough medical history taking and oral cancer screening must rule out these conditions when widened periodontal ligament is observed.
- Root fractures can be related to occlusal trauma or other predisposing factors.
- Pulpal necrosis and development of periapical radiolucencies in absence of caries, failed restorations, and tooth fractures.

The following case (▶Fig. 9.5) illustrates that occlusal trauma can manifest itself in different ways within the same mouth.

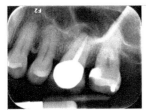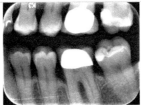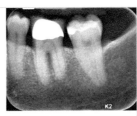

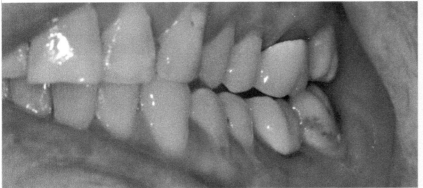

Fig. 9.5 Occlusal trauma may cause different effects on each opposing tooth. Here, there is an interference contact between the first molars caused by the uneven occlusal plane. Bitewings show a bone level mostly parallel to the CEJ of teeth, but the maxillary molar has a large periapical radiolucency related to coronal leakage under a loose crown with strong occlusal wear. The mandibular molar has furcation bone loss and isolated crestal bone loss on the mesial surface. In contrast, the molars on the right side lack occlusal interferences and lack any significant radiographic findings (not shown).

A 60-year-old Caucasian female presents for a consultation requesting a "second opinion on her gum issue." She reports that her dentist recommended gum surgery on the lower right side, which feels fine to her. She is more concerned about the persistent ache on the upper left side and points to tooth no. 14. She recalls that she had a root canal and a crown made for this tooth 10 years ago, and it never felt quite right after that. However, within the last few months, pain developed at this site and it is bothering her more and more. She reports a history of hypertension, for which she takes 100-mg losartan once a day. She has hypothyroidism after surgical removal of an "overactive node," and takes 50-mg levothyroxine to supplement her now low thyroid hormone levels. She also takes 100-mg gabapentin for chronic nerve pain in her right foot. Blood pressure is 117/80 mm Hg and the pulse is 84/min.

There are no remarkable extraoral findings, and there is no intraoral soft tissue pathology other than periodontal disease. Temporomandibular joints (TMJs) function normally with no pain or restriction in mouth opening, but there was some tenderness in the temporalis muscle on the left side upon palpation.

Findings in the periodontal chart are as follows (see ▸ Fig. 9.5, for clinical appearance and radiographs):

Maxilla facial		1	2	3	4	5	6	7	8	9	10	11	12	13	14	15	16
	PD		425	425	423	323	222	212	212	212	213	213	313	314	213	513	
	BOP					1								1			
	CAL		3	3	1	1		1	1	1	1	3	1	2	3		
	GR		1											1	2		
	MGJ		323	434	434	434	434	434	545	545	544	422	423	433	433	434	
	Furc																
	PLQ				1	1			2	2	1	1	1	1	1	2	
Maxilla lingual	PD		424	523	212	313	311	212	211	312	212	212	212	212	424	513	
	BOP		1			1										11	
	CAL			2												2	
	GR		1	2											1		
	Furc																
	Mobil														2		
	PLQ			2										1		2	

Mandible lingual		32	31	30	29	28	27	26	25	24	23	22	21	20	19	18	17
	PD		213	514	313	222	223	212	212	213	312	212	223	313	521	333	
	BOP		1 1	1													
	CAL		1									2	3	2		2	
	GR		1												2		
	MGJ		323	222	212	223	212	212	212	212	222	223	333	334	334	444	
	Furc														2		
	PLQ	2	1	1	1	1	1	1	1	1	1	1	1	1	2		
Mandible facial	PD		213	412	212	212	213	413	213	313	313	313	313	224	593	324	
	BOP			1												1	
	CAL		2	1	2	2	1					1	1		9		
	GR		1	1	2	1	1							1	1		
	MGJ		223	212	222	323	444	655	554	555	655	433	000	101	222	122	
	Furc														2		
	Mobil																
	PLQ	1	1	1	2	2	2	2	1	1	1	1	1	1	2	1	

Abbreviations: BOP, bleeding on probing (1), suppuration (2); CAL, clinical attachment level; Furc, furcation involvement (Glickman class); GR, gingival recession; MGJ, position of mucogingival junction from margin; Mobil, tooth mobility (Miller grade); PD, probing depths; PLQ, plaque level (0 = none, 5 = heavy).

After scaling, root planing, and extractions, probing depths were as follows:

Facial		1	2	3	4	5	6	7	8	9	10	11	12	13	14	15	16
	PD	325	422	323	323	314	313	313	213	323	323	313	312	313	323	223	
	BOP	111							1								
Lingual	PD	435	424	323	323	334	322	323	213	312	212	212	212	212	335	333	
	BOP				111											111	

Lingual		32	31	30	29	28	27	26	25	24	23	22	21	20	19	18	17
	PD	423	323	312	212	212	212	212	212	212	212	313	223	214	413	513	
	BOP																
Facial	PD	414	315	313	212	212	213	312	212	213	213	213	213	313	463	333	
	BOP																

In this case, plaque and calculus removal had some beneficial effect on periodontal health, but the effect was limited as other etiologic factors were not yet removed. The most significant periodontal problem is tooth no. 19 with the deep furcation involvement, furcation-centered bone loss, and persistent deep pocketing at the furcation. While the furcation itself is the likely reason for the persistent pocket, it seems likely that the unique occlusal relationship with no. 14 explains why only no. 19 has furcation involvement, whereas no. 30 does not.

It is possible that when the crown was placed at tooth no. 14, it was in heavy contact with the opposing tooth, producing the "it never felt right" sensation the patient experienced. As both nos. 14 and 19 experienced stronger occlusal forces, it exacerbated inflammation around these teeth causing more severe disease around these teeth than at any other teeth in the mouth. Since no. 14 was root canal treated, heavy occlusal forces may have contributed to cement breakdown and coronal leakage that likely began at the distal open margin as seen on the molar bitewing radiograph. After many years, this lead to contamination of the entire root canal filling, and a reemergence of the periapical infection, which turned out to be the cause of the patient's symptoms.

Neither root canal treatment nor open margin where present at tooth no. 19, but existing periodontal disease produced bone loss that uncovered the buccal furcation entrances. This is evident on the radiographs as there is mild generalized bone loss for the mandible near the furcation level and some shallow interproximal bone defects that suggest a history of chronic periodontitis. Unlike the maxillary molars which in this patient have conical roots with indistinct furcation entrances and long root trunks, the mandibular 1st molars have prominent furcation entrances and normal root trunks in this patient, making them more prone for furcation involvement. As tooth no. 19 also is exposed to more occlusal forces, it exacerbated the existing periodontal disease there and caused more rapid bone loss, which then exposed the furcation, leading to even more bone loss inside the furcation entrance.

9.4.2 Types of Occlusal Trauma

Occlusal trauma can be described by the primary cause of trauma, the duration and the type of forces applied to a tooth.

Primary versus Secondary Occlusal Trauma

Occlusal trauma can happen in the following two ways.

Primary Occlusal Trauma

One way is that excessive force overwhelms normal, healthy periodontal tissue. Here, excessive force applied to a tooth either rips or crushes periodontal fibers, which triggers remodeling of the periodontal attachment that either moves the tooth away from the excessive force or produces a more flexible, wider periodontium that can absorb the excessive force. Generally, primary occlusal trauma causes either tooth fracture, widening of the periodontal ligament, or bone deposition around the involved tooth (see ▶ Table 9.1). If it persists for a long time, it can also contribute to pulpal necrosis and enhanced periodontal disease around teeth exposed to occlusal trauma.

While it is rare to observe primary occlusal trauma in the absence of other conditions, there are cases where primary occlusal trauma seems to be a likely explanation for teeth with isolated deep attachment and bone loss as seen in ▶ Fig. 9.6. Here, isolated deep probing, bone loss, and tooth mobility correspond to an ectopic heavy contact on the buccal side of tooth no. 20, which likely existed for a long time given that the wear facet at this point is the same size as the wear facets at the other contact points.

Pocket depths for the teeth is shown in ▶ Fig. 9.6 (note the isolated deep pocketing at no. 20):

Lingual		24	23	22	21	20	19	18	17
	PD			313	323	733	343		
	BOP					1	1		
Facial	PD			313	413	815	413		
	BOP				1	1	1		

Table 9.1 Symptoms and signs that suggest primary occlusal trauma

- Patient reports pain on occlusion
- Cemental fracture
- Widened periodontal ligament
- Thickening of lamina dura or cortical bone
- Pulpal calcification
- Development of exostoses or lipping at the bone surrounding a tooth exposed to heavy occlusal forces
- Tooth fracture in absence of predisposing factors such as a large restoration
- Restoration fracture in absence of predisposing factors such as poor design and old restoration age
- Root fracture in absence of restorations or endodontic treatment
- Heavy contact or interference contact associated with other signs of occlusal trauma
- Wear facets associated with other signs of occlusal trauma
- Isolated mild to moderate tooth mobility on tooth with heavy occlusal contact
- Fremitus associated with a heavy occlusal contact or interference contact
- Funnel-shaped circumferential bone defect around teeth with heavy occlusal contacts
- Pulpal necrosis or periapical lesion on tooth with heavy occlusal contact and no other contributing factors that explain endodontic infection

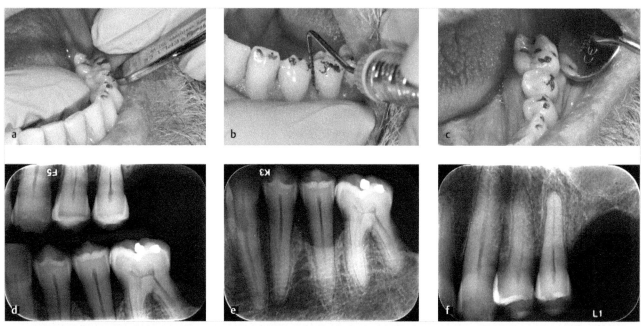

Fig. 9.6 A case where primary occlusal trauma likely lead to locally enhanced periodontal disease. (**a**) This 65-year old male patient with a history of tobacco use has isolated Miller grade I mobility on tooth no. 20, with the tooth being movable in a horizontal direction by about ½ mm as evidenced by the buccal cusp relative to the molar cusps (compare A with C). (**b**) There also are deep pockets around this tooth and nowhere else in the mouth. (**c**) There is a heavy contact on the buccal side of the tooth, but not the cusp tip or fossa. Note that all teeth have large wear facets, and that the aberrant wear facet on the buccal of no. 20 is the same size as the wear facets on the other teeth, suggesting that this occlusal pattern existed for a long time. (**d**) Bitewing radiographs reveal isolated deep bone loss at no. 20, and much less elsewhere. (**e**) Tooth no. 20 has a funnel-shaped circumferential bone defect typical of teeth with periodontal disease and occlusal trauma. (**f**) The opposing no. 13 is also affected by the excessive force but developed a thickened lamina dura instead. Note that the defect at no. 20 is well-delineated and surrounded by dense bone, again suggesting that the lesion and occlusal condition has existed for a long time in a steady state.

Secondary Occlusal Trauma

The other way is that occlusal forces overwhelm a reduced periodontium. Here, either excessive or normal forces keep damaging periodontium that already is damaged by significant periodontal disease, which then accelerates the loss of periodontal tissues. This is the far more common scenario, as periodontitis-induced bone loss will cause loss of tooth support and development of occlusal trauma as part of the normal progression of periodontitis.

Generally, the sign of secondary occlusal trauma is tooth mobility on a tooth with either a short root or much reduced periodontium (▶ Table 9.2).

Typically, if occlusal trauma and periodontitis occur together, periodontal treatment will have reduced effectiveness unless it includes occlusal therapy. A good example of secondary occlusal trauma is shown in this case (▶ Fig. 9.7), where tooth mobility occurs as a consequence of reduced support from very short roots and bone loss from periodontal disease.

Periodontal findings for the maxilla for (▶Fig. 9.7) are as follows:

Maxilla facial		1	2	3	4	5	6	7	8	9	10	11	12	13	14	15	16
	PD		864	634	625	524	524	524	434	434	325	325	523	325	576	654	
	BOP		7	6	5	3	3	4	4	3	3	5	2	2	10	4	
	CAL		1	1 1	1		1 1	1 1	1 1	111	1 1						
	GR		3	113											532		
	MGJ		225	446	656	535	434	535	756	666	656	746	645	535	444	434	
	Furc		2	2											2	2	
	PLQ		1		2										3	3	
Maxilla lingual	PD		535	535	535	535	735	557	735	535	534	434	534	323	326	544	
	BOP																
	CAL																
	GR																
	Furc																
	Mobil		1	1	1	1	1	1	1	1	1			1	2		
	PLQ		2		1	1	2	2	2	2	2	2	2	2	2	2	

Abbreviations: BOP, bleeding on probing (1), suppuration (2); CAL, clinical attachment level; Furc, furcation involvement (Glickman class); GR, gingival recession; MGJ, position of mucogingival junction from margin; Mobil, tooth mobility (Miller grade); PD, probing depths; PLQ, plaque level (0 = none, 5 = heavy).

Table 9.2 Symptoms and signs that suggest secondary occlusal trauma

- Patient reports loosening of teeth along with other symptoms of periodontal disease
- Tooth mobility on teeth with short, conical, or slender roots
- Tooth mobility on teeth with severe bone loss
- Fremitus on teeth with normal occlusal contacts and little bone support
- Tooth mobility tends to be generalized and pervasive
- Occlusal contacts may be normal

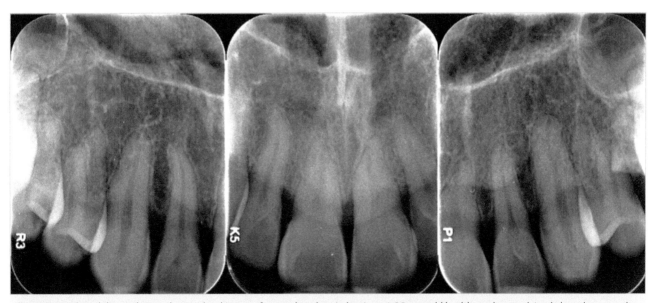

Fig. 9.7 Tooth mobility and secondary occlusal trauma from reduced periodontium. A 36-year old healthy male complained about loose teeth and discomfort when chewing. Periapical radiographs of the maxilla show generalized short, conical root along with periodontal disease-induced bone loss. There is also carries and endodontic infections at teeth nos. 1, 13, and 14. Given the lack of tooth support, development of some mobility is not surprising.

In this case, there is generalized tooth mobility as a result of the periodontitis-induced bone loss on teeth with already short and conical roots. As there is little tooth support, even normal occlusal forces can produce tooth mobility in this case.

Chronic versus Acute

Occlusal trauma can also be classified as chronic or acute. Acute occlusal trauma presents a one-time, short-lived event of occlusal trauma. An example might be a patient accidentally biting on a hard object, which then may either damage the tooth or damage the periodontium. If the periodontium is damaged by acute occlusal trauma, it is often sensitive to percussion and patients may feel a deep, lingering sensation of soreness. Acute occlusal trauma usually leads to tooth fractures or cemental tears, whereas chronic trauma usually produces a widened periodontal ligament or bone defects as these take time to develop. Acute occlusal trauma may not have any lasting consequence as long as there is no pulpal or tooth damage, as the periodontal ligament will heal to its original stage in absence of bacteria.

Chronic occlusal trauma happens with prolonged episodes of repeated or constant occlusal trauma. Examples of chronic occlusal trauma include interference contacts from "high" restorations or bruxism that lead to other signs of occlusal trauma. This type of occlusal trauma is more significant and needs treatment as it may prevent the periodontium from healing normally and be more susceptible to periodontal destruction (▶ Table 9.3).

9.4.3 The Effect of Excessive, Light, and Absent Forces

The amount of force determines the damage done by occlusal trauma.

Obviously, excess force will damage teeth and surrounding bone as seen with a forceful tooth extraction or traumatic tooth avulsion. Sudden excessive force can also develop on a given tooth as a result of accidentally biting on a hard object, or after tooth restoration with a "high" contact. Excessive force can cause a tooth fracture that initiates at a mechanical weak point within the tooth such as the corner of a cavity preparation, caries, root constriction, or a zone where the root has been weakened by root canal preparation. Alternatively, excessive force can damage the surrounding periodontal tissues, especially if the tooth is unrestored and bulky. If excessive force is directed apically, it may crush the blood vessels entering the root apex and lead to pulpal necrosis. Within the periodontal

ligament, fibers opposing the excessive force are torn while the periodontal tissue in the direction of the force is crushed. Similarly, lamina dura bone that stands in the line of excessive force is crushed, destroying associated bone cells within the bone. The crushed bone cannot remodel by itself but needs to be dissolved by newly recruited osteoclasts from the bone marrow outward in a process called "undermining resorption."

Normal or light forces usually do not cause tissue damage, but if persistent in direction, may trigger physiologic remodeling. Remodeling of the supporting fibers and bone may move the tooth in a new position with neutral forcing. This happens on purpose during orthodontic therapy, and accounts for subtle tooth position changes after tooth restoration.

Lack of occlusal forces is also harmful to the periodontium. Without normal mechanical stimulation, fibroblasts and osteoblasts in the supporting periodontal tissues become inactive and fail to remodel collagen and bone matrix. Consequently, the periodontal ligament space narrows and contains less periodontal fibers while the surrounding lamina dura weakens. While this mostly poses a challenge for extraction on unopposed teeth, it may pose a risk for occlusal trauma if previously unopposed teeth suddenly achieve occlusal contact after removal of a load-bearing tooth.

Constant vs. Jiggling Forces

It also matters if forces are constantly directed at a tooth, as with an orthodontic device, or if forces are intermittently applied. Constant forcing is never encountered with occlusal trauma except for orthodontic treatment, where it allows for tooth movement through bone with light forces, or root resorption if forces are excessive. For clinical purposes, intermittent forces are more significant as this happens with "high" restorations or interference contacts. In this case, every time the patient occludes, the tooth with the interference contact concentrates the bite force, which then is directed at portions of the periodontal ligament. With this repetitive, "jiggling" injury, periodontal tissues cannot adapt to the force normally, and typically produce a widened, funnel-shaped periodontal ligament that can absorb the repeated blows.

9.4.4 How to Identify Occlusal Trauma?

Since most signs of occlusal trauma other than fremitus are not diagnostic by themselves, the overall clinical picture needs to be considered in order to judge if occlusal trauma is present:
- Check for signs of occlusal trauma.
- Check occlusion for:
  - Heavy centric occlusal stops.
  - Unwanted excursive contacts during right/left jaw movement, forward slide against opposing teeth.
- Check or review parafunctional habits:
  - Is patient aware of grinding, clenching teeth? Any oral habits?
  - Are others (i.e., spouse) aware of patient grinding, clenching, or other habits?
- Judge how likely occlusal habit history correlate to occlusal trauma signs.
  - Do centric and excursive movements produce fremitus?

Table 9.3 Acute vs. chronic trauma signs and symptoms

Acute	Chronic
Tends to cause tooth damage	• Patient usually does not remember onset. Gradual onset of symptoms • More likely reports tooth mobility than pain • Tends to cause changes in periodontal ligament (widened PDL) or bone (bone loss)

○ Is the level of wear consistent with patient's history of tooth grinding (bruxism)?

○ Is the level of tooth/restoration fractures consistent with clenching history and are affected teeth in heavy contact during clenching?

○ Is the size of the masticatory muscles consistent with the patient's history of parafunction?

○ Do teeth with unusually heavy occlusal contacts or excursive contacts also have enhanced pocketing, attachment loss, bone loss?

○ Do teeth with heavy excursive contacts also have abfraction type lesions?

• If the answer to the above questions is yes, then there likely is a connection between the parafunctional habit, occlusion, and presence of occlusal trauma.

For example, if there is widened periodontal ligament on a mobile tooth with a heavy wear facet, more pronounced bone loss, and a history of bruxism then occlusal trauma likely contributed to the current condition. On the other hand, a patient with small wear facets but no tooth mobility and no locally enhanced bone loss does not likely experience significant occlusal trauma.

9.4.5 How much Does Occlusal Trauma Contribute to Periodontal Destruction?

One of the oldest controversial issues that has been debated in periodontal treatment since the early 1900s is how much occlusal conditions contribute to periodontal destruction. In general, one school of thought subscribes to the idea that occlusion plays a major role in periodontal destruction. Influential early dentists such as Dr Karolyi and Dr Stillman first proposed this idea in the early decades of the 20th century, and a number of renowned researchers and dentists provided evidence for this idea with animal studies, cadaver and clinical studies.[6] Yet, there is another school of thought saying that occlusion plays a minor role in periodontal destruction. Similarly, there are animal, cadaver, and clinical studies that support only a limited role of occlusion in periodontal destruction.

Although the degree of contribution is controversial, the consensus is that occlusal trauma does not initiate, but contributes to periodontal disease. The reason why occlusal evaluation is important during periodontal evaluation is that occlusal findings are related with worsened periodontal findings.

• Patients with untreated occlusal interference contacts will have slowly increasing pocket depth compared to patients without occlusal interference.[7,8]

• Angle Classes II and III are associated with reduced alveolar bone height and gingival recession,[9] but have relationship to periodontal disease severity.[10]

• Fremitus, tooth wear, and tooth mobility are slightly associated with gingival recession.[11]

• Parafunctional habits are weakly associated with periodontitis and tooth loss.

9.4.6 When to Correct Occlusal Trauma?

Since periodontal inflammation causes periodontal tissue swelling that may push teeth toward the occlusal plane and alter occlusal contacts, it is best to treat periodontal inflammation first. Occlusal analysis and treatment should be done after necessary extractions are completed, endodontic infections are treated, caries is controlled, good plaque control is achieved, and SRP is completed.

9.5 Correcting Occlusal Trauma

9.5.1 What Should a Physiologic Occlusion Consist of?

A physiologic occlusion should provide for the lower teeth coming together with the upper teeth in a way that satisfies the following five objectives:

• Centric jaw relation.
• Immediate anterior disclusion.
• Cusp-fossa relationship.
• Stable, even bite from side-to-side, front-to-back.
• Envelope of function.

These objectives are important not only individually, but also collectively. While the first two might be considered most important, achieving all objectives will likely produce superior results, tooth longevity, and patient satisfaction.

Centric Jaw Relation

The first requirement of a physiologic occlusion is to have the mandible condyles centered comfortably in the glenoid fossa, in the anterior-superior position, with the disk interposed between the condyle and the glenoid fossa. At the same time, the teeth can be brought together directly to their habitual position during mouth closing. The centric relation position is the position that the jaw assumes during the about 2,000 swallowing motions that happen each day. If the teeth do not come together evenly, side-to-side, front-to-back while the jaw is in its relaxed swallow position then overload may occur between the joint, the teeth, and the periodontium as the masticatory muscles will attempt to find a stable jaw position through increased force and activity.

Immediate Anterior Disclusion

As soon as the lower jaw is moved from this relaxed centric jaw position forward or side-to-side, the lingual surfaces of the maxillary anterior teeth should cause the mandible to open and separate the occlusal surfaces of the posterior teeth. During closing movement, the back teeth should make contact evenly and simultaneously side-to-side, left, and right with the jaw in its centric jaw position, and relieve the anterior teeth from occlusal forces as masticatory muscles contract with the greatest force. At the same time, the anterior teeth are nestled against each other barely touching, ready to separate the posterior teeth during initial opening movement. This then mutually protects both tooth groups as the anterior teeth with their long conical roots and thin supporting bone are shielded from heavy occlusal force, while the posterior teeth with their short roots are shielded from destructive side-ways and shearing forces.

What Happens if there is no Anterior Disclusion?

If the habitual bite is not the same as the centric jaw position then the occlusal surfaces of the posterior teeth will collide and bounce against each other during the time that the mandible takes to slide forward toward the maxillary anterior teeth during any chewing or swallowing movement. These collisions are referred to as interferences. These interferences over time will cause enamel to wear away forming wear facets, or cause hairline cracks in the enamel that may propagate into larger cracks, chips, and tooth fractures. As the teeth repeatedly are jolted around through these interferences, this may also overload the periodontal ligament fibers or induce degenerative changes in the supporting bone. These changes on teeth, periodontal ligament, and bone produce the clinical signs or "red flags" of occlusal trauma, and may produce a variety of symptoms such as pain on biting.

If there is a lack of anterior disclusion, the signs of occlusal trauma will be concentrated on the posterior teeth as they are closest to the masticatory muscles, experience the greatest force, and lack tooth anatomy that can withstand lateral forces. The rolling or jiggling motion induced by occlusal interferences in this scenario also focuses damage to the periodontium in the form of bone loss and periodontal ligament widening on the posterior teeth.

In addition to local signs of occlusal trauma, there also may be damage to the jaw joint and muscles with time as interferences will prevent a proper fit of the occlusal surfaces and require masticatory muscles use greater force and more frequent muscle contractions to make the occlusal surfaces fit each other. Consequently, the increased muscle activity may lead to excessive muscle growth, muscle tension, and muscle spasms. The increased force of the masticatory muscles will also transmit greater forces to the jaw joint, which then may undergo degenerative changes such as a broken down disk, disk displacement, or arthritic changes in the condyle.

Immediate anterior disclusion therefore provides an ability for teeth to function properly while protecting the posterior teeth from lateral damaging forces. Anterior teeth protecting the posterior teeth from lateral forces and the posterior teeth protecting the anterior teeth from vertical forces are referred to as mutually protected occlusion. Having the jaw positioned anterior and superiorly in the joint in its comfortable "home" with all posterior teeth in simultaneous contact and anterior teeth

poised for disclusion on opening in all directions is referred to as a physiologic bite.

Cusp-Fossa Relationship

This term refers mainly to the way the posterior teeth fit. Cusps of the maxillary teeth should fit into the fossae of mandibular teeth in a precise way, and vice versa for the mandibular cusps fitting into the fossae of maxillary teeth (▶ Fig. 9.8a). The ridges and various grooves on the chewing surface harmonize with the chewing motions of the jaw which are controlled by the slopes of the articular eminence of the glenoid fossa and the angulation of the anterior teeth as the anterior teeth rub against each other during disclusion.

When the jaw has to search for a place to bite from its comfortable centric jaw relation, there is a subconscious urge to clench and grind our teeth in order to find stability. Most patients report that their tendency to clench and grind go away after having their bite "balanced." That change can happen very quickly after having a physiologic bite established.

Should the cusps and fossa "flatten out" from clenching and grinding (bruxism), the occlusal surfaces will look like flat tabletops, which increases the tendency for bruxism even more. Flat teeth cannot chew food well as food may be smashed, but not cut. This leads to an increased need for longer chewing, more muscle activity, more force, and ultimately hypertrophied muscles. It also may lead to an overloaded periodontal ligament and temporomandibular joint.

Importance of a Match between Glenoid Fossa Anatomy and Cusp Design

The angulation and shape of the cusps not only need to fit the opposing occlusal surface, but also need to match with the shape of the glenoid fossa and medial wall of the joint. Rebuilding a tooth with cusps and fossa that are higher or shorter than what the architecture of the joint will allow, introduce problems into the system, and result in breakdown. The reason for this is that the mandible arcs in circles as it

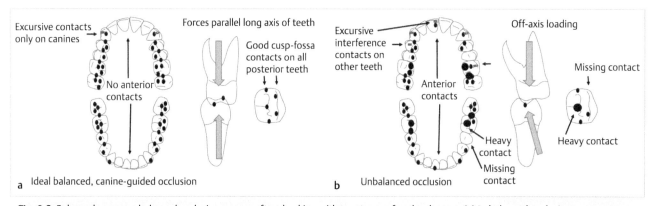

Fig. 9.8 Balanced versus unbalanced occlusion as seen after checking with two types of occlusal paper. (a) In balanced occlusion, every cusp fits into the opposing fossa with equal contact on all posterior teeth in centric occlusion. This results in even "black" contacts on all posterior teeth and the canines when black occlusal paper is applied to the teeth as the patient bites down. With a canine-guided occlusion, the posterior teeth disclude in all excursive movements while the canines guide the jaw movement during initial opening and closing. This results only in excursive "red" marks on the canines and nowhere else as a patient grinds his teeth with red occlusion paper in place. (b) In an unbalanced occlusion, some contacts will be heavy while others are missing, and there will be ectopic centric and excursive contacts. This will result in an uneven and off-axis occlusal forces on teeth which can produce damage to teeth or surrounding tissues.

goes through the chewing motion and that the steepness of this circle is determined by the glenoid fossa anatomy. A steep glenoid fossa must correspond to steep cusps, and a shallow glenoid fossa to shallow cusp inclines. If the glenoid fossa is shallow, but a tooth restored with steep cusps, it sets up the opposing jaw for a collision course against the overly steep cusps as the glenoid fossa will not properly guide the jaw.

These interferences will likely be noticed by the patient during the chewing cycle, creating an uncomfortable bite and producing a risk for clenching and grinding. Occlusal analysis can detect these interferences, and adjustment may help to remove these interferences and improve patient comfort.

In many instances, disregarding occlusal principles may not lead to obvious problems, as patients often can adapt to occlusal problems. Yet, these problems can be detrimental to a patient's oral health long term, and they often can be avoided by achieving proper occlusion.

Stable, Even Bite from Side-to-Side, Front-to-Back

Stable means that when we bring our teeth together in the habitual bite, they should contact all at once without sliding from one to another (▶ Fig. 9.8b). They should meet each other without any shifting or sliding. They should also come together while the condyle stays nestled in the anterior superior part of the glenoid fossa and not cause the condyle to subluxate (the first requirement) out of the joint.

The stability can be detected very easily by having the patient bite on a piece of Mylar shimstock (12 microns thick) and depending on how many "holds" or "tugs" the teeth create as they hold the Mylar shimstock tells us how many teeth are actually in contact in the habitual position. If the four wisdom teeth were not present, and the four incisors did not hold Mylar shimstock, which they should not in centric position, there would be ten sets of Mylar shimstock contacts, five on one side of the mouth, and five on the other. Should there be 10 sets of Mylar shimstock holds, the force that can be created from the masticatory muscles, would be evenly distributed over all of the teeth, and the possibility of breakdown would be dramatically reduced. Combined with proper anterior disclusion and proper cusp-fossa relationships it helps minimize breakdown.

Uneven Occlusion

Even occlusion means that all molars, bicuspids, and cuspids meet at the same time when the jaws close together from a relaxed centric relation position. If one or two teeth contact first followed by a slide to the habitual bite, it is not an even occlusion.

Sometimes, this is hard to achieve, due to the way teeth erupt, or drift when teeth are missing. It is even possible to have one side of the arch higher than the other. In such cases, orthodontic treatment should be considered to reestablish a stable even bite.

Consequences of an Uneven Bite

When one tooth hits before another, it can:
- Damage the tooth over time through wear and risk tooth fracture leading to tooth loss.
- Create a fulcrum which places a force or stress on the TM joint.

- Focus occlusal forces on a small patch of periodontal tissue, possibly irreversibly damaging it and causing gingival recession, abnormal bone formation, enhanced bone loss from periodontal disease, tooth mobility, or a combination of these depending on the direction of the excessive force.

A Common Mistake during Restorative Treatment Leads to Uneven Bites

A common mistake during routine restorative procedures is to forget to obtain a good idea of the original occlusion prior to restoration, and failing to restore the bite to its original pre-restoration position. Commonly, a restoration is created by immediately excavating caries and then filling the cavity preparation with some restorative material, sometimes overfilling it to create a high (hyperocclusion) contact. Then, a piece of articulating paper, many times too thick, and have the anesthetized, "numb" patient tap up and down and grind left and right, and look to see what marks appear on the tooth/restoration that was just placed. If there are marks on the restoration, they adjust those, while many times asking the patient, "How does that feel?"

This of course is problematic as the still "numb" patient will have difficulty producing normal chewing movements on purpose, and will also lack normal sensation in the teeth. It is also problematic as this technique too often leads to a false interpretation of an ideal occlusion, since the original occlusion was never assessed and potentially altered forever during the course of cavity preparation. And last, it is problematic as this technique at best returns the patient back to occlusion the patient started off with prior to placing the restoration.

With all these problems, it is likely that a patient will leave the appointment with a tooth in hyperocclusion, but not be aware of it since the anesthesia masks this sensation. With continued chewing at the next meal, the periodontal ligament supporting this tooth will be injured, and the resulting inflammation will cause severe tooth pain a few hours later, usually in the middle of the night after the appointment.

A Technique to Avoid Uneven Occlusions after Restorative Treatment

To avoid these problems, a quick occlusal analysis with Mylar shimstock is likely helpful:
- Before anesthesia, take Mylar shimstock and find out which teeth hold the Mylar shimstock on both sides of the jaw.
  - This will also provide clues on an existing uneven occlusion, and suggest a need for occlusal adjustment or orthodontic treatment depending on the severity of the occlusal mismatch.
- Record that information for reference.
- Perform local anesthesia and complete the restoration.
- Take the Mylar shimstock and check to see if the original teeth that held it before the restorative procedure, now hold with the same intensity at the end of the procedure.
  - If not, use thin articulating paper, like Accufilm II (24 microns) and check and reduce contacts on the restoration as necessary, until the Mylar shimstock holds as before.
  - As the restoration is adjusted, the original contacts as felt with Mylar shimstock will appear, starting from posterior to anterior.

Restoring the patient's occlusion to the original state will most likely provide for better comfort after the procedure, and eliminate some late night calls from upset patients.

Envelope of Function

The envelope of function refers to the space provided for the chewing stroke. This requirement has several components.

First, the amount of space inside our mouths should be large enough to allow our tongue to develop fully. If there is not enough space then our teeth and bony arches would not allow the teeth to come into their proper places and give us the bite we need.

Second, it refers to the amount of space that exists between the upper and lower jaws, which is called vertical dimension. This space should be great enough to allow for 2 to 3 mm's of room between the relaxed mouth position (VDR, vertical dimension at rest) and the habitual bite.

Third, there are obstacles to the envelope of function, such as misaligned teeth, which cause interferences to the smooth travel of the jaw from up-and-down, and side-to-side. Cross bites are another example. Teeth, which are crowded out of the arch due to a lack of room or jaw size, often move toward the tongue, which can restrict the envelope of function.

Determining Freeway Space

The muscles of the mouth determine the space between the occlusal surfaces during the relaxed jaw position. There are at least three possible methods that determine this space:

- Have the patient lick the lips and swallow, then relax. Next, have the patient bring the teeth together. When observing this patient, was there a little room between the relaxed mouth position and the bite? If this observed space was about 2 to 3 mm, the space is normal.
- Place a small dot on the nose, and another one on the chin and measure the dots from the relaxed position and the bite position. The difference between these measurements is the freeway space.
- Have the patient say "mmm" and measure the two positions.

When masticatory muscles are inflamed from over-activity, like clenching and grinding, freeway space may be restricted. Violating the freeway space with restorations, mouthguards, or splints creates unpredictable results as the muscles may not be able to adapt to the vertical space, and cause significant discomfort and excessive muscle activity.

9.5.2 Occlusal Analysis and Correction

If the habitual bite and the centric jaw position are not coincident, or the habitual bite is not stable or there are obvious signs of breakdown, then an occlusal analysis and correction are necessary.

Preparation

Occlusal analysis requires the following:
- Two sets of study models. One set will be permanently modified during the occlusal analysis model, and it may be helpful to have a record of the original occlusion prior to

treatment so that the areas of modification can be shown to the patient prior to adjustment.
- Accurate study models devoid of blebs and voids on the occlusal surfaces, and properly trimmed.
- The maxillary study model must be mounted in the correct position relative to the temporomandibular joint using a facebow record.
- The mandible model must be mounted relative to the maxillary model using a reliable centric record.

Usually, obtaining a reliable centric record presents the greatest difficulty.

A Method for Obtaining Accurate Centric Records

- With Mylar shimstock, record which teeth touch during centric relation and habitual bite.
- The centric relation position must be captured with the muscles in their relaxed state. If they are tensed or stressed then deprogramming them is necessary. Usually, the muscle that is still in contraction when it should be relaxed is the lateral pterygoid muscle. Place a couple of cotton rolls, one on each side of the jaw, and have the patient hold them for 15 minutes, and recheck to see if the lateral pterygoid muscle has released its hold, so that the centric relation (CR) bite can be taken.
- A centric relation record should not be taken with the patient guiding the jaw into the position. The muscles should not be controlling the closure of the jaw. If the muscles are controlling the jaw, and the patient bites down with any force at all, the teeth that touch first may be intruded, before any of the other teeth come together. Instead, relax the muscles at first with having the patient swallow and relax. Close the jaw with only light hand pressure while giving a verbal command of "relax."
- Repeat the second point as necessary to get a feel for the predictable jaw position in centric relation.
- Repeat once more with a sheet of heat-softened baseplate wax placed between the teeth.
- Let the wax cool, and carefully remove without distorting the wax sheet.
- Observe the wax imprint, making sure that all teeth are clearly imprinted. Repeat wax record if it seems inaccurate or distorted.
- Mount the mandible in relation to the maxilla using the imprinted wax sheet.
- Verify the model and check that model teeth touch in the same way as in the patient in centric relation. Check how the mandible model would have to move to match the patient's habitual bite, and check if this resembles what happens in the patient's mouth.

The Desired, "Ideal" Occlusion in Study Models

With accurate study models mounted with a facebow and reliably taken centric relation records, the canines must hold Mylar shimstock at the same time as the back teeth, while the jaw is in its centric relation position and the four incisors barely touch (meaning Mylar shimstock should be able to "slide" through the incisors, while the Mylar is "holding" in the back).

The Importance of a Healthy Periodontium for Occlusal Analysis

Periodontal ligaments have different degrees of tightness or looseness depending on their health. The ability to intrude a tooth might be as much as 20 microns with a forced bite. So, depending on the health of the gingiva and periodontal ligaments, that 20 microns could vary up to 50 microns. For best accuracy during occlusal analysis and adjustment, the goal is to improve periodontal health as much as possible prior to occlusal analysis so that the periodontal and gingival fibers are as tight as possible. With good periodontal health, patients can detect usually an occlusal discrepancy as small as 10 microns and even 5 microns in some cases.

Benefits of Occlusal Adjustment

From a patient perspective, the benefit of having occlusal discrepancies corrected is a great improvement in everyday comfort. If a patient who has been living for years with a dysfunctional occlusal scheme receives adjustment that creates a good occlusal scheme, the patient will usually say that their bite now feels great. This is a very tangible benefit for the patient, and something patients will notice immediately. At first, the patient may have been touching on only one or two teeth, and then the patient has to "hit and skid," or "shift" their way to their habitual bite, where maybe 16 or 20 teeth are now touching. After adjustment, there is much less force on individual teeth as all teeth touch, and it takes less effort and muscle activity to chew food.

Since less force and muscle activity is required to bring the teeth together to a stable chewing position, it will protect muscles and periodontal tissues from overloading.

This also benefits the jaw joint. Nerve fibers in the periodontal ligament can alert the brain, when biting down, that the bite may be wrong. This will trigger a muscle reflex to move the jaw to a different position where the teeth do not interfere with each other allowing for a better bite for the teeth, but a poorer jaw joint position. While this system is protective of teeth and muscles, it is not as protective for the jaw joint. In other words, when there is a choice of fitting the teeth together in their best, most comfortable position and fitting the jaw into the glenoid fossa in its most comfortable position, the best fit of the teeth always wins. The jaw gets pulled slightly out of joint position as the teeth try to fit into their best position, which can lead to TM joint misalignment, stretched ligaments, and muscles.

Risks of Occlusal Adjustment

Patients may be concerned about losing some of their enamel. In this case, it must be explained that only a small amount is removed, and the model for the "practice run" occlusal adjustment can demonstrate that. It usually helps to reassure patients that the spots that are being removed are preventing the jaw from being able to seat in its normal, relaxed comfortable position. In some cases, the material being subtracted is not enamel but some sort of filling material, amalgam, composite, or crown material.

The procedure should not cause pain, and no anesthesia is needed as no living tissue is removed or exposed. The only exception is that pain can be caused by accidental exposure of dentin (which can be predicted by the "practice run" on models first). Occasionally, there may be some tooth sensitivity, depending on how much enamel is there, and how much has to be removed to achieve the results of a balanced bite. Tooth sensitivity from this procedure will usually subside within a month, but this process can be sped up by applying desensitizing medications (i.e., Gluma, Thermatrol).

Patients may ask if the obstructive tooth structure can wear itself out for a better fit, and it is possible that a patient can wear out tooth structure through grinding. However, it is better for the dentist to do the removal because a dentist can do it in a more conservative manner without the potential for breakdown. This is aptly described in the phrase "the mouth will not wear itself in; it will wear itself out."

In severe cases, occlusal adjustment may require excessive amount of tooth structure removal. In this case, the restoration of many teeth with crowns may be needed, which is considered full mouth reconstruction.

When to Refer? To Whom?

Occlusal problems range from minimal to severe. The occlusal analysis process outlined below will show how much tooth structure has to be removed in order to harmonize the occlusion. If correction of the occlusal problem requires an excessive amount of tooth structure removal, or if it seems likely to damage restorations, consider referring this patient:

- If the occlusal discrepancy seems to be caused by tooth malposition (i.e., tilted, rotated teeth), consider referring to an orthodontist for evaluation and treatment of malpositioned teeth.
- If the teeth appear to be in a normal position, but occlusal correction requires excessive tooth structure removal on many teeth, or is poised to damage complicated prostheses (i.e., large span fixed partial dentures and implant-supported hybrid dentures), consider referring the patient to a prosthodontist for oral rehabilitation.

9.5.3 Occlusal Analysis

The mounted study models are used to show the patient where problems are and corrections should be made. Correction on the chewing surfaces of the teeth involves removing "interferences" to correct the fit of the teeth to coincide with the centric jaw relation of the joint. This is referred to as harmonizing maximum intercuspation position with centric relation to create coincidence.

How is this done? Subtracting small amounts of tooth structure, first from the study model and then from enamel in the patient's mouth, is done a little at a time, until maximum intercuspation position (MIP) is coincident with CR. In some cases, adding small amounts to the teeth may be necessary to bring this coincidence about.

The sequence of tooth structure removal is of some disagreement in the world of occlusion today. In this chapter, we will be evaluating and adjusting centric interferences first, and eccentric interferences second. If eccentric interferences are done first, many clinicians have found too much tooth structure is lost.

9.5.4 Occlusal Correction

Occlusal correction should be considered as one of the first solutions in treating temporomandibular joint problems. Correcting the occlusion to fit the teeth so that it allows the condyle to sit within the anterior superior portion of the glenoid fossa will harmonize the bite with the function of the temporomandibular joint.

The steps for occlusal correction are as follows (see ▶ Fig. 9.9, for clinical case):

- For any but the simplest occlusal discrepancy, perform the following steps on the mounted model prior to the adjustment appointment with the patient. This at a minimum serves as practice run for the patient appointment. More importantly, adjusting the model first allows determination if the patient is suitable for occlusal adjustment.
  - If occlusal adjustment on the model requires excessive tooth structure removal (>0.5 mm of an enamel surface), orthodontic therapy should be considered as an alternative treatment.
  - If occlusal adjustment on the model requires significant adjustment of a filling, crown, or bridge (>0.5 mm), consider fabricating a replacement restoration. If this requires replacement of many restorations (i.e., 6 or more), the patient is likely in need of full mouth rehabilitation, which should only be attempted by experienced dentists.
- Verify with shimstock that occlusion adjustment is needed.
  - Place shimstock foil between the distal most molars on the right side, and have the patient bite down quickly. Tug on shimstock and see if it holds. Repeat for every pair of opposing maxillary and mandibular teeth. Record which teeth hold.
  - If out of a possible 10 sets of teeth that should be holding Mylar shimstock (canines, bicuspids, and molars bilaterally), only have a few sets holding the Mylar shimstock, occlusal adjustment is needed.
- Determine occlusal contacts:
  - Dry teeth.
  - Place articulating paper (blue or black) on the patient's teeth. The articulating paper (i.e., AccuFilm II -24 microns) should be similar in thickness compared to Mylar shimstock.
  - With the patient in a relaxed muscle position, have them tap up and down on their back teeth a few times, while gently holding their jaw in its centric jaw position.
  - Check the occlusal marks and see if it matches what was found with Mylar shimstock. Only few teeth should have contacts. These are the centric interference contacts.

- Remove (subtract) a small amount of enamel or restorative material wherever the marks are by using a fine diamond bur with copious irrigation. With shimstock, check if it holds at the canines when the patient bites down. A short set of rules of where to subtract is as follows:
  - Narrow the cusp that marks instead of deepening the opposing fossa.
  - Substract marks from the side of the cusp that marks.
  - For bucco-lingually tipped teeth, subtract from the side of the mandibular molar cusp that marks as long as it does not shorten the cusp. Avoid grinding the maxillary tooth.
- Repeat the third and fourth points until the canines come together and hold Mylar shimstock. The bite now is balanced in centric occlusion. Continuing to subtract markings after this point would reduce the patient's vertical dimension of occlusion and bring the chin closer to the nose, which is not desired.
- Determine excursive interference contacts:
  - Dry the teeth.
  - Place red occlusal paper on the occlusal surfaces (i.e., AccuFilm II—24 microns).
  - Have the patient move their teeth left and right, keeping the teeth together while they rub with articulating paper between the teeth. Instruct the patient to "rub the teeth side-to-side like sandpaper between the teeth."
  - This should create marks on the incline slopes of the teeth between the central grooves and the cuspal marginal ridges. Once the eccentric movements are marked with the red articulating paper, place the blue or black back in and have the patient tap up down a couple of times.
  - Look for "pure red" marks in the incline slopes of the teeth. These are the excursive interference contacts.
- Subtract "pure red" marks with a fine diamond bur.
- Repeat sixth to seventh points until the eccentric movements can be made without getting any red marks on the incline slopes.
- At this point, the canines or group function (canines, bicuspids, and mesial cusp of the first molar) should be providing the appropriate disclusion to allow the back teeth to separate without provoking any eccentric interference.

The occlusal correction process is now complete. If performing adjustment on a patient, give the patient a 2-week break to allow the muscles to heal and readapt to the new occlusion. Reschedule the patient again to check for further interferences in both centric and eccentric in 2 weeks. Depending on the severity of the case, it may take several occlusal adjustment sessions to get to a stable occlusion.

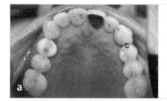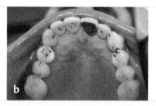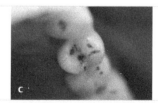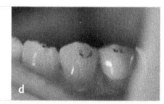

Fig. 9.9 Occlusal analysis and adjustment. (a) Initially, there were heavy contacts on anterior teeth, but no on posterior teeth. (b) Subtracting these lead to a more even distribution of centric contacts (*black*). (c) Excursive movements produced a prominent interference contact (*red*) on the nonfunctional cusp of the maxillary 1st premolar. (d) On the opposing mandibular premolar, this was also seen as a heavy *red* smudge around the normal centric occlusal contact (*black*). This *red* interference contact was then reduced, which markedly improved patient comfort and over time reduced tooth mobility in the area.

9.5.5 What to Expect after Treatment

Once the bite has been harmonized into centric relation position, what can be expected? The first thing patients probably will notice is the ease of which the teeth can be closed together into habitual bite with the jaw in its centric relation position. The jaw joint should feel good with the condyle nestled in its anterior superior position of the glenoid fossa and the teeth being able to swing close to their habitual or MIP position without any "hits" or "skids" along the way. Patients may notice a louder than usual chewing noise as the teeth touch because more teeth are now contacting in the MIP position. If a patient were to try to clench together, the patient would notice that the teeth do not shift anymore. Everything fits together comfortably. Many patients say, "This is the first time that my teeth fit together like this. It feels great!" The patient also feels that the facial muscles and muscles around the joint feel more relaxed.

With the new bite aligned with the centric jaw position, healing may be noticed. The disk interposed between the condyle and the glenoid fossa is not compressed like it was before. Teeth, which were receiving too much force before, now feel better because more of them contact when the close the jaws are closed. The load is more evenly dispersed. Teeth that were feeling mobile before, now feel more stable. On radiographs it may be noticed that the periodontal ligament spaces are reducing in width.

By using procedures to harmonize the bite with the centric jaw position, dental treatment is improved. Periodontal disease responds better to treatment after occlusal adjustment, mobile teeth become more stable, tooth grinding habits tend to go away, and temporomandibular joint problems subside. As stated before, there is more to these corrective procedures than the scope of this book allows. The most important thing that a dentist can give to patients is a physiologic occlusion that is in harmony with a centric related jaw position.

9.6 Alleviating Tooth Mobility

Tooth mobility is caused by the loss of support, occlusal trauma, or inflammation in the supporting tissues. Generally, the treatment for tooth mobility follows the cause of tooth mobility:

- If occlusal trauma caused tooth mobility, occlusal adjustment, and correction is needed.
- If periodontal or periapical inflammation caused tooth mobility, periodontal, or endodontic treatment is needed.
- If tooth mobility is caused by the loss of support, little can be done unless regenerative therapy can regenerate lost bone, which is unlikely in most cases of tooth mobility.

As tooth mobility caused by the loss of support usually cannot be reversed, the goal is to make the patient more comfortable and lessen the load on a single tooth by splinting teeth together. Here, teeth with reduced support are linked to teeth with good bony tissue support, such as canines.

This usually eliminates the sensation of tooth mobility, even though the underlying cause of tooth mobility has not been corrected.

There are several splint types that can be categorized as (see ▶ Fig. 9.10, for various types):
- Diagnostic, provisional, or definite.
- Extra-coronal or intra-coronal.

9.6.1 Splint Types

Extra-coronal Splints

Splinting materials are attached to a group of teeth by bonding to the enamel, making them more rigid. This is the most commonly seen splint in a general practice setting. Benefits are as follows:
- *Noninvasive:* No tooth preparation is required.
- The splint can be removed with relative ease.
- Splinting procedure is relatively easy.

Disadvantages are as follows:
- Splint results in a different feel afterward. Usually, this is done on mandibular incisors and the splint will be felt as a bar running across the teeth.
- Splint makes oral hygiene more difficult. Splinted teeth cannot be flossed, but need an interproximal brush for hygiene. Splints also tend to accumulate calculus.
- Splint does not last long. Usually, the splint will break down and debond from some teeth about every few years. Debonded areas may be prone to caries.

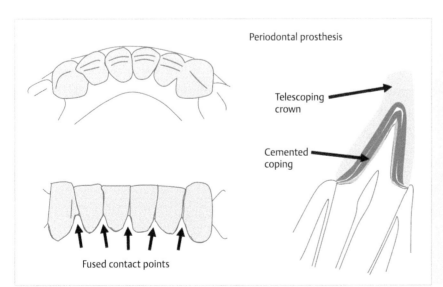

Periodontal prosthesis

Telescoping crown

Cemented coping

Fused contact points

Fig. 9.10 Periodontal prosthesis using a fixed partial denture fitted over cemented copings on individual teeth. Since there is no cement between the copings and the fixed partial denture, it allows for slight individual tooth movement while preventing cement breakdown and recurrent caries. These type of prostheses can be very esthetic and long-lasting with good periodontal maintenance, but they are also expensive and require a laboratory technician capable of precise work.

- Difficult to splint maxillary anterior teeth as the splint usually is highly visible on the facial side. The lingual side of these teeth cannot be splinted in most cases as this will interfere with occlusion.

Intra-coronal Splints

These involve cutting a small channel into the teeth, inserting a rigid custom formed metal splint and bonding or cementing it in place to stabilize the teeth. Here, the reinforcing element is placed inside a groove that is cut into the teeth.

Advantages are as follows:
- Can be quite esthetic as splint is hidden intra-coronally.
- Less intrusive to occlusion and oral hygiene, although interproximal flossing cannot be done.

Disadvantages are as follows:
- Only works if teeth line up in a good arch form.
- More challenging technically.

Diagnostic Splints

These are simply splints made of orthodontic wire that is ligated to the teeth. This can be done to temporarily immobilize teeth or test if splinting improves comfort. They are usually taken off within a few weeks and replaced with other splint types.

Provisional Splints

These are the most commonly seen splint. They are usually made with flowable composite that is bonded to the lingual surfaces of mandibular incisors and reinforced with a bit of orthodontic archwire or a bit of fiber band.

Permanent, Definite, or Fixed Splints

These permanently "fixe" loose teeth together by crowning the affected teeth and fabricating a splint in which the crowns are joined or fused together.

Occlusal Splint or Guards

If parafunctional clenching or grinding habits are evident then a removable occlusal splint or bite guard may further protect the teeth from the consequences of too much biting force. Since parafunctional forces and habits tend to be stress related, these removable guards can be used during times of tension, stress, or when these bad habits are evident.

Periodontal Prosthesis

This is a definite splint that is used to restore and stabilize teeth with reduced bone support. These are challenging and expensive to create as they require fabrication of individual metal copings and a fixed partial denture that overlays all copings. While the copings are cemented to the teeth, the fixed partial denture is held through precise fit to the copings without interfering cement (▶ Fig. 9.11). This allows slight individual tooth movement while preventing cement washout under individual copings and recurrent caries. Needless to say, patients with periodontal prostheses need to perform diligent oral hygiene and frequent periodontal maintenance. However, the reward of these prostheses is that they can possibly maintain compromised dentitions for decades with good hygiene and maintenance, and are a good alternative to full mouth rehabilitation with implant-supported overdentures.

9.6.2 When to Remove Mobile Teeth?

Mobile teeth generally do not need to be removed because of tooth mobility. As long as the periodontal tissue is healthy and there are no other dental problems such as caries associated with a mobile tooth, a mobile tooth may be retained indefinitely.

Instead, the decision to remove a mobile tooth rests on the following:
- Presence of acute infection (i.e., caries, recurrent periodontal abscess, and endodontic infection) that cannot be managed because of the tooth's mobility.
- Patient does not want to keep tooth because it is bothersome, and the patient does not want to attempt splinting it.
- The tooth is not restorable.
- Presence of the mobile tooth prevents necessary restoration of other teeth in the area.

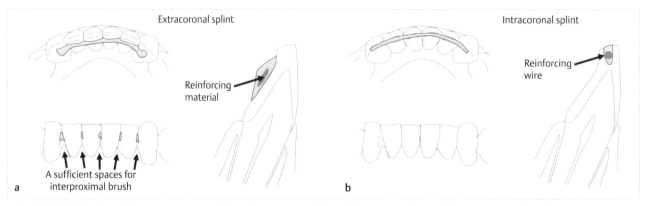

Fig. 9.11 (a, b) Various splint types. A common splint is the extra-coronal splint, where a piece of wire or fiber strip is bonded to the mobile teeth and adjacent firm teeth. Clinical view of such extra-coronal splint. It is important to leave enough space between gingiva and splint to allow easy interproximal cleaning with a small interproximal brush. A temporary wire splint can be used to see if splinting improves patient comfort. For this a pair of orthodontic wires is adapted to the facial and lingual surfaces of the teeth to be splinted, and fixated with soft ligation wire that is tied over and under the orthodontic wire and contact point with the ends tucked under the contact point. If this improves patient comfort, more definite splinting should be considered. If mandibular incisors or posterior teeth line up well, a small groove can be cut into the incisal edges or existing restorations and a wire embedded into this groove, linking all teeth together. This is very comfortable to a patient and nearly invisible, but it is only possible in select cases.

9.7 Key Takeaways

- Tooth mobility is readily understood by patients and often requires an interdisciplinary approach. Effective periodontal therapy will be compromised without occlusal therapy.
- Mobility can be caused by excessive occlusal forces (primary occlusal traumatism) or reduced periodontal support (secondary occlusal traumatism).
- Occlusal trauma accelerates bone loss in periodontal disease; but without inflammation, mobility will not worsen.
- Fremitus, percussion sensitivity, root fracture, wear facets, and excessive attrition are signs of occlusal trauma. Other signs include exostosis development, cemental tears, widened periodontal ligament (PDL), and vertical bone defects.
- Physiologic occlusion protects all teeth from harmful occlusal forces; the anterior teeth protect the posterior teeth and vice versa in a mutually protected occlusion.
- A balanced occlusion supports the jaw joint and the muscles of mastication and provides a stable bite; the teeth anatomy should harmonize with the glenoid fossa anatomy.
- Proper occlusal adjustment relieves any interferences and allows maximum intercuspation in a relaxed, stable-centric jaw relation.
- Splints can be used for patient comfort but with diligent care mobile teeth may be retained indefinitely.

9.8 Review Questions

A 52-year old healthy female presents to you complaining about her teeth being loose and wanting a "cleaning." She has no known allergies and only takes a multivitamin supplement. She travels frequently back and forth between the local area and another country, and has most of her dental treatment done outside of the country because of cost. However, she noticed some of her teeth becoming loose within the last year, and thought she needed more tooth cleanings. She originally sought treatment at a hygiene clinic, but was referred to you since her periodontal disease was "too difficult" to be treated there. She brushes her teeth now three times daily and flosses once daily. The patient denies grinding or clenching her teeth.

Extraoral exam is unremarkable with no signs of pathology noted in the lymph nodes, craniofacial musculature, skin, and TMJ area. Other than signs of dental conditions such as caries and periodontal disease, intraoral tissues including salivary glands appeared healthy.

You notice that the patient habitually slides the mandible anteriorly. As a result, there are little to no occlusal contacts on posterior teeth, but heavy contacts between the incisors. However, when you ask the patient to swallow and you guide the patient's relaxed mandible posteriorly, you notice that the occlusal contacts shift to the molars. The patient, however, reports that she does not like this position as it feels uncomfortable.

Blood pressure is 103/55 mm Hg and the pulse is 63/min.

Clinical and radiographic presentation is as follows (see ▶ Fig. 9.12, for clinical presentation, ▶ Fig. 9.13, for radiographs):

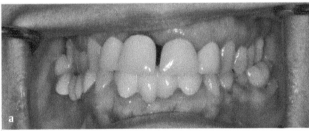
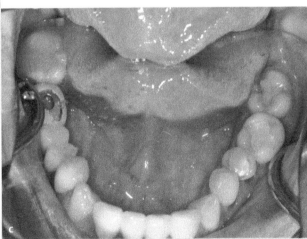
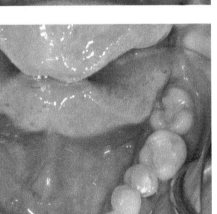
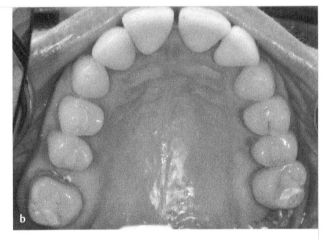

Fig. 9.12 (a–c) Facial view and occlusal views.

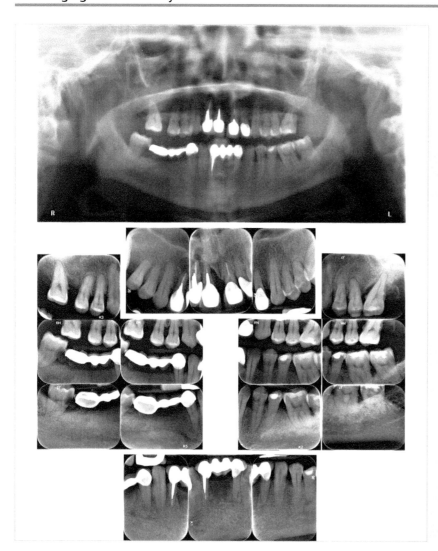

Fig. 9.13 Radiographic series.

After scaling, root planing, and extractions, probing depths were as follows:

Facial		1	2	3	4	5	6	7	8	9	10	11	12	13	14	15	16
	PD		323		423	524	423	636	725	414	313	341	352	627		1433	
	BOP							1						111		1	
Lingual	PD		425		422	423	423	514	557	433	535	512	436	536		316	
	BOP							1									
	Mobil							1	1		1						

Lingual		32	31	30	29	28	27	26	25	24	23	22	21	20	19	18	17
	PD		434			215	324	612			215	412	323	323	425	324	
	BOP																
Facial	PD		434			215	324	512			215	412	323	323	426	324	
	BOP																
	Mobil		1			1		1			1						

Learning Objective: Recognize causes of tooth mobility.

1. This patient complains of tooth no. 8 being loose. What is the likely cause of tooth mobility here?
   A. Occlusion
   B. Loss of support
   C. Previous facial trauma
   D. Abnormal tooth development

2. Tooth no. 7 has mobility and an apparent endodontic infection. What is the relationship between these findings? Endodontic infections …
   A. Cause inflammation in the periodontal ligament leading to tooth mobility
   B. Are usually triggered by tooth mobility
   C. Are the end result of severe periodontal disease that also cause tooth mobility
   D. Are typically caused by occlusal trauma

3. What is the likely explanation for tooth mobility on tooth no. 28?
   A. Occlusion
   B. Loss of support
   C. Previous facial trauma
   D. Abnormal tooth development

Learning Objective: Identify occlusal trauma.

4. Evaluate the following statements:
   Statement 1: Since tooth no. 8 is mobile, it must also display fremitus.
   Statement 2: Since no. 7 has an endodontic infection, it is pointless to check for fremitus.
   A. Both statements are correct
   B. Neither statement is correct
   C. Only the first statement is correct
   D. Only the second statement is correct

5. What sign of occlusal trauma is NOT present in the maxilla?
   A. Cemental fracture
   B. Funnel-shaped bone defects
   C. Restoration fracture
   D. Wear facets

6. The damage seen in the anterior dentition was most likely exacerbated by
   A. Constant force in primary occlusal trauma
   B. Constant force in secondary occlusal trauma
   C. Jiggling force in primary occlusal trauma
   D. Jiggling force in secondary occlusal trauma

7. This patient has _____
   A. Acute occlusal trauma caused by severe endodontic infections
   B. Acute occlusal trauma caused by poor restorations
   C. Chronic occlusal trauma caused by constant pressure from the fixed partial denture
   D. Chronic occlusal trauma caused by an imbalanced occlusal scheme

Learning Objective: Correcting occlusal trauma.

8. In this patient, which of the patient's exam findings MOST strongly suggests that occlusal analysis and adjustment is necessary?
   i. Crossbite on the right side
   ii. Severe periodontal disease
   iii Curved occlusal plane
   iv. Discrepancy between habitual bite and centric relation
   v. Abfractions
   vi. Vertical bone defects
   vii. Canine wear facets
   A. i and ii
   B. ii and iii
   C. iv and v
   D. vi and vii

9. In this patient, occlusal adjustment should achieve what:
   A. Immediate anterior disclusion
   B. Only contacts on the molars in centric relation
   C. Centric occlusion similar to current bite
   D. Molar contacts during excursion

10. What is the most important step in reducing tooth mobility of tooth no. 28?
    A. Perform occlusal analysis and adjustment
    B. Eliminate pocketing
    C. Shorten crown by occlusal reduction
    D. Remove attached pontic

Learning Objective: Alleviating tooth mobility.

11. The patient complaints that the maxillary incisors are loose. What treatment could help address this complaint?
    A. Intracoronal fixed splint
    B. Extracoronal fixed splint
    C. Removable splint
    D. Splinting is not indicated

12. If this patient had no periodontal bone loss around the maxillary incisors and there was no root canal infection, but the patient still had mobile incisors, what splint would be appropriate?
    A. Extracoronal fixed
    B. Intracoronal fixed
    C. Extracoronal removable
    D. Intracoronal removable

9.9 Answers

1. **B.** Loss of support is the most proximal cause of tooth mobility. The tooth is associated with deep vertical defects reaching near the apex, and the remaining root structure within the bone is conical and slender. At the same time, this tooth supports a large crown. The crown-to-root ratio is exceedingly poor, and the loss of support likely causes the mobility. Occlusal trauma may have been the more distant cause as there is a linear radiopaque object near the tooth suggesting a cemental

fracture, and the bone loss may have been accentuated by this fracture. The heavy occlusal contact may have triggered this fracture. Other causes such as root canal infection or root fracture are possible explanations as well, although the case description so far does not provide evidence for this.

2. **A.** Endodontic infections usually produce periapical and periodontal inflammation, which weakens periodontal fibers and supporting bone, leading to tooth mobility. Tooth mobility by itself usually does not cause root canal infections. It is possible that root canal infections can be triggered by severe periodontal disease, but in this case it appears that the endodontic infection developed first as evidenced by the large periapical lesion.

3. **A.** Tooth no. 28 likely experiences severe occlusal forces in centric relation as it is the only remaining abutment of the long-span fixed partial denture in this area. All posterior occlusal forces of the right side are concentrated on this partial denture, which in turn acts as lever on the small premolar. Even though there is pocketing at this tooth, the crown-to-root ratio is still acceptable, and there is no sign of endodontic disease at this tooth.

4. **B.** Neither is correct. While fremitus requires that a tooth is capable of movement, it does not mean that all mobile teeth display fremitus. A tooth can be mobile, but will not display fremitus if there is no occlusal force or if the occlusal force is directed toward sound periodontium. Since endodontic infections and occlusal trauma can independently occur on the same tooth, you should check for presence of both for all teeth.

5. **C.** Multiple signs of occlusal trauma are present. There is a cemental fracture at tooth no. 8 (**A**). There are funnel-shaped bone defects at teeth nos. 8 and 15 (**B**). Wear facets can be seen at some teeth, especially the left maxillary canine where tooth wear has exposed darker dentin at the tip.

6. **C.** The anterior restorations seem large and given the patient's habitual anterior occlusion, lead to excessive jiggling forces on the tooth leading to tooth fracture and periodontal breakdown. Since the patient does not constantly keep the teeth in occlusion, it is not a constant force (**A-B**). The presence of vertical defect tells you that occlusal trauma accentuated bone loss in this case, and the loss of support did not precede occlusal trauma (**D**).

7. **D.** It is unlikely that the patient has acute occlusal trauma as the history does not suggest a bite accident or sudden onset of symptoms. Even though restorations can exert constant pressure if the contact points are made tight, this effect is limited to a few days after placement and stopped once teeth adapt to the new restoration.

8. **C.** Generally, occlusal adjustment is indicated if there is signs of tissue breakdown and an occlusal imbalance. Of the pairs presented, wear facets, vertical bone defects, and abfractions most clearly are associated with occlusal trauma, and a discrepancy between centric relation and habitual bite is most conducive for the development of abnormal and traumatic bite patterns. The occlusal plane normally is slightly curved, and cross bites may occur

with no deleterious effect. Periodontal disease can be severe without occlusal trauma.

9. **A.** In a balanced, mutually protective occlusion, posterior teeth should provide centric contacts (not just molars-**B**) and contacts should cease during excursive movements (**A**, not **D**). The habitual anterior bite contributes to the patient's signs of occlusal trauma (**C**).

10. **D.** The tooth's mobility is caused by primary occlusal trauma as the nonfunctional fixed partial denture acts as crow bar on this tooth magnifying occlusal forces. Therefore, eliminating the pontic will help most in stopping occlusal trauma and allowing the periodontal ligament to heal. Occlusal analysis and adjustment likely needs to be done in this patient, but lower in priority as the occlusal scheme for this tooth may not be affected by the cross bite of nos. 3 and 4 once the pontic is removed. Pocket depth reduction is important but again not as high of a priority as removing the pontic since no treatment has been rendered yet and SRP will be simplified without the pontic. Occlusal reduction will not help in this case as the tooth is not protruding above the occlusal plane.

11. **D.** Teeth nos. 7 and 8 have too severe disease for conventional endodontic and periodontic treatment to be predictable, and splinting will likely not prolong tooth survival. Splinting is indicated for mobile, but stable teeth where splinting improves patient comfort.

12. **B.** In the absence of bone loss and endodontic infection, splinting can help reduce mobility of maxillary teeth. Extracoronal splinting will not work in this patient as a lingual bar will interfere with occlusion and a facial bar connecting the teeth will be unsightly. A removable appliance will function as an occlusal guard in this patient as it covers the incisal edge and opens the bite. However useful this may be for some patients, it is not indicated here for mobility reduction. An intra-coronal splint could work, especially if it is a periodontal prosthesis as it would preserve the occlusal surface, but link the teeth together for improved supported in an esthetically pleasing fashion.

9.10 Evidence-based Activities

- Debate if occlusal trauma has a major or minor role in periodontal disease based on scientific literature (see references).
- Go to the University of Texas Health Science Center School of Dentistry at San Antonio's library of critically appraised topics (CAT) at https://cats.uthscsa.edu/ and search for a review on occlusion-related topics. Read any CAT you can find, and debate if the conclusion is still correct based on current literature.
- Create a current CAT on using occlusion or off-axis loading of implants or any other topic not currently covered following the outline provided by Sauve S et al in "The critically appraised topic: a practical approach to learning critical appraisal" (Ann R Coll Physicians Surg Can: 1995; 28:396–398).

References

[1] American Academy of Periodontology. Parameter on comprehensive periodontal examination. J Periodontol 2000;71(5, Suppl):847–848

[2] Sneed WD. Noncarious cervical lesions: why on the facial? A theory. J Esthet Restor Dent 2011;23(4):197–200

[3] Fennis WM, Kuijs RH, Kreulen CM, Roeters FJ, Creugers NH, Burgersdijk RC. A survey of cusp fractures in a population of general dental practices. Int J Prosthodont 2002;15(6):559–563

[4] Zhou SY, Mahmood H, Cao CF, Jin LJ. Teeth under high occlusal force may reflect occlusal trauma-associated periodontal conditions in subjects with untreated chronic periodontitis. Chin J Dent Res 2017;20(1):19–26

[5] Mortazavi H, Baharvand M. Review of common conditions associated with periodontal ligament widening. Imaging Sci Dent 2016;46(4):229–237

[6] Harrel SK, Nunn ME, Hallmon WW. Is there an association between occlusion and periodontal destruction?: Yes—occlusal forces can contribute to

periodontal destruction. J Am Dent Assoc 2006;137(10):1380–, 1382, 1384 passim

[7] Harrel SK, Nunn ME. The association of occlusal contacts with the presence of increased periodontal probing depth. J Clin Periodontol 2009;36(12):1035–1042

[8] Harrel SK, Nunn ME. The effect of occlusal discrepancies on periodontitis. II. Relationship of occlusal treatment to the progression of periodontal disease. J Periodontol 2001;72(4):495–505

[9] Ustun K, Sari Z, Orucoglu H, Duran I, Hakki SS. Severe gingival recession caused by traumatic occlusion and mucogingival stress: a case report. Eur J Dent 2008;2(2):127–133

[10] Geiger AM. Malocclusion as an etiologic factor in periodontal disease: a retrospective essay. Am J Orthod Dentofacial Orthop 2001;120(2):112–115

[11] Kundapur PP, Bhat KM, Bhat GS. Association of trauma from occlusion with localized gingival recession in mandibular anterior teeth. Dent Res J (Isfahan) 2009;6(2):71–74

Index

Note: Page numbers set in **bold** or *italic* indicate headings or figures, respectively.